Biochemistry and Pharmacology
of Platelets

The Ciba Foundation for the promotion of international cooperation in
medical and chemical research is a scientific and educational charity established by
CIBA Limited – now CIBA-GEIGY Limited – of Basle. The Foundation operates
independently in London under English trust law.

Ciba Foundation Symposia are published in collaboration with
Elsevier Scientific Publishing Company, Excerpta Medica, North-Holland Publishing Company
in Amsterdam.

Elsevier / Excerpta Medica / North-Holland, P. O. Box 211, Amsterdam

Biochemistry and Pharmacology of Platelets

Ciba Foundation Symposium 35   (new series)

1975

Elsevier · Excerpta Medica · North-Holland
Amsterdam · Oxford · New York

ISBN Excerpta Medica 90 219 4039 6
ISBN American Elsevier 0-444-15183-4

Published in December 1975 by Elsevier/Excerpta Medica/North-Holland, P.O. Box 211, Amsterdam and
American Elsevier, 52 Vanderbilt Avenue, New York, N.Y. 10017.

Suggested series entry for library catalogues: Ciba Foundation Symposia.
Suggested publisher's entry for library catalogues: Elsevier/Excerpta Medica/North-Holland

Ciba Foundation Symposium 35 (new series)

Printed in The Netherlands by Van Gorcum, Assen

Contents

Participants

Symposium on Biochemistry and Pharmacology of Platelets, held at the Ciba Foundation, London, 21st–23rd January, 1975

Chairman: G. V. R. BORN Department of Pharmacology, University of Cambridge, Medical School, Hills Road, Cambridge CB2 2QD

R. S. ADELSTEIN Section on Molecular Cardiology, National Heart and Lung Institute, Building 10, Room 7B-15, Bethesda, Maryland 20014, USA

J. CAEN Laboratoire d'Hémostase, Hôpital St Louis, 2 Place du Dr Alfred Fournier, 75475 Paris, Cedex 10, France

I. COHEN Tel Aviv University Medical School and The Rogoff-Wellcome Medical Research Institute, Beilinson Medical Center, Petah Tiqva, Israel

N. CRAWFORD Department of Biochemistry, The University of Birmingham, PO Box 363, Birmingham B15 2TT

T. C. DETWILER Department of Biochemistry, Downstate Medical Center, State University of New York, 450 Clarkson Avenue, Brooklyn, New York 11203, USA

A. DE VRIES Beilinson Medical Center, POB 85, Petah Tiqva, Israel

H. FEINBERG Department of Pharmacology, University of Illinois at the Medical Center, 835 South Wolcott Avenue, PO Box 6998, Chicago, Illinois 60680, USA

R. M. HARDISTY Department of Haematology, The Hospital for Sick Children, Great Ormond Street, London WC1N 3JH

R. J. HASLAM Department of Pathology, McMaster University, 1200 Main Street West, Hamilton, Ontario, Canada L8S 4J9

H. HOLMSEN   Specialized Center for Thrombosis Research, Temple University Health Sciences Center, Philadelphia, Pennsylvania 19140, USA

E. F. LÜSCHER   Department of Biochemistry, Theodor Kocher Institut, Universität Bern, Freiestrasse 1, 3000 Bern, Switzerland

A. J. MARCUS   Hematology Section, 13 West, New York VA Hospital, 408 First Avenue, New York, NY 10010, USA

F. MICHAL   Department of Pharmacology, University of Cambridge, Medical School, Hills Road, Cambridge CB2 2QD

D. C. B. MILLS   Department of Medicine, Temple University Health Sciences Center, Philadelphia, Pennsylvania 19140, USA

J. F. MUSTARD   Faculty of Health Sciences, McMaster University, 1200 Main Street West, Hamilton, Ontario, Canada L8S 4J9

R. L. NACHMAN   Department of Medicine, Division of Hematology, The New York Hospital–Cornell Medical Center, 525 East 68th Street, New York, NY 10021, USA

A. NURDEN   Nuffield Institute of Comparative Medicine, The Zoological Society, Regent's Park, London NW1 4RY

MARIAN A. PACKHAM   Department of Biochemistry, University of Toronto, Toronto, Canada M5S 1A8

A. PLETSCHER   Research Department, F. Hoffmann-La Roche & Co. Ltd, 4002 Basle, Switzerland

W. SCHNEIDER   Medizinische Universitäts-Klinik und Poliklinik, D-665 Homburg/Saar, Germany

D. SHEPRO   *Microvascular Research*, 2 Cummington Street, Boston, Massachusetts 02215 (and Departments of Biology and Surgery, Boston University)

R. J. SKAER   Department of Medicine, University of Cambridge, Hills Road, Cambridge CB2 2QL

J. B. SMITH   Department of Medicine, Cardeza Foundation for Hematologic Research, Jefferson Medical College of Thomas Jefferson University, Philadelphia, Pennsylvania 19107, USA

J. M. SNEDDON   Department of Pharmacology, University of Bristol, The Medical School, University Walk, Bristol BS8 1TD

A. M. WHITE   Research Division, CIBA Laboratories, Horsham, Sussex RH12 4AB

Editors: KATHERINE ELLIOTT *(Organizer)* and JULIE KNIGHT

Introduction

G. V. R. BORN

Department of Pharmacology, University of Cambridge

Haemostasis is one of the essential survival mechanisms in all animals and, as such, has a very long and fascinating evolutionary history. In man and other mammals haemostasis depends on the clotting of the blood plasma and on the aggregation of a particular type of circulating cell, the platelet. Platelets have only two well-established physiological functions, to form haemostatic plugs in injured vessels and to provide a phospholipid material that greatly accelerates plasma coagulation. About ten years ago, the late Michael Cross produced evidence that the latter depends to some extent on the former, and this conclusion has been thoroughly confirmed (Hardisty & Hutton 1966). Therefore, the primary event underlying the function of platelets is their change from a non-adhesive to an adhesive state in which they adhere both to the vessel wall and to each other to form aggregates. The biochemical reactions which cause platelet aggregation are still not clear but, as this symposium will show, so much intelligent effort is being devoted to the problem that it is reasonable to expect its solution, at least in outline, in another decade or so. Indeed, during the past ten years platelet research has contributed considerably to the research explosion in biology generally. Principally, of course, this has been because the developmental mechanisms which allow different cell types to adhere selectively to each other have been essential to the evolution of multicellular organisms. It turns out, however, that platelets are highly specialized and efficient in this respect, which is not surprising in view of the fact that adhesion is their *raison d'être*. Clearly, mutual adhesion is important to the cells of the liver, for example, or to those of the central nervous system; but no-one would claim that the functional investigation of those cells was exhausted with the elucidation of their adhesion mechanisms.

This should make biologists specializing in platelets rather narrow and possibly boring to other biologists. Fortunately that seems not to be so. The

1

main reason for this happy state of affairs is, of course, the unity of the fundamental biochemical machinery of all cells, plant as well as animal. That has meant that, as usual, investigations of platelet biochemistry are to a considerable extent derivative. On the other hand, where we do discover differences—that is, components or processes that seem special to platelets—it commonly turns out that these differences are not so different but are thereupon profitably searched for in other cell types and are indeed often found there.

Good examples of such fruitful research interaction are the two discoveries, made independently but clearly related, which can be considered to have initiated the recent avalanche in platelet research. First it was found that platelets contain extraordinarily high concentrations of adenine nucleotides and that, during clotting, some of the ATP is rapidly broken down (Born 1958). Then it was shown that ADP which is, of course, the first breakdown product of ATP specifically causes platelets to aggregate (Gaarder *et al.* 1961).

At about the same time it became possible to quantify and analyse the functional behaviour of platelets *in vitro* through the introduction of a simple photometric method (Born 1962). This was merely an adaptation of a method long used by bacteriologists to follow the growth of microorganisms and by biochemists to follow the progress of reactions in suspensions. Nevertheless, this technique appears to have been responsible for most of the major discoveries with platelets since then.

It is necessary to stress that these discoveries concern the behaviour of platelets *in vitro*, because our ignorance about the processes that bring about platelet aggregation *in vivo* is still almost complete. Probably the main reason for this is that it is much more difficult to devise satisfactory quantitative methods for investigating the processes *in vivo* than *in vitro*. The difficulty will be clear to anyone who has ever watched the experimental production of a haemostatic plug of platelets: everything happens almost incredibly fast. Once again, the adaptation of a well-established technique, namely microiontophoresis, has begun to provide quantitative information about the formation of platelet aggregates—that is, thrombi—in small blood vessels (Begent & Born 1970; Begent *et al.* 1972). This, fortunately perhaps, is not the aspect of platelet research to which this symposium will be devoted; but it seems right to draw attention to the proposition that when the biochemical problems facing us have been solved there will still be plenty to do.

Even within the subject of this symposium, Bernard Shaw's dictum applies that science never solves a problem without creating ten more. In fishing from the crowded problem pool a few of those that happen to be near the surface just now, I am bound to expose limitations of awareness of recent achievements as well as personal preferences.

To quote from Professor Lüscher's abstract: 'Platelets are triggered into activity by an astonishing variety of different agents'. These agents include some of the common biogenic amines which activate many other tissues as well. Therefore, a current problem of the greatest interest common to pharmacologists and biochemists is the isolation and characterization of the membrane receptors for these amines; the mechanisms of the initial interactions; and the transduction of these interactions into other systems, notably into the adenylate cyclase system. Activation by ADP is of special interest for platelet research although ADP (and related substances) act pharmacologically also on other tissues, such as smooth muscle. The identification of binding sites for ADP and related substances in various proteins is advancing in great strides at present; and so are the evolutionary implications of the similarities and differences in these sites (see e.g. Rossmann *et al.* 1974). An enzyme, glutamate dehydrogenase from beef liver, exists which has at least two and probably three nucleotide binding sites on a single folded polypeptide chain. It is an allosteric enzyme, its activity being modulated by the concentration of the key nucleotides ADP and GTP (Engel 1973). In contrast with such isolated proteins almost nothing is known about the site or sites with which added or released ADP reacts when it activates platelets or other cells. What these sites are like, and whether they are similar to or even identical with those of intracellular proteins, is a current problem to which several of us here, including Dr Nachman and myself with Dr Noel Cusack, are giving close attention.

A related problem is the molecular mechanism by which adenosine and a number of related substances inhibit platelet aggregation. The discovery of this inhibition (Born & Cross 1963), shortly after that of platelet activation by ADP, initiated a great effort aimed at finding selective inhibitors of platelets, because platelet aggregation is the immediate cause of a considerable proportion of acute arterial thromboses. The discovery of an effective, selective inhibitor would also solve a major problem hindering the development of artificial organs, such as oxygenators which serve as temporary lungs; for the flow of blood through them tends to be arrested by the formation of platelet thrombi (Richardson 1972). In spite of excellent work by many, including particularly Dr Haslam and Dr Holmsen here, the exact mechanism of inhibition by adenosine is still not completely understood. This is not surprising because much, though not all, of the evidence indicates the mediation of cyclic AMP in inhibition produced by adenosine; and similar puzzles are facing those who work on cyclic AMP in other tissues. In this context it is hardly necessary to recall the close but un-understood relationship between cyclic AMP and calcium. Calcium ions are clearly involved in the platelet activation process but exactly how is still uncertain, to judge from our calcium contributors—Professor Lüscher, Dr Skaer and Dr Haslam.

I am myself particularly intrigued by the formation of the long, thin spikes which stick out of the platelets within a few hundred milliseconds of activation. Where do these spikes come from and, which is almost the same question, what are they made of? Many cell types are able to produce spikes but all those of which I am aware take much longer to form and remain much shorter. The function of the rapidly formed spikes on platelets seems clear: they increase the effective collision diameter of platelets, thereby helping them to fulfil their biological purpose, namely adhesion to other cells.

I began by pointing out this purpose; and I can now end by asserting that even when, after much further work, we have found out how platelets produce these spikes we shall be faced again with another question. The proposition that these spikes promote effective collisions implies that their surfaces have sites for mutual adhesion. That question will have to be answered next and no doubt the answer will raise further questions.

These and many other questions are posed by the central problem of the biochemical mechanism by which non-adhesive platelets become adhesive. What evidence there is suggests that the mechanism represents a specialized adaptation of the excitation→contraction→secretion sequence common to various types of cell. This evidence will be discussed in this symposium which, it may be hoped, should therefore be of some interest to cell biologists generally.

References

BEGENT, N. & BORN, G. V. R. (1970) Growth rate *in vivo* of platelet thrombi, produced by ionto-phoresis of ADP, as a function of mean blood flow velocity. *Nature (Lond.)* 227, 926-930

BEGENT, N. A. BORN, G. V. R. & SHARP, D. E. (1972) The initiation of platelet thrombi in normal venules and its acceleration by histamine. *J. Physiol. (Lond.)* 223, 229-242

BORN, G. V. R. (1958) Changes in the distribution of phosphorus in platelet-rich plasma during clotting. *Biochem. J.* 68, 695-704

BORN, G. V. R. (1962) Quantitative investigations into the aggregation of blood platelets. *J. Physiol. (Lond.)* 162, 67P

BORN, G. V. R. & CROSS, M. J. (1963) The aggregation of blood platelets. *J. Physiol. (Lond.)* 168, 178-195

ENGEL, P. C. (1973) Evolution of enzyme regulator sites: evidence for partial gene duplication from amino-acid sequences of bovine glutamate dehydrogenase. *Nature (Lond.)* 241, 118-120

GAARDER, A., JONSEN, J., LALAND, S., HELLEM, A. & OWREN, P. A. (1961) Adenosine diphos-phate in red cells as a factor in the adhesiveness of human blood platelets. *Nature (Lond.)* 192, 531-532

HARDISTY, R. S. & HUTTON, R. A. (1966) The kaolin clotting time of platelet-rich plasma: a test of platelet factor-3 availability. *Br. J. Haematol. 11*, 258-268

RICHARDSON, P. (1972) The performance of membranes in vascular prosthetic devices. *Bull. N.Y. Acad. Med. 48*, 379-405

ROSSMANN, M. G., MORAS, D. & OLSEN, K. W. (1974) Chemical and biological evolution of a nucleotide-binding protein. *Nature (Lond.)* 250, 194-199

Common pathways of membrane reactivity after stimulation of platelets by different agents

ERNST F. LÜSCHER and P. MASSINI

Theodor Kocher Institute, University of Berne

Abstract Platelets are triggered into activity by an astonishing variety of different agents, which can be roughly subdivided into three classes, namely proteolytic enzymes, 'large molecules', and small molecules, such as ADP, adrenaline, 5-hydroxytryptamine, and vasopressin. The 'large molecules' include collagen, certain aggregated immunoglobulins, and bovine and porcine factor VIII complex. All of them display activity only if present in a polymerized form characterized by a repetitive structure.

The response of the platelet to these variable stimuli consists always of the same sequence of events, which mostly starts with a 'rapid shape change', that is, a disk → 'spiny sphere' transformation, and includes aggregation, the release of materials stored in storage organelles, and manifestations of contractility.

The uniformity of this response implies that every type of stimulation either leads to the same membrane alteration, or always activates the same 'second messenger' system.

Since the sequential reactions of stimulation are prevented by measures which increase the level of cyclic AMP, and since the cyclic AMP synthesizing enzyme, adenylate cyclase, shows a decreased activity after stimulation, it seems reasonable to assume that cyclic AMP is somehow—perhaps quite indirectly—involved in the upkeep of a normal, resting membrane.

The stimulation of platelets is linked to an increase in the cytoplasmic Ca^{2+} level. These cations can be mobilized from storage organelles inside the platelet, as well as by influx through the plasma membrane, which acquires an increased Ca^{2+} permeability upon stimulation. The appearance of calcium ions in the cytoplasm accounts for most of the morphological manifestations of platelet activation. Experiments with ionophores, capable of transporting Ca^{2+} ions across membranes, have shown the release reaction also to be calcium-dependent.

Possible mechanisms which could explain the mode of action of the different initiators of platelet activation on the plasma membrane are discussed. The possibility of an 'intramembrane aggregation' of specific receptor molecules, leading to the formation of cation-permeable channels, is envisaged. Such a mechanism would explain the need for a repetitive structure of the class of 'large molecule'-type inducers, and could account for the effect of proteinases in terms of a removal of parts of essential molecules which normally prevent for steric or other reasons the formation of cation-permeable clusters.

It is emphasized that the ideas developed, although in part supported by experimental evidence and by analogies to other cell systems, are largely speculative and must be considered mainly as a stimulus for further work and discussion.

The inert, resting platelet can be activated by a remarkable variety of external stimuli. In each case, the end result of such stimulation is the same and it is obvious, therefore, that all primary effects on the platelet surface lead to a common sequence of events. Since the vast majority of the stimulating agents will not penetrate into the platelet, it must be assumed either that they always bring about the same typical alteration of the structure of the plasma membrane, or that a variety of such alterations is always capable of eliciting the same signal which triggers cellular activity.

The subject discussed here deals with a problem of general importance for any type of cell. In fact, the mechanisms involved are not only of importance in relation to the reactivity of 'excitable' cells—that is, cells destined to perform a specific function upon well-defined external signals—but are, in the widest sense, responsible for the reactivity of cells to the multitude of stimuli which must govern their behaviour in a given surrounding medium or tissue. Again, the platelet as an isolated, easily obtainable 'cell' may serve as a very useful model and studies of its reactivity, besides being important for a better understanding of platelet function in haemostasis and thrombosis, may shed some light on the problem of cellular stimulation in general.

INDUCERS OF PLATELET ACTIVITY

The agents capable of triggering platelets into activity may be subdivided into three classes, namely: proteolytic enzymes, 'large molecules' or complexes of molecules, and low molecular weight substances.

Proteolytic enzymes

Davey & Lüscher (1965) were the first to point out that besides thrombin, several other enzymes are capable of activating platelets and that all of them have a specificity resembling that of trypsin. This and more recent work has also shown that there is a distinct specificity involved which is best illustrated by the finding that thrombin is a most powerful inducer, whereas staphylocoagulase-thrombin, although it clots fibrinogen, is inactive towards platelets (Davey & Lüscher 1967). This makes it likely that certain steric requirements must be fulfilled for activity and it might be that this is in direct relation to the fact that the thrombin substrate on platelets appears to be a glycoprotein (cf. Phillips & Agin 1974). Although thrombin also combines with another receptor on the platelet, which binds the enzyme with a higher affinity than the substrate proper (Phillips 1974), there can be no doubt that hydrolytic cleavage is the essential step in the activation of platelets by this enzyme and by certain specific proteinases. It is remarkable that this quite limited alteration of one (or very few) membrane constituent(s) is sufficient for the induction of the whole sequence of secondary reactions, the more so since considerable proteolytic degradation of platelet membrane proteins by other proteinases, such as chymotrypsin, has no such comparable effect.

Large molecules

Besides thrombin, the most important physiological inducer of platelet alterations is undoubtedly *collagen*. Platelets *in vivo* and *in vitro* adhere to collagen fibres (Hugues 1960; Hovig 1963) and thereby undergo alterations which are typical for their activation. It is noteworthy that neither gelatin nor tropocollagen are inducers: it is essential that a polymerized form is available. In the light of more recent findings it seems unlikely that the carbohydrate moiety of the collagen molecule is of importance in the reaction with platelets (cf. Muggli & Baumgartner 1973); it must be assumed that the platelet has specific, non-enzymic receptors for certain sites of the collagen molecule and that only the simultaneous engagement of a multitude of such receptors leads to platelet activation.

Bovine and porcine (but not human) factor VIII preparations will also activate human platelets (Forbes & Prentice 1973). It is of considerable interest that here again the activity is linked to the high molecular weight part of the molecule (Brown *et al.* 1975).

Immune complexes and *aggregated human IgG* will induce alterations, comparable to those observed after collagen or thrombin treatment, in washed human platelets. 'Monomeric', i.e. normal, circulating IgG will inhibit this reaction (Pfueller & Lüscher 1972). This again demonstrates the dependence of the effect on a larger complex and strongly suggests that only the simultaneous involvement of several receptor sites on the platelet membrane leads to platelet stimulation. In this context it is noteworthy that zymosan, a known activator of the alternate pathway of complement activation, is capable of inducing platelet activation in a platelet-rich plasma (PRP) (Pfueller & Lüscher 1974; Zucker & Grant 1974). Interestingly enough, it does so only when fibrinogen is present at the same time. This suggests that human platelets possess a multi-receptor system which will react only if all its parts become involved. Endotoxin and inulin, other efficient C3 activators, are unable to induce alterations in human platelets and the reason for this might be that they are less able to bind fibrinogen (Pfueller & Lüscher 1974).

Finally, it has been reported that platelets activated in PRP by adenosine 5′-diphosphate (ADP) will not show a release reaction, one of the typical manifestations of 'activated' platelets, unless they are allowed to aggregate first (Zucker & Peterson 1967). This might be interpreted to mean that under these circumstances the platelet–platelet contact is the trigger for the induction of far-reaching platelet alterations (cf. Massini & Lüscher 1972). It seems as if ADP is capable of inducing in platelets a membrane alteration which is linked to the acquisition of surface properties which resemble closely those of the class of active 'large molecules' described above.

In summary, it is established that certain high molecular weight materials are capable of 'activating' platelets, provided they have repetitive structures, as realized in their aggregated or polymeric forms. The platelet obviously reacts only when a multitude of its specific receptors for a given type of such an inducer are engaged at the same time (cf. Lüscher et al. 1973).

Low molecular weight molecules

These include adrenaline, 5-hydroxytryptamine and ADP, all of them released from activated platelets, as well as vasopressin (cf. Mustard & Packham 1970). It is noteworthy that all of them are vasoactive compounds and, therefore, obviously capable of triggering other cells, besides the platelets, into activity. Pharmacologists have postulated specific receptors for the vasoactive hormones: accordingly, α- and β-receptors have also been described in platelets and the blockers of such receptors are inhibitors of platelet activation (cf. Mustard & Packham 1970; Thomas 1968).

THE PLATELET'S RESPONSE TO STIMULATION

Although there are certain inducer-specific differences, the general scheme of events after stimulation of platelets is always the same. Within seconds 'rapid shape change' takes place: the disk-shaped platelet is transformed, without increase in volume, into a 'spiny sphere', displaying very long and thin protrusions (Born 1972). This is followed by aggregation, which, depending upon the amount of inducer added, remains spontaneously reversible, or leads to subsequent alterations; these include the release reaction, that is, the release of material contained in specific storage organelles (cf. Holmsen et al.

1969), and gross manifestations of contractile activity, such as the contraction of platelet aggregates and clot retraction.

These morphological changes are accompanied by a series of biochemical alterations, including a sudden 'metabolic burst', involving both glycolysis and oxidative metabolism (Mürer et al. 1967; Mürer 1968: Karpatkin & Langer 1968; Kuramoto et al. 1969), followed by a decrease in metabolically active ATP and the appearance of the products of nucleotide metabolism, such as ADP, AMP, IMP, and hypoxanthine (Holmsen et al. 1972). Concomitantly a rapid fall in the activity of adenylate cyclase is observed (Brodie et al. 1972; Salzman & Neri 1969; Marquis et al. 1970; Zieve & Greenough 1969) and it seems likely that, although the overall level of cyclic 3':5'-adenosine mono-phosphate (cyclic AMP) does not show pronounced changes (Haslam & Taylor 1971), this corresponds to the depletion of the cyclic nucleotide in certain compartments.

The remarkable monotony of the platelet's response implies that the primary membrane alteration, independent of how it is brought about, invariably leads to a common pathway of secondary events which in turn are responsible for the observed manifestations of the platelet's functional activity.

A COMMON PATHWAY OF MEMBRANE REACTIVITY

A possible role of cyclic AMP

The problem of transforming a membrane-bound reaction into a signal capable of triggering a cell into a specific activity is a very general one and some years ago led to the development of the 'second messenger' concept. Cyclic AMP in many instances, particularly in hormone-stimulated cells, has been proposed for such a role. It has been pointed out before that cyclic AMP synthesis is reduced in activated platelets: furthermore, measures taken to increase cyclic AMP levels in platelets, be it by stimulation of synthesis or by interference with degradation, for example by the application of inhibitors of phosphodiesterase, will lead to a pronounced increase in the resistance of platelets to activation (Salzman & Levine 1971; Vigdahl et al. 1971). The question then arises of in what way cyclic AMP exerts its 'stabilizing' effect, a question which, in view of the many possible activities of this compound, is as yet rather difficult to answer. It is obvious, though, that any explanation must take into account that the final result of such an effect must consist in the prevention of membrane disturbances which occur at the origin of aggregation, release and other events in the activation sequence. Looked at in this way, cyclic AMP must be directly or indirectly involved in the upkeep of membrane integrity, or in the restoration to normal of a disturbed membrane structure (cf. Lüscher 1973). We are thus faced with the rather particular situation that in the blood platelet cyclic AMP seems to play a passive role in the propagation of cellular stimulation, which in fact is made possible by its decreased availability. It can be mentioned in this context, though, that in other cells the transformation from the active, mobile to the resting form is also linked to an increase in intracellular cyclic AMP (cf. Johnson *et al.* 1972).

The role of calcium ions

It must be assumed that in the resting platelet, the concentration of Ca^{2+}ions is as low as in the resting muscle; that is, about $10^{-7}M$ (Cohen & de Vries 1973). Very early in the course of activation, this concentration increases, perhaps first only in certain compartments of the cell. Proof for this statement comes from the rapid breakdown of the microtubules, which is essential for the disk→sphere transformation in rapid shape change. Microtubules are present in intact form only at very low Ca^{2+} concentrations: they depolymerize whenever the level of the cation is raised (Weisenberg 1972). Furthermore, contractility, which forms the basis for most morphological manifestations of the activated platelet, again depends upon the availability of Ca^{2+}ions (cf. Cohen & de Vries 1973: Bottecchia & Fantin 1973).

All this implies that membrane stimulation invariably leads to the availability of Ca^{2+} ions within the platelet. There are, under physiological conditions, two potential sources for this cation, namely storage organelles inside the platelet and the surrounding medium.

Calcium storage organelles, comparable to the 'relaxing factor' or sarcoplasmic reticulum of muscle, have been described several times in platelets (Grette 1963; Statland *et al.* 1969). They are not to be confused with other storage organelles, such as the dense bodies, which secrete considerable amounts of calcium *to the outside* in the course of the release reaction (Skaer *et al.* 1974; Mürer & Holme 1970).

The availability of Ca^{2+} ions from the outside implies that upon stimulation, the platelet's plasma membrane becomes permeable to this cation. This is indeed the case. Fig. 1 shows that upon the addition of thrombin, there is a rapid uptake of Ca^{2+} by human platelets. Part of this uptake is accounted for by adsorption (perhaps to newly available binding sites on the altered membrane): but there is also a significant influx into the cytoplasmic compartment. Ionophores, which selectively transport divalent cations through biomembranes, offer the possibility of testing the effects of Ca^{2+} ions which are transported into the cytoplasm. As shown by Massini & Lüscher (1974), the iono-

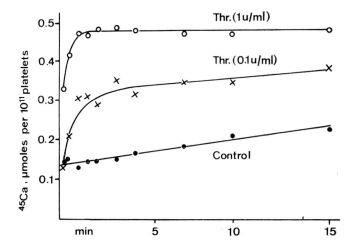

Fig. 1. Thrombin-induced uptake of ^{45}Ca by human platelets. 0.6 ml aliquots of a suspension of washed platelets were incubated with ^{45}Ca and ^{3}H-labelled acetylated bovine serum albumin at 37 °C; thrombin was then added. After 0 to 15 min the platelets were centrifuged through a barrier of separating oil. The sediments were analysed for ^{45}Ca and ^{3}H and the amount of external calcium taken up was calculated. The ^{45}Ca contained in the external space was corrected for by means of the ^{3}H content of the sediment ('albumin space'). (P. Massini & E. F. Lüscher 1974). Final concentrations: 34 mM-Tris-+ 8 mM-TES-buffer, pH = 7.4 at 37 °C; 0.3 mM-CaCl$_2$; 0.5 mM-KCl; 4 mM-glucose; 1 mg/ml albumin: 0.7 μCi/ml ^{3}H-labelled albumin; 0.04 μCi/ml ^{45}C; 10^9 platelets per ml.

phore A 23187, when applied to human platelets suspended in a calcium-containing medium, will induce platelet aggregation, the retraction of platelet-containing fibrin clots produced by reptilase (which does not by itself activate platelets), and the release reaction. It is of particular interest that the release reaction therefore must also be considered a calcium-dependent process (cf. also Feinman & Detwiler 1974; White *et al.* 1974; Gerrard *et al.* 1974). The same ionophore will also induce release in an EDTA-containing suspension medium, because it will transport internal calcium from storage organelles into the cytoplasm (cf. in this context Scarpa & Inesi 1972; Massini & Lüscher 1974).

In summary, it is evident that a remarkable variety of events which follow platelet stimulation, such as aggregation, the release reaction, contractility, and the related morphological changes, are explained by the availability of calcium ions within the cell. Calcium is also known to activate or to inhibit enzyme systems, such as adenylate cyclase and some phosphodiesterases (Shio *et al.* 1970; Vigdahl *et al.* 1969: see also McMahon 1974), and therefore is very likely to be responsible for many other, indirect effects as well.

Thus, the evidence that Ca^{2+} ions play a key role in the activation of blood platelets by an external stimulus appears quite convincing.

How does calcium availability relate to membrane reactivity?

Here again, the two different pathways of Ca^{2+} mobilization must be considered. Perhaps the release from storage organelles inside the cell must be explained against the background of the information available on the induction of the release reaction in general. According to Lucy (1970) a disturbance in one membrane (in most cases the plasma membrane) is capable of inducing alterations in a neighbouring membrane system (e.g. of an organelle). This disturbance is seen as the transformation of the bilayer to a micellar structure, with a concomitant tendency to membrane fusion, and, most likely, altered permeability properties. A second, attractive hypothesis is based on the observation by Entman *et al.* (1969) that cyclic AMP is involved in the pump system which actively accumulates Ca^{2+} in cardiac sarcoplasmic reticulum. It is tempting to speculate that in the platelet the decreased production of cyclic AMP which follows stimulation affects a comparable transport system, resulting in the leakage of calcium into the cytoplasm. This hypothesis would indeed link together the cyclic AMP metabolism and calcium availability in a most satisfactory way. It must be pointed out, though, that experimental proof for these ideas is as yet missing.

Any attempt at explaining the increased calcium permeability of the stimulated membrane must take into account that stimulation is mediated by a great variety of agents. If cation permeability is the result of the formation of hydrophilic channels due to the 'intramembrane' aggregation of suitable, most likely quite specific proteins, then the effect of the large molecules, as outlined above, becomes understandable: these are repetitive structures capable of arranging membrane receptor molecules in such a way that 'hydrophilic clusters' will form through which calcium ions will penetrate. Proteolytic effects are then perhaps explained by the removal of fragments from essential molecules which for steric or other reasons prevent the latter from spontaneous intramembrane aggregation. These ideas are in part supported by observations on other cell types: stimulated lymphocytes, for example are known to show a 'capping phenomenon' due to the lateral displacement of protein constituents within the membrane (Taylor *et al.* 1971).

It is realized that this explanation may be an oversimplification; it does not take into account the effects of small molecules such as adrenaline, 5-hydroxytryptamine, or vasopressin. Furthermore, Weissmann *et al.* (1974) have recently shown that synthetic lipid membranes, without any protein content, will react with an increased permeability to stimulation with aggregated immunoglobulin. Such liposomes are even able to discriminate between different types of immunoglobulin.

CONCLUSIONS

The stereotyped response of the platelet to a wide variety of external stimuli suggests a common pathway of membrane reactivity. The induced membrane alterations, independent of the stimulating agent, can either be always of the same type, or must invariably lead to the same sequential reaction, most likely via a common 'second messenger'. It has been shown that the availability of calcium ions within the cytoplasm accounts for many of the typical manifestations of the activated platelet. It is also well established that measures taken to increase intracellular cyclic AMP will prevent the onset of platelet alterations, including those due to calcium availability. An attempt has been made to assign to cyclic AMP a role which is directly or indirectly concerned with the upkeep of membrane integrity and therefore with preventing the mobilization of calcium from internal organelles, as well as the influx of the cation through an altered, permeable membrane.

At the present time, all such explanations invariably have a speculative character; they are, only in part, supported by observations made on other cells or in other experimental systems. The main purpose of this brief review, therefore, is to stimulate thoughts and discussion on a particularly fascinating and important aspect of platelet activity.

References

BORN, G. V. R. (1972) in *Erythrocytes, Thrombocytes, Leukocytes* (Gerlach, E., Moser, K., Deutsch, E. & Wilmans, W., eds.), pp. 253-257, Thieme, Stuttgart

BOTTECCHIA, D. & FANTIN, G. (1973) Platelets and clot retraction. Effect of divalent cations and several drugs. *Thromb. Diath. Haemorrh. 30*, 567-576

BRODIE, G. N., BAENZIGER, N. L., CHASE, L. R. & MAJERUS, P. W. (1972) The effects of thrombin on adenyl cyclase activity and a membrane protein from human platelets. *J. Clin. Invest. 51*, 81-88

BROWN, J. E., BAUGH, R. F., SARGEANT, R. B. & HOUGIE, C. (1975) Separation of bovine factor VIII-related antigen (platelet aggregating factor) from bovine antihemophilic activity. *Proc. Soc. Exp. Biol. Med. 147*, 608-611

COHEN, I. & DE VRIES, A. (1973) Platelet contractile regulation in an isometric system. *Nature (Lond.) 246*, 32-37

DAVEY, M. G. & LÜSCHER, E. F. (1965) Actions of some coagulant snake venoms on blood platelets. *Nature (Lond.) 207*, 730-732

DAVEY, M. G. & LÜSCHER, E. F. (1967) Actions of thrombin and other coagulant and proteolytic enzymes on blood platelets. *Nature (Lond.) 216*, 857-858

ENTMAN, M. L., LEVEY, G. S. & EPSTEIN, S. E. (1969) Demonstration of adenyl cyclase activity in canine cardiac sarcoplasmic reticulum. *Biochem. Biophys. Res. Commun. 35*, 728-733

FEINMAN, R. D. & DETWILER, T. C. (1974) Platelet secretion induced by divalent cation ionophores. *Nature (Lond.) 249*, 172-173

FORBES, C. D. & PRENTICE, C. R. M. (1973) Aggregation of human platelets by purified porcine and bovine antihaemophilic factor. *Nature New Biol. 241*, 149-150

GERRARD, J. M., WHITE, J. G. & RAO, G. H. R. (1974) Effects of the ionophore A 23187 on blood platelets. 2. Influence on ultrastructure. *Am. J. Pathol. 77*, 151-166

GRETTE, K. (1963) Relaxing factor in extracts of blood platelets and its function in the cells. *Nature (Lond.) 198*, 488-489

HASLAM, R. J. & TAYLOR, A. (1971) Role of cyclic 3′,5′-adenosine monophosphate in platelet aggregation. In *Platelet Aggregation* (Caen, J., ed.), pp. 85-93, Masson, Paris

HOLMSEN, H., DAY, H. J. & STORMORKEN, H. (1969) The blood platelet release reaction. *Scand. J. Haematol.* Suppl. 8

HOLMSEN, H., DAY, H. J. & SETKOWSKY, C. A. (1972) Secretory mechanisms. Behaviour of adenine nucleotides during the platelet release reaction induced by adenosine diphosphate and adrenaline. *Biochem. J. 129*, 67-82

HOVIG, T. (1963) Aggregation of rabbit blood platelets produced in vitro by saline 'extracts' of tendons. *Thromb. Diath. Haemorrh. 9*, 248-263

HUGUES, J. (1960) Accolement des plaquettes au collagène. *C. R. Séances Soc. Biol. 154*, 866-868

JOHNSON, G. S., MORGAN, W. D. & PASTAN, I. (1972) Regulation of cell motility by cyclic AMP. *Nature (Lond.) 235*, 54-56

KARPATKIN, S. & LANGER, R. M. (1968) Biochemical energetics of stimulated platelet plug formation. Effect of thrombin, adenine diphosphate and epinephrine on intra-and extra-cellular adenine nucleotide kinetics. *J. Clin. Invest. 47*, 2158-2168

KURAMOTO, A., STEINER, M. & BALDINI, M. (1969) Stimulation of platelet glycolysis. *Blood 34*, 522

LUCY, J. A. (1970) The fusion of biological membranes. *Nature (Lond.) 227*, 815-817

LÜSCHER, E. F. (1973) Function of platelets in relation to cell membranes. In *Thrombosis: Mechanism and Control* (Brinkhous, K. M. & Hinnom, S., eds.), pp. 251-260, Schattauer, Stuttgart

LÜSCHER, E. F., PFUELLER, S. L. & MASSINI, P. (1973) Platelet aggregation by large molecules. *Ser. Haematol. 6*, 382-391

MARQUIS, N. R., BECKER, J. A. & VIGDAHL, R. L. (1970) Platelet aggregation III. An epinephrine induced decrease in cyclic AMP synthesis. *Biochem. Biophys. Res. Commun. 39*, 783-789

MASSINI, P. & LÜSCHER, E. F. (1972) On the mechanism by which cell contact induces the release reaction of blood platelets; the effect of cationic polymers. *Thromb. Diath. Haemorrh. 27*, 121-133

MASSINI, P. & LÜSCHER, E. F. (1974) Some effects of ionophores for divalent cations on blood platelets—comparison with the effects of thrombin. *Biochem. Biophys. Acta 372*, 109-121

MCMAHON, D. (1974) Chemical messengers in development: a hypothesis. *Science (Wash. D.C.) 185*, 1012-1021

MUGGLI, R. & BAUMGARTNER, H. R. (1973) Collagen-induced platelet aggregation: requirement for tropocollagen multimers. *Thromb. Res. 3*, 715–728

MÜRER, E. H. (1968) Release reaction and energy metabolism in blood platelets with special reference to the burst in oxygen uptake. *Biochim. Biophys. Acta 162*, 320-326

MÜRER, E. H. & HOLME, R. (1970) A study of the release of calcium from human blood platelets and its inhibition by metabolic inhibitors, N-ethylmaleimide and aspirin. *Biochim. Biophys. Acta 222*, 197-205

MÜRER, E., HELLEM, A. J. & ROZENBERG, M. C. (1967) Energy metabolism and platelet function. *Scand. J. Clin. Lab. Invest. 19*, 280-282

MUSTARD, J. F. & PACKHAM, M. A. (1970) Factors influencing platelet function: adhesion, release and aggregation. *Pharmacol. Rev. 22*, 97-187

PHILLIPS, D. R. (1974) Thrombin interaction with human platelets. Potentiation of thrombin-induced aggregation and release by inactivated thrombin. *Thromb. Diath. Haemorrh. 32*, 207-215

PHILLIPS, D. R. & AGIN, P. P. (1974) Thrombin substrates and the proteolytic site of thrombin action on human platelet plasma membranes. *Biochim. Biophys Acta 352*, 218-227

PFUELLER, S. L. & LÜSCHER, E. F. (1972) The effects of aggregated immunoglobulins on human blood platelets in relation to their complement-fixing abilities. I. Studies of immunoglobulins of different types. *J. Immunol. 109*, 517-525

PFUELLER, S. L. & LÜSCHER, E. F. (1974) Studies on the mechanism of the human platelet reaction induced by immunological stimuli. II. The effects of zymosan. *J. Immunol. 112*, 1211-1218

SALZMAN, E. W. & LEVINE, L. (1971) Cyclic 3',5'-adenosine monophosphate in human blood platelets. II. Effect of N^6-2'-O-dibutyryl cyclic 3',5'-adenosine monophosphate on platelet function. *J. Clin. Invest. 50*, 131-141

SALZMAN, E. W. & NERI, L. L. (1969) Cyclic 3',5'-adenosine monophosphate in human blood platelets. *Nature (Lond.) 224*, 609-610

SCARPA, A. & INESI, G. (1972) Ionophore mediated equilibration of calcium ion gradients in fragmented sarcoplasmic reticulum. *FEBS Lett. 22*, 273-276

SHIO, H., PLASSE, A. M. & RAMWELL, P. W. (1970) Platelet swelling and prostaglandins. *Microvasc. Res. 2*, 294-301

SKAER, R. J., PETERS, P. D. & EMMINES, J. P. (1974) The localization of calcium and phosphorus in human platelets. *J. Cell Sci. 15*, 679-692

STATLAND, B. E., HEAGAN, B. M. & WHITE, J. G. (1969) Uptake of calcium by platelet relaxing factor. *Nature (Lond.) 223*, 521-522

TAYLOR, R. B., DUFFUS, W. P. H., RAFF, M. B. & DE PETRIS, S. (1971) Redistribution and pinocytosis of lymphocyte surface immunoglobulin molecules induced by anti-immunoglobulin antibody. *Nature New Biol. 233*, 225-229

THOMAS, D. P. (1968) The role of platelet catecholamines in the aggregation of platelets by collagen and thrombin. In *Platelets in Haemostasis (Exp. Biol. Med. 3)*, pp. 129-134, Karger, Basel & New York

VIGDAHL, R. L., MARQUIS, N. R. & TAVORMINA, P. A. (1969) Platelet aggregation II. Adenyl cyclase, prostaglandin E_1, and calcium. *Biochem. Biophys. Res. Commun. 37*, 409-415

VIGDAHL, R. L., MONGIN, JR., J. & MARQUIS, N. R. (1971) Platelet aggregation. IV. Platelet phosphodiesterase and its inhibition by vasodilators. *Biochem. Biophys. Res. Commun. 42*, 1088-1094

WEISENBERG, R. (1972) Microtubule formation in vitro in solutions containing low calcium concentrations. *Science (Wash. D.C.) 177*, 1104-1105

WEISSMANN, G., BRAND, A. & FRANKLIN, E. C. (1974) Interaction of immunoglobulins with liposomes. *J. Clin. Invest. 53*, 536-543

WHITE, J. G., RAO, G. H. R. & GERRARD, J. M. (1974) Effects of the ionophore A 23187 on blood platelets. 1. Influence on aggregation and secretion. *Am. J. Pathol. 77*, 135-150

ZIEVE, P. D. & GREENOUGH, W. B. III (1969) Adenyl cyclase in human platelets: activity and responsiveness. *Biochem. Biophys. Res. Commun. 35*, 462-466

ZUCKER, M. B. & GRANT, R. A. (1974) Aggregation and release reaction induced in human platelets by zymosan. *J. Immunol. 112*, 1219-1227

ZUCKER, M. B. & PETERSON, J. (1967) Serotonin, platelet factor 3 activity and platelet aggregating agent released by ADP. *Blood 30*, 556

Discussion

Cohen: I would like to comment on the effect of extracellular calcium on platelets. In the sequence of events in the activation of platelets, aggregating agents may cause a change in the conformation of the fluid membrane, by binding to a receptor or by a proteolytic process. A change of the platelet membrane protein conformation might occur and affect the local lipid structure. This may induce the availability of internal Ca^{2+} to actomyosin sites, and the shape change would be triggered. This change in shape happens in the presence or in the absence of extracellular calcium.

In respect of the requirement for extracellular Ca^{2+} for aggregation, I suggest the following. If extracellular Ca^{2+} is present, it may bind to the phospholipid heads of the lipid bilayers, neutralize their charges, and produce a compression wave which is effective at long distances. This has been shown in synthetic lipid bilayers (Rubalcava *et al.* 1969; Vanderkooi & Martonosi 1969; Singer 1971). If the same phenomenon occurs in platelet membranes, the Ca^{2+}-generated compression waves might cause structural changes in proteins embedded in the lipid bilayers. This causes some kind of disturbance—let us imagine it as a whirlpool—in the fluid membrane which somehow favours aggregation if the platelets are stirred and therefore contact each other. Then the storm calms down, everything goes back into order, apparently, and if pronounced alterations and the release reaction do not occur, first aggregation and then the shape change reverse, giving the original disk shape.

Haslam: There is indirect evidence from our work that extracellular calcium does penetrate into platelets of some species in the presence of aggregating agents in addition to thrombin. For example, as I shall describe later (see p. 140), in dog platelets extracellular calcium is necessary for the intracellular formation of cyclic GMP in response to acetylcholine. It is likely that Ca^{2+} ions enter the platelets and then activate guanylate cyclase in the cytosol (A. F. Adams & R. J. Haslam, unpublished work). With human platelets we can also measure substantial increases in cyclic GMP on stimulation by aggregating agents but it is less clear at present whether the calcium we assume mediates this effect enters the cytoplasm from outside the platelet or from internal stores.

Born: Is there evidence that the extra calcium comes from outside? It could simply be released from somewhere inside the platelet.

Haslam: In the dog platelet we believe the calcium enters from outside. In the human platelet a large proportion may come from internal stores, as suggested by several types of experiments including those done with A23187 in the absence of extracellular calcium (Feinman & Detwiler 1974).

Detwiler: We showed that the divalent cation ionophore A23187 induced the normal platelet secretory response, even in the presence of EGTA. Thus, if Ca^{2+} is the agent involved, it must come from an intracellular source.

Lüscher: If you accept that release is also calcium-dependent (which in fact has been shown for the mast cell; cf. Foreman *et al.* 1973; Cochrane & Douglas 1974), then it becomes obvious that both possibilities must be considered. The induction of the release reaction by thrombin is perfectly possible in a medium containing EDTA; thus, calcium must be mobilized from the inside. On the other hand, clot retraction, as shown by Cohen & de Vries (1973), is entirely dependent upon the external calcium concentration. The same is observed after the induction of retraction by an ionophore which transports calcium out of the cell as well as into it. Thus, under conditions where only intracellular calcium is mobilized, only a very short-lived stimulation of the contractile system is to be expected, which then tapers off because calcium leaks out through the plasma membrane.

With respect to the suggested disturbance of the membrane, which is a prerequisite for aggregation, the platelet model is unique in that it offers direct proof for such a far-reaching rearrangement within the lipid bilayer; procoagulant membrane phospholipids, in fact, become available only in the activated platelet.

According to C. Bouvier & G. Gabbiani (personal communication), antiactin antisera will react with the platelet surface shortly after the onset of stimulation by ADP. Since there is good reason to believe that actomyosin is attached to the inner side of the membrane, this again supports the idea of a drastic rearrangement of the latter's constituents. All these observations seem to fit in with the ideas developed by Lucy (1970) in relation to membrane fusion. According to him, this process is preceded by the transformation of the membrane bilayer into a micellar structure. This would correspond to a local inside-out reorientation of membrane constituents.

Feinberg: In support of Dr Cohen's contention, we found (LeBreton & Feinberg 1974) that ^{45}Ca does not enter the platelet during stimulation of shape change by ADP.

Cohen: I was suggesting that the external calcium, by somehow changing the conformation of the membrane, might trigger the mobilization of internal calcium. In this case, the extracellular calcium, or at least part of it, might bind to the phospholipid heads of lipid bilayers without necessarily penetrating the membrane.

Born: In smooth muscle, binding of external calcium to the membrane releases calcium from its inner side. There is, therefore, some sort of transduction mechanism.

White: One wonders to what extent the cytoplasmic calcium stores might change in the isolation process, and whether such changes might depend on the anticoagulant used.

Detwiler: The question of whether calcium goes into the platelet seems quite clear. Although you see an uptake of ^{45}Ca when you stimulate the platelet, there is a net efflux, so this must just be an exchange. It seems to be clear that all the responses that one observes in a platelet can occur in the absence of extracellular calcium, with the exception of aggregation. So with human platelets at least there is no question about whether or not there is a requirement for extracellular calcium. Am I over-simplifying this?

Born: I don't think so. In 1968 I suggested a model for aggregation showing how calcium may come into it (Born 1968). The suggestion was that when the shape change occurs new sites are exposed to which fibrinogen binds via calcium. The calcium could form bridges from a negative group on the fibrinogen, for example a sialic acid carboxyl, to a negative group on the platelet surface. This would make the adhesion reaction similar to pharmacological reactions in which an agonist binds to a specific receptor in a reaction involving calcium. The calcium provides electrostatic forces acting over comparatively long distances but, of course, no specificity; that is provided by secondary forces acting over much shorter distances which depend on the closeness of fit of many groups. This suggestion does not appear to have been refuted.

Mustard: The cation in the granules of pig and rabbit platelets is magnesium, not calcium; hence, during the release reaction, magnesium is released and it is possible to determine whether or not calcium is taken up (Kinlough-Rathbone *et al.* 1973). If the uptake of calcium is prevented by adding a chelating agent to the external medium, the release reaction is inhibited (Kinlough-Rathbone *et al.* 1974; Sneddon 1972). This does not occur to the same extent with human platelets. The species difference is apparent, but it may be important in another way also. If the granules in the human platelets discharge into a canalicular system which is not immediately accessible to the chelating agent, the calcium in the canalicular system may affect the platelet reactions.

A further question is: what proof exists that chelating agents can take calcium from the platelet membrane? If the chelating agents do not remove calcium from the membrane, it may be available for the release reaction.

Born: Someone should investigate this, using agents such as EGTA with enormously high affinities for calcium.

Mills: It has been done with red cells where the problem is simpler because most of the cell's calcium is in the membrane. Harrison & Long (1968) have shown that the red cell membrane can be depleted of calcium by treatment with chelating agents.

Mustard: Concerning your calcium–fibrinogen model, Dr Born, if one uses suspensions of washed human platelets and adds fibrinogen before adding ADP, the aggregation response is normal. If one adds fibrinogen with ADP it is also normal. However, if one adds fibrinogen *after* the ADP-induced shape change has occurred, the aggregation response is weak. It appears that fibrinogen has to be present during the initial shape change. These observations may be in keeping with your hypothesis. For some unknown reason, after the change in shape has taken place, fibrinogen does not augment aggregation. Perhaps, if it binds to the membrane, it can only do so before the shape change.

Born: One could still look at it either way, however.

Feinberg: It is clear that external calcium is not required for shape change; however, shape change may be associated with a redistribution of calcium within the platelet such that calcium ion increases. The rise in intraplatelet calcium ion might then be the basis of contractile activation. On the other hand, aggregation requires external calcium which seems to be involved in platelet–platelet interaction—for example, Professor Lüscher's suggestion of externalized actomyosin or Professor Born's fibrinogen hypothesis. Dr Haslam points out that the cytoplasmic location of guanylate cyclase and the rise of cyclic GMP argues for the entry of calcium. As shown by Mürer (1969), thrombin induced an efflux of calcium associated with granule release and, as shown by Robblee *et al.* (1973) using ^{45}Ca, granule release is followed by calcium influx. Efflux of calcium followed by an influx also represents a redistribution of intraplatelet calcium and the activation of adhesiveness might be associated with either the calcium efflux or influx or both.

Haslam: We found with human platelets two distinct divalent cation requirements for aggregation by ADP or vasopressin (Haslam & Rosson 1972). Firstly, calcium was required, in the sense that aggregation could be inhibited after incubation with EGTA for a period. This calcium was presumably coming not from the external medium, where it would have been bound immediately by EGTA, but either from the membrane or from within the platelets. Secondly, there was an additional requirement for an extracellular divalent cation which could be either calcium or magnesium. I tend to invoke some sort of charge neutralization role for this divalent cation, but I don't know exactly what is being neutralized. Thus, I suggest that there are two distinct cationic requirements for the aggregation of human platelets and that the only calcium that is essential is platelet calcium.

Lüscher: On closer analysis, the calcium uptake by thrombin-stimulated platelets is found to result from the superposition of two different phenomena. The first one is accounted for by absorption, whereas the second one consists of a steady influx of the cation. Thus, it is established that the activated plasma membrane is capable of binding more calcium and that it also becomes permeable to calcium. It may be that the appearance of new calcium-binding is intimately linked to aggregation.

Holmsen: The uptake of calcium from the medium by platelets induced by thrombin is a matter of dispute. Mürer & Holme (1970) have shown that 95 % of the ^{45}Ca associated with platelets treated with thrombin in the presence of extracellular ^{45}Ca could be washed off with EDTA-containing saline. Furthermore, Robblee *et al.* (1973) suggest that the calcium taken up by platelets during the thrombin–platelet interaction is preferentially bound to the membrane, in particular to proteins adsorbed to the *outside* of the membrane. It seems, therefore, from these results as if calcium does not enter the platelet cytoplasm. I don't know of other data suggesting the entry of calcium to the cytoplasm during the thrombin-induced release reaction.

Born: The possibility of two types of calcium action is interesting, because in excitable tissues there is apparently a movement of calcium across the membrane; but it is so small that it can only be demonstrated by electrophysiological methods. Thus it can be shown that a slow current remaining after sodium and potassium currents are excluded depends on calcium concentration (Reuter 1967; Reuter & Seitz 1968). Perhaps the *slow* influx, which may still be large enough to affect the intracellular machinery, is a calcium current of this kind; it would be much more difficult to demonstrate in platelets than in muscle.

Nachman: An interesting point here is the geography of the membrane. Professor Lüscher mentioned the actin becoming available later. I take it that with your immunological techniques you are not able to detect actin or myosin before any aggregation?

Lüscher: No, never.

References

BORN, G. V. R. (1968) in *Metabolism and Permeability of Erythrocytes and Thrombocytes* (Deutsch, E., Gerlach, E. & Moser, K., eds.), pp. 294-302, Thieme, Stuttgart

COCHRANE, D. E. & DOUGLAS, W. W. (1974) Calcium-induced extrusion of secretory granules (exocytosis) in mast cells exposed to 48/80 or the ionophores A-23187 and X-537A. *Proc. Natl. Acad. Sci. U.S.A. 71*, 408-412

COHEN, I. & DE VRIES, A. (1973) Platelet contractile regulation in an isometric system. *Nature (Lond.) 246*, 32-37

FEINMAN, R. D. & DETWILER, T. C. (1974) Platelet secretion induced by divalent cation ionophores. *Nature (Lond.) 249*, 172-173

FOREMAN, J., MONGAR, J. L. & GOMPERTS, B. D. (1973) Calcium ionophores and movement of calcium ions following the physiological stimulus to a secretory process. *Nature (Lond.) 245*, 249-251

HASLAM, R. J. & ROSSON, G. M. (1972) Aggregation of human blood platelets by vasopressin. *Am. J. Physiol. 223*, 958-967

HARRISON, D. A. & LONG, C. (1968) The calcium content of human erythrocytes. *J. Physiol. (Lond.) 199*, 367–381

KINLOUGH-RATHBONE, R. L., CHAHIL, A. & MUSTARD, J. F. (1973) Effect of external calcium and magnesium on thrombin-induced changes in calcium and magnesium of pig platelets. *Am. J. Physiol. 224*, 941-945

KINLOUGH-RATHBONE, R. L., CHAHIL, A. & MUSTARD, J. F. (1974) Divalent cations and the release reaction of pig platelets. *Am. J. Physiol. 226*, 235-239

LEBRETON, G. & FEINBERG, H. (1974) ADP-induced changes in intraplatelet Ca^{2+} ion concentration. *Pharmacologist 16*, 313

LUCY, J. A. (1970) The fusion of biological membranes. *Nature (Lond.) 227*, 815-817

MÜRER, E. H. (1969) Thrombin-induced release of calcium from blood platelets. *Science (Wash. D.C.) 166*, 623

MÜRER, E. H. & HOLME, R. (1970) A study of the release of calcium from human blood platelets and its inhibition by metabolic inhibitors, N-ethylmaleimide and aspirin. *Biochim. Biophys. Acta 222*, 197-205

REUTER, H. (1967) The dependence of slow inward current in Purkinje fibres on the extracellular calcium concentration. *J. Physiol. (Lond.) 192*, 472-492

REUTER, H. & SEITZ, N. (1968) The dependence of calcium efflux from cardiac muscle on temperature and external ion composition. *J. Physiol. (Lond.) 195*, 457-470

ROBBLEE, L. S., SHEPRO, D., BELAMARICH, F. A. & TOWLE, C. (1973) Platelet calcium flux and the release reaction. *Ser. Haematol. 6*, 311-316

RUBALCAVA, B., MARTINEZ DE MUÑOZ, D. & GITLER, C. (1969) Interaction of fluorescent probes with membranes. I. Effect of ions on erythrocyte membranes. *Biochemistry 8*, 2742-2747

SINGER, S. J. (1971) The molecular organization of biological membranes. In *Structure and Function of Biological Membranes* (Rothfield, L. I., ed.), pp. 145-250, Academic Press, New York

SNEDDON, J. M. (1972) Divalent cations and the blood platelet release reaction. *Nature New Biol. 236*, 103-104

VANDERKOOI, J. & MARTONOSI, A. (1969) Sarcoplasmic reticulum. VIII. Use of 8-anilino-1-naphthalene sulfonate as conformational probe on biophysical membranes. *Arch. Biochem. Biophys. 133*, 153-163

Binding of adenosine diphosphate by human platelet membrane

RALPH L. NACHMAN

New York Hospital—Cornell Medical Center, New York

Abstract Isolated membranes from human platelets bind adenosine diphosphate. The process is reversible, temperature and divalent cation dependent, and related to membrane protein thiol groups. Exposure of the isolated membranes to trypsin, chymotrypsin or pronase inhibited [^{14}C]ADP uptake. Extraction of the bound radioactivity and subsequent thin layer chromatographic analysis revealed that the ADP was unchanged. AMP, ATP and 2-chloroadenosine, known inhibitors of platelet aggregation, blocked [^{14}C]ADP membrane binding whereas cyclic AMP, adenosine and prostaglandin E_1 had no effect. Monovalent Fab fragments of rabbit antibodies prepared to human platelet membranes interfered with ADP-induced platelet aggregation and 5-hydroxytryptamine release; however, there was no inhibition of [^{14}C]ADP uptake by the isolated membrane vesicles. A soluble protein preparation from frozen–thawed washed human platelets also binds [^{14}C]ADP with the same apparent kinetics as the isolated membrane vesicles. Extraction of the bound radioactivity from the soluble protein mixture revealed that the ADP was unchanged. The soluble preparation retained a high degree of specificity for ADP binding comparable to that shown by the isolated membrane particles. It has not yet been possible to relate the ADP binding at the platelet surface to any of the previously described membrane enzyme systems or to a known platelet protein complex.

Significant progress has been made in recent years leading to the identification of membrane-bound receptors for hormones such as insulin (Cuatrecasas 1972), corticotropin (Lefkowitz *et al.* 1970), gonadotropin (Dufau *et al.* 1973), growth hormone (Gavin *et al.* 1972) and glucagon (Rodbell *et al.* 1971) in mammalian tissues, and cholinergic receptors in the electric organs of fish and eel (Hall 1972). These studies are based on the use of radioactive molecules which selectively bind to specific receptor sites. In general, three criteria should be fulfilled before radioactive binding should be considered as a valid characterization and identification of a membrane receptor. (1) The receptor should

23

have a high specificity for the bound agent, (2) the process should be saturable and characterized by a finite and generally small number of receptor sites, and (3) the affinity and rate constants for the binding reaction should correlate with known biological properties of the receptor stimulant or antagonist molecule (Cuatrecasas 1974).

Using these principles we have attempted to identify and characterize the adenosine diphosphate receptor on human platelet membranes. ADP is a major initiator of platelet aggregation, which is an important step in physiological haemostasis and pathological thrombosis. The precise mechanism by which ADP induces the aggregation response is unknown. Studies in other laboratories have examined the metabolic fate of radioactive ADP following interaction with the intact platelet surface (Salzman *et al.* 1966; Spaet & Lejnieks 1966). Born (1965) proposed that there was a specific ADP receptor site on the platelet membrane which triggered the aggregation reaction. Boullin *et al.* (1972) reported that bound labelled ADP was demonstrable in washed platelet aggregates after the addition of the ADP to platelet-rich plasma suspensions.

This report presents our studies on the binding of [^{14}C]ADP to isolated human platelet membrane vesicles. Specific ADP binding sites are present on the platelet membrane. In addition, solubilized preparations obtained from whole platelets bind ADP. Inhibition studies using structurally analogous nucleotides known to interfere with platelet aggregation support the premise that the binding of ADP to these receptors is an early event which initiates the aggregation response (Nachman & Ferris 1974).

STUDIES ON ISOLATED MEMBRANES

Isolated human platelet membranes obtained by sucrose density gradient ultracentrifugation of cell homogenates (Marcus *et al.* 1966) when analysed by sodium dodecyl sulphate (SDS) acrylamide gel electrophoresis contain a heterogeneous group of polypeptides of different molecular weight classes ranging from 10 000 to over 250 000 (Nachman & Ferris 1972). Three major glycoproteins have also been identified in the platelet membrane (Fig. 1). When isolated platelet membrane vesicles were incubated with [^{14}C]ADP, washed, solubilized and then subjected to SDS acrylamide gel electrophoresis, no [^{14}C]ADP label was clearly associated with any of the membrane polypeptides. The strongly denaturing conditions used in solubilizing the membrane material in SDS urea apparently did not allow detection of any ADP receptor relationships. Therefore binding studies were performed using isolated human platelet

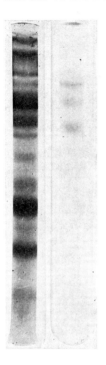

FIG. 1. Sodium dodecyl sulphate-acrylamide gel analysis of human platelet membrane protein. *Left*: Coomassie blue stained gel for proteins. *Right*: PAS stain for glycoproteins. Anode at the bottom.

membrane vesicles in an aqueous buffer system with [^{14}C]ADP. The binding of labelled ADP to platelet membranes was measured by three methods (Nachman & Ferris 1974). In the centrifugation method, [^{14}C]ADP was incubated with a membrane suspension (200 to 300 μg) in a 1 ml volume for 60 minutes at 37 °C with shaking. The suspension was diluted with buffer and ultracentrifuged. The membrane pellet was resuspended in buffer, washed twice and then measured for the amount of retained radioactivity. A second method for assaying binding involved the separation of particle-bound tracer from unbound tracer using Millipore filtration. A third method for assaying binding involved equilibrium dialysis of [^{14}C]ADP-labelled membranes. Incubation of human platelet membranes with the radioactive nucleotide resulted in binding as measured in these three different assay systems (Table 1). For convenience, because of the rapidity and reproducibility of the method, the Millipore filtration system was used in subsequent studies. To determine the number of binding sites and the binding constant for ADP, we measured the amount of ADP bound to membrane particles as a function of the free ADP

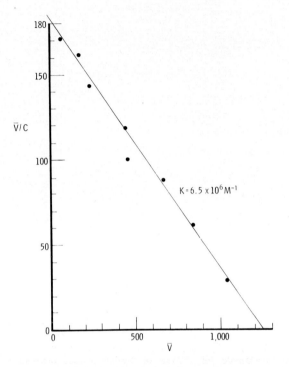

Fɪɢ. 2. Scatchard plot. With [^{14}C]ADP at 3.6×10^{-6}ᴍ, unlabelled ADP from 10^{-7}ᴍ to 10^{-3}ᴍ was added. Incubations were carried out at 37 °C for 1 hour in buffer containing 300 µg of membrane particles. Particle-bound and free [^{14}C]ADP were separated by Millipore filtration. $\bar{V}$, amount of bound ADP (pmol per mg of membrane protein); C, molar concentration of ADP. K, affinity constant. (Modified from Nachman & Ferris 1974, with permission of the Editor of *The Journal of Biological Chemistry*.)

TABLE 1

Binding of [^{14}C]ADP to platelet membranes

Method	[^{14}C]ADP bound (pmol/mg)
Centrifugation	64 ± 8 (6)
Millipore filter	106 ± 6 (6)
Equilibrium dialysis	117 ± 12 (3)

[^{14}C]ADP (372 pmol) was incubated with membrane vesicles ($\sim$ 300 µg of particle per ml) in buffer for 1 hour at 37 °C with vigorous shaking. Values indicate means $\pm$ s.ᴅ. The number of experiments is indicated in parentheses.
(From Nachman & Ferris 1974, with permission of the Editor of *The Journal of Biological Chemistry*.)

TABLE 2

Dissociation of membrane-bound [^{14}C]ADP

Membrane incubation	[^{14}C]ADP bound (%)
Buffer	100
ADP	
10^{-6}M	48
10^{-5}M	24
10^{-4}M	0

[^{14}C]ADP (372 pmol) was incubated with membrane vesicles ($\sim$ 300 μg of particle per ml) in buffer for 1 hour at 37 °C with vigorous shaking. Non-radioactive ADP was added to separate suspensions in the amounts indicated and incubation continued for an additional 30 min. Particle-bound [^{14}C]ADP was isolated by Millipore filtration. (From Nachman & Ferris 1974, with permission of the Editor of *The Journal of Biological Chemistry*.)

added and analysed the data by a Scatchard plot (Fig. 2). The calculations suggest that there is a major population of membrane binding sites with an association constant K for the interaction with [^{14}C]ADP of 6.5×10^6M^{-1} and approximately 50 000–100 000 ADP binding sites per platelet.

The membrane binding was temperature-dependent. When membranes were heated to 100 °C for 5 minutes [^{14}C]ADP binding was totally abolished. Maximal binding occurred after 60 minutes of incubation at 37 °C and binding was reversible, as seen in Table 2. Extraction of the bound radioactivity and subsequent thin layer chromatographic analysis revealed that the ADP was unchanged. Binding was calcium- and magnesium-dependent, influenced by the integrity of membrane protein thiol groups and inhibited by prior exposure of the isolated membranes to trypsin, chymotrypsin or pronase.

In order to correlate the binding of the [^{14}C]ADP by the membrane vesicles with physiologically induced platelet aggregation, we studied the relative inhibitory effects of various agents known to interfere with ADP-induced platelet aggregation. For these studies varying amounts of non-radioactive agents known to influence platelet function were preincubated with the membrane vesicle suspension, after which [^{14}C]ADP was added (Fig. 3). ADP and 2-chloroadenosine were the most potent inhibitors of membrane [^{14}C]ADP binding. ATP and AMP were intermediate in their capacity to inhibit the binding reaction. Adenosine showed only a slight inhibitory effect at high concentrations. Prostaglandin E$_1$ (PGE$_1$) had no effect on [^{14}C]ADP binding even at high (10^{-4}M) concentrations. These studies lend some support to the role of the binding sites in physiological ADP aggregation. It appeared that those agents which are known to competitively inhibit ADP-induced platelet

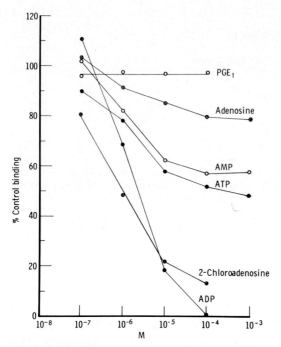

F<small>IG</small>. 3. Inhibition of [^{14}C]ADP binding by agents known to affect platelet function. The reagents were added at the indicated concentrations for 30 min at 37 °C, followed by [^{14}C]-ADP. (From Nachman & Ferris 1974, with permission of the Editor of *The Journal of Biological Chemistry*.)

aggregation also inhibited [^{14}C]ADP membrane binding. Adenosine and PGE$_1$, potent inhibitors of aggregation, had no effect on binding. These agents interfere with ADP-mediated platelet aggregation via interactions with the cyclic AMP system (Mills & Smith 1971). 2-Chloroadenosine, a highly potent inhibitor of ADP-induced platelet aggregation, through interaction with the cyclic AMP system (Mills & Smith 1971), also markedly inhibited [^{14}C]ADP binding. Thus it would appear that this agent also acts as a competitive inhibitor at the membrane binding site. Inhibition experiments were also performed with various nucleoside diphosphates; only GDP at high concentrations (10^{-4}M) inhibited [^{14}C]ADP binding. Preincubation of membrane particles with dibutyryl cyclic AMP had no effect on [^{14}C]ADP binding.

STUDIES ON SOLUBLE RECEPTORS

In order to characterize the ADP receptor mechanism in more precise bio-

TABLE 3

Binding of [^{14}C]ADP to platelet membranes

Method	[^{14}C]ADP bound (pmol/mg)
Membrane	97 ± 7 (7)
Membrane (frozen–thawed cells)	0 (4)

[^{14}C]ADP (372 pmol) was incubated with membrane vesicles (300 μg of particle per ml) in buffer for 1 hour at 37 °C with vigorous shaking. Values indicate means ± s.d. Number of experiments in parentheses.

chemical terms, we attempted to solubilize the binding protein(s). It was of some interest that binding of [^{14}C]ADP was abolished when membranes were obtained from frozen–thawed cells (Table 3). These observations raised the possibility that freeze–thawing released a receptor molecule(s) into solution. A soluble preparation was obtained by washing platelets from several units of whole blood, incubating them in an equal volume of buffer, and freeze–thawing them three times. The cells were removed by centrifugation and the supernate from the frozen–thawed cells was utilized. An ultracentrifuged, dialysed, and concentrated soluble preparation obtained from the frozen–thawed cells was subsequently assayed for [^{14}C]ADP binding. Small Sephadex G-25 columns were used to separate receptor-bound and free [^{14}C]ADP (Lefkowitz et al. 1972). Significant [^{14}C]ADP binding by the soluble fraction was demonstrated using column displacement as well as equilibrium dialysis methods (Table 4). An example of the binding of [^{14}C]ADP by the platelet soluble fraction is shown in Fig. 4. A significant portion of the [^{14}C]ADP in experiment (a) emerged with the protein in the soluble fraction. When the protein from this region of the chromatogram was extensively dialysed, 94% of the counts remained with the protein. In contrast no [^{14}C]ADP was bound

TABLE 4

Binding of [^{14}C]ADP to soluble fraction

Method	[^{14}C]ADP bound (pmol/mg)
Column	204 ± 14 (8)
Equilibrium dialysis	316 ± 24 (4)

[^{14}C]ADP was incubated with 1 mg of soluble receptor and binding determined by column displacement using small G-25 columns or equilibrium dialysis. Values indicate means ± s.d. Numbers of experiment in parentheses.

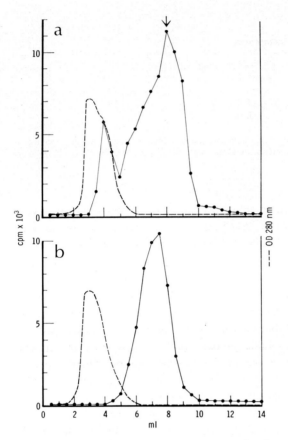

FIG. 4. Binding of [^{14}C]ADP by soluble preparation from frozen–thawed cells. (a) Two mg of soluble protein incubated with [^{14}C]ADP (670 pmol) at 37 °C for 1 hour. The mixture was then passed down a G-25 Sephadex column (1.5 cm × 28.5 cm) and fractions were monitored for protein and radioactivity. Arrow indicates position of free [^{14}C]ADP marker. (b) Same as above, using 2 mg of human albumin as protein solution.

by the control albumin column (experiment b). Gel chromatography of the soluble ADP receptor for determining the molecular weight of the binding species was performed on Sephadex G-150. A small aliquot of receptor solution was incubated with [^{14}C]ADP and then applied to the column (Fig. 5). The collected fractions were monitored for protein content as well as radio-activity. Free unbound ADP emerged after 50 ml of buffer had passed through the column while the bound nucleotide emerged earlier with a group of proteins in the molecular weight range of 160 000. The soluble receptor binding of [^{14}C]ADP, similar to the membrane vesicle binding reaction, was saturable,

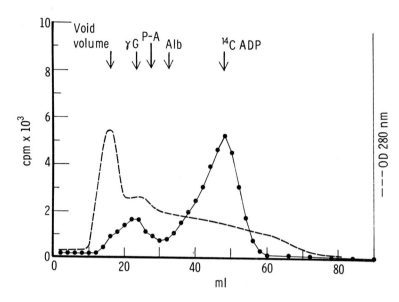

FIG. 5. Binding of [¹⁴C]ADP by soluble preparation from frozen–thawed cells using a G-150 column (1.5 cm × 28.5 cm). Two mg of soluble protein were incubated with [¹⁴C]ADP (670 pmol) at 37 °C for 1 hour. The mixture was then passed down the column and fractions were monitored for protein and radioactivity. Molecular weight marker protein elutions are indicated: γ-globulin, 160000; phosphorylase *a* (P-A), 94000; albumin (alb), 60000; and free [¹⁴C]ADP.

reversible, temperature-dependent, and supported by calcium or magnesium ions. Extraction of the bound radioactivity and subsequent thin layer chromatographic analysis revealed that the ADP was unchanged. The dissociation constant for ADP was determined by estimating the amount of ADP bound to the soluble receptor as a function of the total free ADP added (Fig. 6).

It is essential that the receptors solubilized from the particulate membranes or whole cells retain their specificity for the binding ligand. The comparative binding of several radioactive platelet-active agents is shown in Table 5. It is apparent that the platelet soluble receptor preparation retained a high specificity for ADP comparable to that shown by the isolated membrane particles.

In order to correlate the binding of [¹⁴C]ADP by the soluble receptor fraction with physiologically induced platelet aggregation, we studied the relative inhibitory effects of various agents known to interfere with ADP-induced aggregation (Fig. 7). These studies, which were done in a manner analogous to those using membrane vesicles, revealed that non-radioactive ADP was a potent inhibitor of [¹⁴C]ADP uptake. AMP was intermediate in its capacity

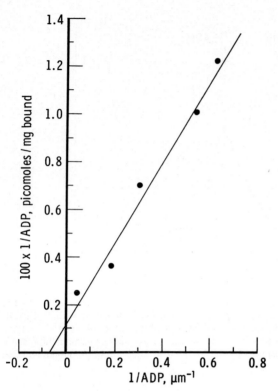

FIG. 6. Binding of [^{14}C]ADP to the soluble receptor preparation. Sips plot. With [^{14}C]ADP at 3.6×10^{-6}M, unlabelled ADP from 10^{-7}M to 10^{-3}M was added to mixtures of the soluble preparation. After incubation at 37 °C for 1 hour binding was determined using small G-25 columns. The intercept on the x axis provides an estimate of the dissociation constant. $K_d = 1 \times 10^5$M^{-1}.

TABLE 5

Comparative binding of platelet-active reagents

Material	ADP bound (pmol/mg)
[^{14}C]ADP	184
[^{14}C]ATP	10
[^{14}C] PGE$_1$	0
[^{14}C]Adrenaline	0
[^{14}C]AMP	2

The radioactive materials (1×10^{-6}M) were incubated with the soluble preparation for 1 hour at 37 °C. Binding was determined using small G-25 columns. Values indicate means of duplicate experiments.

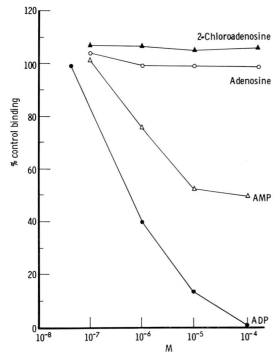

FIG. 7. Inhibition of [^{14}C]ADP binding by the soluble preparation with agents known to affect platelet function. The reagents were added at the indicated concentrations for 30 min at 37 °C, followed by [^{14}C]ADP.

to inhibit the binding reaction. Adenosine and 2-chloroadenosine were not inhibitory. The effect of 2-chloroadenosine was significantly different from the effect observed with isolated vesicles, where inhibition of [^{14}C]ADP binding was marked (Fig. 3, p. 28). The possibility thus exists that the molecular mechanisms involved in ADP binding by the soluble preparation differ from those operating in the membrane vesicle preparation. Whether this difference represents interactions by different molecular species from different subcellular sites or aberrant responses due to alterations of the same binding system by physical manipulation remains to be determined. As with the membrane particles, the various nucleoside diphosphates had no significant effect in inhibiting [^{14}C]ADP binding. Cyclic AMP also had no effect on [^{14}C]ADP binding by the soluble receptor preparation.

ATTEMPTS TO IDENTIFY THE MEMBRANE ADP BINDING SYSTEM

It would be of some importance if it were possible to relate the ADP binding at the platelet surface to any of the previously described membrane enzyme systems or to a known platelet protein complex such as thrombosthenin. In other cell systems, such as ox brain cell membranes, it has been demonstrated that ADP binds to a sodium-activated ATPase (Kaniike *et al.* 1973). A sodium-dependent potassium-stimulated ATPase is present at the platelet surface (Aledort *et al.* 1968), but ouabain, a known inhibitor of this system, had no effect on [^{14}C]ADP binding (Nachman & Ferris 1974). Other surface enzyme activities have been implicated as possible mediators of ADP-induced platelet aggregation. Various nucleoside diphosphates such as CDP, UDP and IDP in high concentrations lead to platelet shape changes and aggregation (Salzman *et al.* 1967). Platelet membrane nucleosidediphosphate kinase (E.C.2.7.4.6) catalyses the conversion of [^{14}C]ADP to [^{14}C]ATP (Guccione *et al.* 1971). Mustard & Perry (1973) have presented evidence supporting the role of platelet membrane nucleosidediphosphate kinase as a potential receptor for ADP in the aggregation reaction. Our observations that radioactive ADP remains unchanged after binding by the membrane vesicles or the soluble receptor preparation, and that UDP, CDP and IDP at high concentrations (10^{-3}M) failed to inhibit membrane particle or the soluble receptor [^{14}C]ADP binding, suggest that the receptor mechanism characterized in these studies is probably not related to the nucleosidediphosphate kinase system. Several studies have implicated cyclic AMP as a regulating factor in platelet aggregation (Ardlie *et al.* 1967; Salzman *et al.* 1972). Agents which increase platelet cyclic AMP inhibit platelet aggregation while agents which induce the aggregation response are associated with a decrease in cyclic AMP. Cyclic AMP had no effect on [^{14}C]ADP binding by either the membrane vesicles or the soluble receptor preparation. Preincubation of membrane vesicles with PGE$_1$, which increases membrane adenylate cyclase and platelet cyclic AMP, had no effect on [^{14}C]ADP binding. In addition there was no evidence of binding of [^{14}C]PGE$_1$ by the soluble preparation or the membrane vesicles. These observations suggest that the membrane ADP binding is probably not directly a function of the cyclic AMP system.

The platelet actomyosin complex may be sterically available at the platelet surface (Nachman *et al.* 1967; Booyse *et al.* 1971). Several hypotheses have been predicated on the premise that ADP-altered thrombosthenin ATPase acts as a trigger for the induction of platelet changes leading to aggregation. The demonstration that ADP binds to F-actin (Bárány *et al.* 1964) adds circumstantial evidence for the possible relationship of membrane ADP

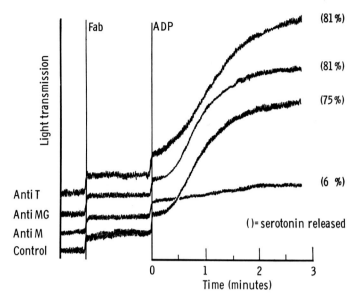

Fig. 8. Immuno interference with ADP-induced platelet aggregation and 5HT (serotonin) release. Platelets were labelled with [^{14}C] 5HT in platelet-rich plasma. Antibody fragments were added at a final concentration of 0.35 mg/ml. ADP final concentration was 4.4 μM. Anti T, anti-thrombosthenin; anti MG, anti-membrane glycoprotein; anti M, anti-membrane.

binding and surface thrombosthenin. In addition our data suggest that intact thiol groups are necessary for membrane ADP binding as well as thrombosthenin ATPase activity (Nachman *et al.* 1967). If surface thrombosthenin were involved in membrane ADP binding, it might be possible to interfere with this process with appropriate blocking antibodies. In order to explore these potential relationships, we have incubated platelets with non-agglutinating Fab fragments of antibodies to various platelet proteins including thrombosthenin, and the major platelet membrane glycoprotein (Nachman *et al.* 1973). In addition we used Fab fragments from a potent antibody raised to isolated platelet membranes (Kaplan & Nachman 1974). The influence of these antibody fragments on the ADP-induced platelet aggregation response as well as 5-hydroxytryptamine (5HT) release was studied. Anti-thrombosthenin and anti-membrane glycoprotein had no significant effects on ADP-induced platelet aggregation. The polyvalent membrane antibody interfered with the aggregation response as well as 5HT release (Fig. 8). None of these antibody fragments inhibited [^{14}C]ADP binding by isolated membrane vesicles. Thus it has not been possible by these immunological techniques to unambiguously identify the membrane receptor.

It is probable that the process of ADP-induced platelet aggregation involves a complex series of membrane-mediated events which may include an inter-related series of different membrane protein systems. The integrated functions of these separate membrane proteins probably lead to rapid modification of the ADP at the surface of the intact cell. By utilizing membrane vesicles as well as a soluble preparation we have been able to isolate and demonstrate an early event in this sequence—ADP binding. The purification and identification of a specific molecular entity which serves as the ADP 'trigger' at the platelet surface should greatly amplify our present understanding of haemostatic events.

ACKNOWLEDGEMENT

This work was supported by NIH Grant HL 14810 and a grant from the Krakower Hematology Foundation.

References

ALEDORT, L. M., TROUP, S. B. & WEED, R. I. (1968) Inhibition of sulfhydryl dependent platelet functions by penetrating and non penetrating analogues of parachloromercuri-benzene. *Blood 31*, 471-479

ARDLIE, N. G., GLEN, G. & SCHWARTZ, C. J. (1967) Inhibition and reversal of platelet aggregation by methylxanthines. *Thromb. Diath. Haemorrh. 18*, 670

BARÁNY, M., KOSHLAND, D. E., JR, SPRINGHORN, S. S., FINKELMAN, F. & THERATTILI-ANTHONY, T. (1964) Adenosine triphosphate cleavage during the G-actin to F-actin transformation and the binding of adenosine diphosphate to F-actin. *J. Biol. Chem. 239*, 1917-1919

BOOYSE, F. M., STERNBERGER, L. A., ZSCHOCKE, D. & RAFFELSON, M. E., JR (1971) Ultrastructural localization of contractile protein (thrombosthenin) in human platelets using an unlabelled antibody peroxidase staining technique. *J. Histochem. Cytochem. 19*, 540-550

BORN, G. V. R. (1965) Uptake of adenosine and adenosine diphosphate by human blood platelets. *Nature (Lond.) 206*, 1121-1122

BOULLIN, D. J., GREEN, A. R. & PRICE, K. S. (1972) The mechanism of adenosine diphosphate induced platelet aggregation: binding to platelet receptors and inhibition of binding and aggregation by prostaglandin E_1. *J. Physiol. (Lond.) 221*, 415-426

CUATRECASAS, P. (1972) Properties of the insulin receptor isolated from liver and fat cell membranes. *J. Biol. Chem. 247*, 1980-1991

CUATRECASAS, P. (1974) Membrane receptors. *Ann. Rev. Biochem. 43*, 844

DUFAU, M. L., CHARREAU, E. H. & CATT, K. J. (1973) Characteristics of a soluble gonadotropin receptor from the rat testis. *J. Biol. Chem. 248*, 6973-6982

GAVIN, J. R., ARCHER, J. A. & LESNIAH, M. A. (1972) Hormone receptor interactions in circulating cells: studies in normal and pathologic states in man. *J. Clin. Invest. 51*, 35a

GUCCIONE, M. A., PACKHAM, M. A., KINLOUGH-RATHBONE, R. L. & MUSTARD, J. F. (1971) Reactions of ^{14}C-ADP and ^{14}C-ATP with washed platelets from rabbits. *Blood 37*, 542-555

HALL, Z. N. (1972) Release of neurotransmitters and their interaction with receptors. *Ann. Rev. Biochem. 41*, 925-952

KAPLAN, K. & NACHMAN, R. L. (1974) The effect of platelet membrane antibodies on aggregation and release. *Br. J. Haematol. 28*, 551-560

KANIIKE, K., ENDMAN, E. & SCHINER, W. (1973) ADP binding to $(Na^+ + K^+)$ activated ATPase. *Biochim. Biophys. Acta 298*, 901-905

LEFKOWITZ, R. J., ROTH, J., PRICER, W. & PASTAN, I. (1970) ACTH receptors. The adrenal specific binding of ACTH ^{125}I and its relation to adenylcyclase. *Proc. Natl. Acad. Sci. U.S.A. 65*, 745-752

LEFKOWITZ, R. J., HABER, E. & O'HARA, O. (1972) Identification of the cardiac beta-adrenergic receptor: solubilization and purification by affinity chromatography. *Proc. Natl. Acad. Sci. U.S.A. 69*, 2828-2832

MARCUS, A. J., ZUCKER-FRANKLIN, D., SAFIER, L. B. & ULLMAN, H. L. (1966) Studies on human platelet granules and membranes. *J. Clin. Invest. 45*, 14-28

MILLS, D. C. B. & SMITH, J. B. (1971) The influence on platelet aggregation of drugs that affect the accumulation of adenosine $3':5'$-cyclic monophosphate in platelets. *Biochem. J. 121*, 185-196

MUSTARD, J. F. & PERRY, D. W. (1973) Interaction of platelets with nucleoside diphosphates. *Fed. Proc. 32*, 844abs

NACHMAN, R. & FERRIS, B. (1972) Studies on the proteins of human platelet membranes. *J. Biol. Chem. 247*, 4468-4475

NACHMAN, R. & FERRIS, B. (1974) Binding of adenosine diphosphate by isolated membranes from human platelets. *J. Biol. Chem. 249*, 704-710

NACHMAN, R. L., MARCUS, A. J. & SAFIER, L. B. (1967) Platelet thrombosthenin: subcellular localization and function. *J. Clin. Invest. 46*, 1380-1389

NACHMAN, R. L., HUBBARD, A. & FERRIS, B. (1973) Iodination of the human platelet membrane. *J. Biol. Chem. 248*, 2928-2936

RODBELL, M., KRANS, H., POHL, S. C. & BIRNBAUMER, L. (1971) The glucagon sensitive adenyl cyclase system in plasma membranes of rat liver. *J. Biol. Chem. 246*, 1861-1871

SALZMAN, E. W., CHAMBERS, D. A. & NERI, L. L. (1966) Incorporation of labelled nucleotides and aggregation of human blood platelets. *Thromb. Diath. Haemorrh. 15*, 52-68

SALZMAN, E. W., CHAMBERS, D. A. & NERI, L. L. (1967) Platelet aggregation by non-adenine nucleotides. *Fed. Proc. 26*, 759

SALZMAN, E. W., KENSLER, P. C. & LEVINE, L. (1972) Cyclic $3'5'$-adenosine monophosphate in human blood platelets. *Ann. N.Y. Acad. Sci. 201*, 61-71

SPAET, T. H. & LEJNIEKS, I. (1966) Studies on the mechanism whereby platelets are clumped by adenosine diphosphate. *Thromb. Diath. Haemorrh. 15*, 36-51

Discussion

Feinberg: With Professor Born I have studied ADP binding by intact human platelets (Feinberg 1973). Platelets in plasma containing [^{14}C]ADP or [^{3}H]ADP and ^{125}I-labelled human serum albumin were sedimented through silicone oil (Feinberg *et al.* 1974). The uptake of radioactivity from labelled ADP by the platelets was calculated from the determination of the total uptake of ADP radioactivity and that occurring in the plasma trapped between the platelets. At 10 seconds (the earliest time interval after the addition of labelled ADP) there was significant uptake of radioactivity and it increased with further incubation (Fig. 1). In agreement with Dr Nachman, we found that PGE$_2$, in concentrations which inhibited platelet aggregation, did not inhibit the uptake

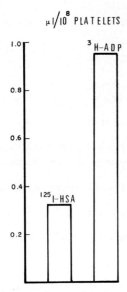

FIG. 1. (Feinberg). Uptake of radioactivity from ^{125}I-labelled human serum albumin and [³H]ADP. Human platelets in plasma were incubated at 37 °C with ^{125}I-labelled human serum albumin and with [³H]ADP. A sample was taken 10 seconds after the addition of labelled compounds and centrifuged over silicone oil. Radioactivity was measured in the platelet-free plasma and in the platelet pellet. The uptake was calculated as the volume occupied by the radioactive compound relative to its concentration in plasma.

of ADP radioactivity and that very little uptake occurred using other labelled nucleoside diphosphates (GDP, IDP and UDP).

Earlier work by Professor Born (1965) showed that the continuing uptake of ADP radioactivity represented the uptake of ADP metabolites, principally adenosine. Incubation at 18 °C, 27 °C and 37 °C resulted in significant differences in the slope of uptake of radioactivity; however, the three uptake curves extrapolated to a common value which we took as an indication of ADP binding.

We resuspended platelets in plasma that had been heated at 56 °C for 30 minutes to decrease the metabolism of ADP. We found that the uptake of radioactivity remained fairly constant for about five minutes and only then began to increase. When non-isotopic adenosine was present there was hardly any effect on the initial kinetics of radioactivity uptake from ADP but the subsequent increase in radioactivity was depressed. On the other hand, unlabelled ADP depressed both the initial kinetics and the subsequent rise in uptake. Dipyridamole, which inhibits the uptake of adenosine, had no effect on the initial uptake of ADP radioactivity but did decrease the subsequent rise in uptake.

Salzman *et al.* (1969) had shown earlier, using [α-^{32}P]ADP and a filtration method, that no radioactivity was taken up, and concluded that ADP is not bound to platelets. With our technique we found an uptake of radioactivity which did not increase with further incubation.

Using different concentrations of ADP we obtained evidence for several sites (that is, the Scatchard binding plot was not linear). We estimated that about 88 000 molecules of ADP could bind per platelet and that the high-affinity sites had an affinity constant of about $10^5 M^{-1}$.

It is interesting that despite the widely differing techniques there is good agreement between Dr Nachman's study and ours on the number of ADP binding sites. I think the difference in affinity constant and the fact that Dr Nachman finds only one class of sites might be due to the long equilibration time (one hour) used in his study.

Born: I attempted to measure this first several years ago (Born 1965) but I am still doubtful about the relevance of the results we and others have obtained to the binding of ADP to specific receptors for it on the platelets. The doubts are based on an excellent paper by Burgen (1966) in which the agonist–receptor interaction is subjected to an exceptionally fundamental analysis. In our system ADP behaves as a pharmacological agonist. ADP is a highly charged molecule, like other pharmacological agonists including acetyl-choline and the biogenic amines. These agonists interact with the receptors for them in such a way that by all ordinary methods binding cannot be demonstrated, because the dissociation constants are such that the duration of each molecular interaction is of the order of 10^{-8} second. So we have to consider association and dissociation rates of ADP at the receptor molecule. These may be so fast that the comparatively crude techniques used so far for demonstrating binding may be irrelevant to the analysis of the reaction mechanism. All sorts of tricks are being used to discover specific binding reactions of this kind; for example, molecular modifications for affinity labelling.

Adelstein: Dr Nachman, I noticed that in Table 1 (p. 26), the binding of [^{14}C]ADP to platelet membranes was about 100 pmol/mg whereas the binding of [^{14}C]ADP to the soluble fraction from the frozen–thawed cells (Table 2, p. 27) was 200-300 pmol/mg. One might have hoped that if you were concentrating the receptor proteins the binding might have increased much more. Do you think the procedure used in preparing the soluble fraction resulted in denaturation of the binding sites?

Nachman: The frozen–thawed supernatant is a molecular mixture, and unfortunately it contains proteinases. My present working premise is that there is proteolytic denaturation during processing. We have been able recently, by doing the isolation in the presence of better inhibitor systems, to get higher specific activities for binding.

Adelstein: Were you able to obtain a specific activity for the material eluted by Sephadex gel filtration?

Nachman: Yes. The specific activity was significantly higher than that of the material put on the Sephadex G-150 column.

Mills: You appear to imply an absence of nucleosidediphosphate kinase activity in the supernatant from frozen–thawed platelets. This is surprising, as it is a soluble cytoplasmic enzyme.

Nachman: We were able to retrieve labelled ADP from the soluble 'receptor' and show that it was not altered, so we inferred that the specific binding had nothing to do with nucleosidediphosphate kinase. We didn't measure the enzyme in the soluble receptor preparation.

Mustard: If [^{14}C]ADP is added to the supernatant from a platelet suspension, it is not converted to [^{14}C]ATP unless a source of phosphoryl donor in the form of ATP or another nucleoside triphosphate is added (Guccione *et al.* 1971). One cannot exclude the possibility that nucleosidediphosphate kinase was present in the preparations unless one does an experiment of this sort.

Nachman: We did that assay with the membrane particles, and there was no conversion of labelled ADP to ATP. We didn't do this with the frozen–thawed supernatant.

Holmsen: What chromatographic system was used to demonstrate that the radioactivity bound to membrane and supernatant protein was authentic [^{14}C]ADP? In your figures you showed only that the peak of radioactivity coincided with that of added ADP. Where in your system did other known ADP metabolites migrate, such as ATP, AMP, IMP and adenosine?

Nachman: The system is fully described in our publication (Nachman & Ferris 1974). ATP, AMP and adenosine appear in different spots. They all move in clearly different areas in the chromatogram.

Holmsen: In Fig. 7 (p. 33), which showed that 'known' inhibitors of ADP-induced platelet aggregation also interfere with ADP binding, AMP in 10^{-5}M concentration was used. Rozenberg and I (1968) have shown that AMP *per se* is absolutely *without* effect on ADP-induced platelet aggregation at this concentration. It has first to be broken down to adenosine before inhibition occurs. Therefore, your demonstration of inhibition of ADP binding by AMP speaks *against* the binding mechanism that you have described here, representing the ADP-'receptor' binding which possibly is involved in the aggregation mechanism.

Nachman: Actually the concentration of AMP used in these experiments varied from 10^{-7}M to 10^{-3}M. Maximum inhibition of binding occurred at the higher concentrations, although, as you noted, significant inhibition took place at 10^{-5}M. We are aware of your studies. Other studies (Packham *et al.* 1969) suggest that AMP even at low concentrations such as 8.5×10^{-6}M can inhibit platelet aggregation significantly if the platelets are preincubated with the inhibitor for 5 or 10 minutes. Thus, under some circumstances AMP might very well compete for the membrane receptor. We don't know yet how adenosine, present as a contaminant of AMP, affects this reaction.

Holmsen: Your Fig. 7 showed that adenosine gave far less inhibition than AMP, so the presence of the usual 5–15% adenosine in commercial AMP preparations cannot explain your AMP effect as being due to adenosine. Moreover, it has now been established that most, if not all, of the inhibitory effect of adenosine can be accounted for by the formation of cyclic AMP *inside* the platelet membrane (Haslam 1975), and one should therefore expect that adenosine does not inhibit aggregation through binding to the ectocellular 'ADP receptor'.

Concerning a possible binding of ADP to surface-located thrombosthenin, I would add that we have demonstrated binding of considerable amounts of metabolic ADP to the ethanol-insoluble fraction of platelets (Holmsen 1972). Recently, French & Wachowicz (1974) have identified actomyosin as the major ADP-binding protein in this fraction. ADP in this complex does not exchange with externally added ADP. In your experiments ADP was added to freeze–thaw platelet lysate, and you showed binding. We also used freeze–thaw lysates, but added radioactive ADP did not bind (or exchange with endogenous, bound ADP) to proteins precipitable with ethanol.

Nachman: Your material contained subcellular material. Our soluble 'receptor' material was freed of subcellular material in the ultracentrifuge and then dialysed into a buffer system.

Holmsen: Centrifugation of our freeze–thaw lysates yields a particle-free supernatant that contains ethanol-precipitable ADP-protein complex.

Nachman: How was actomyosin soluble in your buffer system?

Holmsen: Washed platelets were suspended in 0.6 M-KCl and then frozen and thawed. What I am trying to get at is what connection may exist between your ADP-binding substance(s) in the soluble fraction and our ethanol-insoluble ADP (Holmsen 1972). So, is the bond(s) between ADP and your ADP-binding component(s) destroyed by ethanol?

Nachman: We haven't tried that; but, as you know, 0.6 M-KCl buffer will extract actomyosin, whereas our buffer system did not contain 0.6 M-KCl.

Haslam: I am concerned, as I suspect you are too, Dr Nachman, about the soluble 'receptor'. Is there really any good evidence that this is derived from the plasma membrane?

Nachman: None directly: except that we have been able to take membrane from large amounts of platelets and make a frozen–thawed preparation. We obtain a small amount of protein which behaves the same, with respect to ADP binding, as the large amount of protein obtained from whole cells.

Mills: Of course, ADP inside the platelet will react with several different known materials. What we are looking for as an ADP receptor is something located on the outside of the membrane, so perhaps we should direct ourselves towards phenomena which can be specifically related to external membrane function. I am particularly interested in the effect of mersalyl in your system. At a concentration which completely inhibits the binding of ADP in your soluble receptor system, mersalyl does not inhibit the first action of ADP on the intact platelet—the initiation of the shape change.

Nachman: At 10^{-5}M.

Mills: We found this also at 10^{-4}M.

Nachman: I agree; and I cannot explain the difference!

Haslam: Are the systems comparable, since in one there are a lot of plasma proteins present, and the other is an isolated system? Plasma proteins will react with thiol reagents.

Nachman: We can argue that an isolated membrane or an isolated soluble 'receptor' behaves differently under the conditions tested.

Crawford: I too am a bit concerned about the heterogeneity of your membrane fraction, Dr Nachman, since almost certainly this will be a mixture of both surface and intracellular membrane components. I would support Dr Mills' comments about the need to establish the surface localization of the ADP receptor.

In this context, perhaps I could refer to our own studies on platelet subcellular fractionation and our demonstration of the ubiquitous presence of F-actin associated with all the particulate elements of the cell (Taylor & Crawford 1975).

As you know, from studies with muscle actins, G-actin is now believed to be an 'ATP-actin' and F-actin an 'ADP-actin'. Dephosphorylation of the bound ATP occurs during polymerization. In both forms of actin the nucleotide is not apparently covalently linked and is to some extent exchangeable (Laki 1971). In our subcellular fractionation studies we use zonal rotor ultracentrifugation and we have one procedure for isolating the membrane and granular organelles (lysosome-like granules, mitochondria, 5-hydroxytryptamine storage bodies) in one single gradient run (Taylor & Crawford 1974a) and another which separates the mixed membrane fraction into surface and intracellular membrane vesicles (Taylor & Crawford 1974b). The surface membrane fraction has been identified by lactoperoxidase covalent radioiodination and by ^{125}I-labelled anti-platelet membrane antibody. The two membrane fractions are also analytically and enzymically distinguishable. Using sodium dodecyl sulphate/urea solubilized platelet fractions, and SDS acrylamide gel electrophoresis, we find that actin is present as a prominent 43000 mol.wt. band in all the platelet fractions. This band co-electrophoreses with muscle and platelet actins (Taylor & Crawford 1975). In the membrane fractions we refer to this actin as 'membrane-associated actin' since establishing it as an integral or intrinsic protein is quite difficult, although it survives two long sucrose density gradient procedures and up to a week's dialysis. However, that some of this actin, or perhaps even all of it, is present as F-actin was indicated by its combination with skeletal muscle myosin to produce a 3–4-fold enhancement of the Mg^{2+}-ATPase activity. We do not have any evidence yet to suggest that it is surface-oriented in the whole platelet but perhaps we should at least entertain the possibility that it may participate in ADP-mediated phenomena, if not at an exteriorized site, perhaps at some location subadjacent to the surface membrane.

Nachman: We have looked at membrane particles derived from the granule fraction of a platelet homogenate. This granule membrane fraction binds ADP, but we have not fully characterized this process. The cytosol or soluble material at the top of the gradient derived by subcellular fraction does not react with ADP.

Crawford: This is an interesting point, since in our fractions although the actin subunit which co-electrophoreses with authentic muscle and platelet actin is present in all platelet fractions including the 6×10^6 *g* min soluble phase, only the particulate bound actin is combinable with skeletal muscle myosin with increased Mg^{2+}-ATPase activity. We have assumed that the cytosol actin is in the G-form (Taylor & Crawford 1975).

Cohen: In relation to the physiological significance of the binding of ADP by the membrane, you mentioned that this binding depends on calcium. Since shape change can occur in the absence of calcium, the binding of ADP to the receptor is evidently not necessary for the change in shape.

Nachman: It is true that calcium influences the membrane particle [^{14}C]ADP binding. This effect is less marked in the soluble receptor system.

Marcus: I would like to make some general comments on attempts to isolate platelet receptors for substances such as 5HT, ADP or adrenaline. Professor Born's points about receptor mechanisms are well taken. When one is studying the pharmacology of the uptake of 5HT by whole platelets, considerable information can be obtained about receptor mechanisms. On the other hand, when one is studying an isolated platelet fraction with the potential of binding ADP or 5HT, the term 'receptor' may not be entirely accurate. Perhaps the term 'acceptor' would be better. In other tissues it has been possible to obtain

subcellular particles—in the form of either membranes or soluble fractions—
which take up hormones in a reversible manner, and it has been possible to
study kinetics and other properties of the uptake. In these instances it is
appropriate to talk about a 'receptor'. When one attempts to apply such
approaches to platelets, the difficulties are considerable. Whole platelets take
up 5HT by a clearly defined mechanism. On the other hand, a platelet homogenate does not take up 5HT. If platelets are labelled with radioactive 5HT
and a homogenate is prepared therefrom, all the radioactivity appears in the
supernatant. Therefore, if we have isolated a particle or soluble fraction from
platelets which can take up 5HT, nucleotides, adrenaline, and so on, in a
manner similar to but not identical with uptake in the whole platelet, it might
be more suitable to call this an 'acceptor'. However, if someone isolates a
platelet derivative which takes up adenine nucleotides, 5HT, etc. in the same
time sequence and with the same kinetics as whole platelets, it might then be appropriate to call this substance a 'receptor'.

Born: I don't entirely agree. Our techniques may still be inadequate but
improvements should enable us to isolate a receptor or receptors for 5HT;
for example, through the design of affinity analogues. This is being done for
other biogenic amines and has to be applied to 5HT. One has to start from the
premise that there are specific receptors for 5HT on the platelet membrane.

Marcus: What you say about receptor mechanisms in other cells is certainly
true, but so far I don't think this methodology has been successfully applied
to platelets. I do believe, however, that refinements in methodology will
eventually allow the isolation of platelet receptors in the true sense of the term.

Lüscher: It is very difficult to provide experimental evidence for the binding
of aggregated IgG to washed platelets: but since the release- and aggregation-
inducing effect of the IgG aggregates is inhibited by monomeric IgG, a specific
receptor with a low binding affinity must be postulated.

Born: It may be relevant to recall that adrenaline is antagonized by phenoxy-
benzamine at the α-receptor, where the dissociation constant of the antagonist
is much lower.

Marcus: Again we are switching back from whole platelets in plasma or
buffer to subcellular platelet particles. So far in platelet research it has not
been possible to transpose thinking about 'receptor mechanisms' in living
platelets to subcellular platelet particles, whereas with liver cells or adipose
tissue it has been possible to do so.

Caen: We have been studying the molecular defect in thrombasthenia
(Degos *et al.* 1975). An IgG antibody found in the serum of a thrombasthenic
patient reacted in complement fixation with platelets from 350 normal individuals but was unreactive with platelets from eight other thrombasthenic

patients. ADP-induced aggregation of normal platelets was inhibited by the patient's antibody.

Family studies using the quantitative complement fixation test showed that healthy heterozygotes were easily distinguishable from normal or thrombasthenic individuals since their platelets had an intermediate amount of the reactive antigen.

Indirect immunoprecipitation tests using this serum and soluble membrane antigens labelled with ^{125}I that had been extracted from normal platelets by the detergent Nonidet P-40 gave a single radioactive peak at a molecular weight of 120000 in SDS polyacrylamide gel electrophoresis. A similar estimate of the molecular weight was obtained from Sephadex G-200 filtration of the soluble antigens extracted from normal platelets by spontaneous release or by chaotropic agents and tested in complement fixation with the patient's own serum.

These findings strongly suggest that the molecule recognized by this antibody is absent from, or structurally modified in, thrombasthenic patients, and that it may be involved in platelet aggregation.

Nachman: Is this a surface antigen?

Caen: It seems to be.

Nachman: Do you have any kinetic studies on the relative affinity of the receptor for ADP?

Caen: Not yet.

References

BORN, G. V. R. (1965) Uptake of adenosine and of adenosine diphosphate by human blood platelets. *Nature (Lond.) 206*, 1121-1122

BURGEN, A. S. V. (1966) The drug-receptor complex. *J. Pharm. Pharmacol. 18*, 137-149

DEGOS, L., DAUTIGNY, A., BROUET, J. C., COLOMBANI, M., ARDAILLOU, N., CAEN, J. P. & COLOMBANI, J. (1975) A molecular defect in thrombasthenic platelets. *J. Clin. Invest. 56*, 236-240

FEINBERG, H. (1973) Interaction of ADP with platelets. *Br. J. Pharmacol. 47*, 654P

FEINBERG, H., MICHEL, H. & BORN, G. V. R. (1974) Determination of the fluid volume of platelets by their separation through silicone oil. *J. Lab. Clin. Med. 84*, 926-934

FRENCH, P. C. & WACHOWICZ, B. (1974) Investigations of the binding component of the ethanol insoluble metabolic ADP of human platelets and its relation to the release reaction. *Haemostasis 3*, 271-281

GUCCIONE, M. A., PACKHAM, M. A., KINLOUGH-RATHBONE, R. L. & MUSTARD, J. F. (1971) Reactions of ^{14}C-ADP and ^{14}C-ATP with washed platelets from rabbits. *Blood 37*, 542-555

HASLAM, R. J. (1975) This volume, pp. 121-143

HOLMSEN, H. (1972) Ethanol-insoluble adenine nucleotides in platelets and their possible role in platelet function. *Ann. N.Y. Acad. Sci. 201*, 109-121

LAKI, K. (1971) in *Contractile Proteins and Muscle* (Laki, K., ed.), pp. 97-113, Marcel Dekker, New York

NACHMAN, R. & FERRIS, B. (1974) Binding of adenosine diphosphate by isolated membranes from human platelets. *J. Biol. Chem. 249*, 704-710

PACKHAM, M. A., ARDLIE, M. G. & MUSTARD, J. F. (1969) Effect of adenine compounds on platelet aggregation. *Am. J. Physiol. 217*, 1009

ROZENBERG, M. C. & HOLMSEN, H. (1968) Adenine nucleotide metabolism of blood platelets. II. Uptake of adenosine and inhibition of ADP-induced platelet aggregation. *Biochim. Biophys. Acta 155*, 342-352

SALZMAN, E. W., ASHFORD, T. P., CHAMBERS, D. A. & NERI, L. L. (1969) Platelet incorporation of labelled adenosine and adenosine diphosphate. *Thromb. Diath. Haemorrh. 22*, 304-315

TAYLOR, D. G. & CRAWFORD, N. (1974a) The subcellular fractionation of pig platelets by zonal centrifugation. In *Methodological Developments in Biochemistry*, vol. 4: *Subcellular Studies* (Reid, E., ed.), pp. 319-326, Longmans, London

TAYLOR, D. G. & CRAWFORD, N. (1974b) The subfractionation of platelet membranes by zonal centrifugation: identification of surface membranes. *FEBS Lett. 41*, 317-322

TAYLOR, D. G. & CRAWFORD, N. (1975) The identification of actin associated with pig platelet membranes and granules. *Biochem. Soc. Trans. 3*, 161-164

Enzyme activities on the platelet surface in relation to the action of adenosine diphosphate

J. FRASER MUSTARD, M. A. PACKHAM, D. W. PERRY, M. A. GUCCIONE and R. L. KINLOUGH-RATHBONE

Department of Pathology, McMaster University, Hamilton, Ontario and Department of Biochemistry, University of Toronto, Ontario

Abstract With suspensions of washed platelets from rabbits, we have demonstrated that ADP reacts with a nucleosidediphosphate kinase on the platelet surface. Several observations relate to the hypothesis that this enzyme takes part in ADP-induced shape change and aggregation. In high concentrations other nucleoside diphosphates (GDP, CDP, IDP, UDP) cause platelet shape change and weak aggregation; they also inhibit ADP-induced aggregation. [^{14}C]GDP and [^{14}C]CDP are converted to the corresponding [^{14}C]nucleoside triphosphates, but to a lesser extent than is [^{14}C]ADP. Nucleoside triphosphates, added to the suspending medium, enhance the conversion of [^{14}C]nucleoside diphosphates to [^{14}C]nucleoside triphosphates. All the nucleoside triphosphates inhibit ADP-induced aggregation, but ATP (which has the greatest enhancing effect) is most inhibitory. AMP inhibits ADP-induced shape change and aggregation and inhibits nucleosidediphosphate kinase both in the presence and absence of externally added ATP. Prostaglandin E$_1$ and hydroxylamine inhibit ADP-induced shape change and aggregation but inhibit the nucleosidediphosphate kinase activity only in the absence of external ATP. ADP-induced shape change without aggregation occurs in the presence of EGTA or EDTA but during the first minute after [^{14}C]ADP addition, only about half as much [^{14}C]ADP is converted to [^{14}C]ATP as in the absence of EGTA or EDTA. EGTA does not inhibit nucleosidediphosphate kinase in the presence of external ATP although EDTA does. Thus all compounds tested which inhibit nucleosidediphosphate kinase also inhibit ADP-induced aggregation. After the addition of ADP to suspensions of washed rabbit platelets, increased amounts of ATP appear in the suspending fluid. Membrane-bound or internal nucleoside triphosphate may donate the phosphoryl group. Prostaglandin E$_1$ (but not acetylsalicylic acid) inhibits this increase in ATP in the medium. Acetylsalicylic acid does not inhibit nucleosidediphosphate kinase activity. With platelets prelabelled by incubation with [^{14}C]adenosine, there is no ADP-induced increase in [^{14}C]ATP in the medium, nor is ^{51}Cr lost from platelets prelabelled with this isotope. When platelets are prelabelled with ^{32}P, addition of ADP leads to the appearance of [^{32}P]ATP in the suspending fluid. The evidence indicates that ADP interacts with nucleosidediphosphate kinase on the platelet surface which donates a phosphoryl group to form ATP in the suspending fluid.

47

As a result of his early studies of the effects of ADP on platelets, Born (1965) suggested that there was a specific receptor on the platelet membrane which was responsible for inducing the aggregation reaction. Attempts to demonstrate ADP binding to intact platelets in plasma with [^{14}C]ADP (Born 1965; Boullin *et al.* 1972) are open to criticism because of the possibility of adenosine formation or contamination in the system. The radioactivity that becomes associated with the platelets when [^{14}C]ADP is added to platelet-rich plasma is probably due to the formation of [^{14}C]adenosine that is then taken up by the platelets and converted to radioactive ADP (Spaet & Lejnieks 1966; Salzman *et al.* 1969). Nachman & Ferris (1974) have recently described the binding of [^{14}C]ADP to isolated platelet membranes over a period of 60 minutes. The uptake of the radioactive label was inhibited by compounds which are structurally similar to ADP and would compete for the same binding site. They concluded that there are approximately 100 000 ADP binding sites per platelet. Born (1965) proposed from his studies of the uptake of adenosine and ADP by platelets that there are approximately 200 000 ADP receptor sites per platelet. Hampton & Mitchell (1966) examined the effect of ADP on the electrophoretic mobility of platelets and came to the conclusion that there are 85 000 receptor sites for ADP per platelet.

Several hypotheses concerning ADP-induced platelet aggregation are based on the premise that ADP inhibits an ATPase associated with platelet membrane contractile protein (thrombosthenin). Chambers and associates (1967) proposed that ADP-induced aggregation occurs because of inhibition of an ecto-ATPase on the platelet surface and that continuous activity of this enzyme is required to maintain the platelets in a non-adhesive state. They presented evidence that ecto-ATPase is similar to or identical with the ATPase associated with platelet actomyosin. Booyse & Rafelson (1969) suggested that ATPase inhibition by ADP causes reversible dissociation of the contractile protein into actin and myosin which then cross-link adjacent platelets. The proposals involving an ecto-ATPase would have to include the assumption that ATP could be transferred from the membrane to the ecto-ATPase or that there is a continuous source of ATP available in the suspending medium of platelets.

Another enzyme with which ADP can interact on the platelet surface is nucleosidediphosphate kinase (E.C. 2.7.4.6). Mourad & Pert (1967) reported that platelets exhibited nucleosidediphosphate kinase activity and Chambers and associates (1968) observed that the nucleosidediphosphate kinase of human platelets was capable of interacting with other nucleoside diphosphates as well as with ADP. Gaarder *et al.* (1961) showed that GDP and CDP in high concentrations caused aggregation in citrated human platelet-rich plasma. Chambers *et al.* (1968) reported similar results with GDP, CDP, IDP and UDP.

We found that when [^{14}C]ADP is added to suspensions of washed platelets from rabbits, from 10 to 20% of the label appears as [^{14}C]ATP within 5 to 10 minutes (Guccione *et al.* 1971). (We had established in these studies and in earlier experiments (Packham *et al.* 1969) that [^{14}C]ADP is not converted to [^{14}C]adenosine by these washed platelets suspended in an artificial medium and that the platelets do not take up radioactivity under these conditions; there was no evidence of loss of adenylate kinase from the platelets in these suspensions.) It was evident that the original source of the phosphoryl group required for the conversion reaction must be the platelets, but it was not established whether ATP *per se* was released or lost from the platelets or whether only the phosphoryl group was transferred directly from the platelets to the [^{14}C]ADP. Feinberg *et al.* (1973) obtained similar results with suspensions of washed rabbit or human platelets. They also found that when [γ-^{32}P]ATP is added to a platelet suspension, the labelled phosphoryl group is transferred to the platelets.

MATERIALS AND METHODS

Platelet suspensions

Suspensions of twice-washed platelets from rabbits or humans were prepared as previously described (Ardlie *et al.* 1970; Mustard *et al.* 1972). The final suspending medium was Tyrode solution containing 0.35% albumin; the platelet count was adjusted to 700000 per mm^3. Platelet suspensions were kept at room temperature and the samples were warmed at 37 °C for five minutes before use in the studies involving the luciferin–luciferase assay of adenine nucleotides, or the conversion of labelled nucleoside diphosphates to the corresponding nucleoside triphosphates. For some of the aggregation experiments, apyrase was included in the suspending medium and the suspensions were stored at 37 °C (Ardlie *et al.* 1971).

Reagents

Nucleoside mono-, di-, and triphosphates, L-adrenaline, dibutyryl cyclic AMP and hydroxylamine were obtained from Sigma Chemical Company, St. Louis, Mo. Both synthetic CDP and CDP isolated from yeast were used. Acetylsalicylic acid (ASA) was from British Drug Houses, Toronto, Canada. Prostaglandin E$_1$ (PGE$_1$) was a generous gift of the Upjohn Company, Kalamazoo, Michigan; it was dissolved and diluted as described elsewhere (Kinlough-Rathbone *et al.* 1970). Human lyophilized fibrinogen, grade 1, was obtained from A. B. Kabi, Stockholm, Sweden. It was treated with DFP as described by Packham *et al.* (1974) and used at a final concentration of 0.1 % in the platelet suspending medium in the experiments in which aggregation was studied. Apyrase was prepared from potatoes by the method of Molnar & Lorand (1961). All materials to be added to platelet suspensions were dissolved in Tyrode solution and adjusted to pH 7.35. All concentrations given are final concentrations after all additions.

Radioactive compounds

[8-^{14}C]Adenosine 5'-diphosphate, trisodium salt ([^{14}C]ADP) and [U-^{14}C]-guanosine 5'-diphosphate, trisodium salt ([^{14}C]GDP) were from New England Nuclear Corp., Boston, Mass. [U-^{14}C]Cytidine 5'-diphosphate, ammonium salt ([^{14}C]CDP), [8-^{14}C]adenosine ([^{14}C]adenosine) 52 mCi/mmol, and sodium [^{51}Cr]chromate (^{51}Cr), 100–300 mCi/mg Cr, 1 μCi/μl, were from Amersham/Searle, Arlington Heights, Ill. Orthophosphate labelled with ^{32}P (carrier-free) was from Atomic Energy of Canada Ltd., Ottawa, Canada. Platelets were prelabelled with ^{51}Cr, ^{32}P, or [^{14}C] adenosine as described elsewhere (Cazenave *et al.* 1973; Lloyd *et al.* 1972; Reimers *et al.* 1973).

Platelet aggregation was studied as described by Packham *et al.* (1974).

Conversion of [^{14}*C*]*nucleoside diphosphates to* [^{14}*C*]*nucleoside triphosphates* (and the slight conversion to [^{14}C]nucleoside monophosphates) was measured at 37 °C as described elsewhere (Packham *et al.* 1974). ^{32}P-labelled adenine nucleotides were separated from each other and from [^{32}P]orthophosphate by low voltage paper electrophoresis at 4 °C using 0.12 M-citrate buffer at pH 4.8. All nucleotide-containing spots were found by illuminating the chromatograms or electrophoretograms with ultraviolet light. The spots were cut out and counted by liquid scintillation counting.

Measurement of materials in platelet suspending fluid

The amounts of materials in the platelet suspending fluid following the addition of ADP or Tyrode solution (controls) were determined by centrifuging the suspensions at 12 000 × *g* for 1 minute in an Eppendorf centrifuge (Brinkmann, Rexdale, Ont.) The supernatant solution was removed for assay. Measurements of ATP and ADP were done immediately or after storage at −20 °C for 18 hours.

ATP and ADP in the platelet suspending fluid were assayed by a modification (Jenkins *et al.* 1971) of the luciferin–luciferase (firefly) assay of Kalbhen &

TABLE 1

Conversion of [^{14}C]ADP, [^{14}C]GDP or [^{14}C]CDP to the corresponding nucleoside triphosphates (NTP) by a suspension of washed rabbit platelets in the presence and absence of
external ATP

Labelled compound added[a]	Added external ATP (μM)	% of label as NTP after incubation with platelets[b]		
		2 min	5 min	10 min
[^{14}C]ADP	0	1.8	5.9	10.2
[^{14}C]ADP	9	6.1	17.1	23.4
[^{14}C]ADP	90	19.7	42.1	61.6
[^{14}C]GDP	0	0	0.7	1.4
[^{14}C]GDP	9	2.1	7.4	12.8
[^{14}C]GDP	90	12.0	33.0	55.7
[^{14}C]CDP	0	0	0.5	1.1
[^{14}C]CDP	9	3.1	3.2	6.3
[^{14}C]CDP	90	3.3	3.7	8.8

[a] The final concentration of the labelled nucleoside diphosphates was 5μM.
[b] Mean values of two experiments.

Koch (1967) using the Dupont Luminescence biometer reagent kit (E. I.
Dupont de Nemours and Co., Wilmington, Del.).

^{51}Cr in the supernatant solutions or in samples of the platelet suspensions
was counted in a well-type crystal scintillation counter.

RESULTS

The addition of [^{14}C]ADP to a suspension of washed rabbit platelets led
to the formation of [^{14}C]ATP (Table 1). At equimolar concentrations, much
less [^{14}C]GDP and [^{14}C]CDP were converted to their triphosphates than was
[^{14}C]ADP to its triphosphate. Also shown in this table is the effect of adding
ATP to the suspending medium. This caused markedly enhanced conversion
of [^{14}C]ADP to [^{14}C]ATP and of [^{14}C]GDP to [^{14}C]GTP, but only slightly
enhanced the conversion of [^{14}C]CDP to [^{14}C]CTP.

The effect of nucleoside mono-, di- and triphosphates on rabbit platelets
is summarized in Table 2. Results of experiments on the aggregation of platelets
are also included. With the exception of AMP, the nucleoside monophosphates had little effect on ADP-induced platelet aggregation or on the conversion of [^{14}C]ADP to [^{14}C]ATP. At the concentrations tested, only AMP

TABLE 2

Summary of effects of nucleoside mono-, di-, and triphosphates on rabbit platelets[a]

Compound	Platelet aggregation		Effect on ADP-induced aggregation	Effect on conversion of [^{14}C]ADP to [^{14}C]ATP
	Rabbit	Human		
GMP	no	no	very slight inhibition	no effect
CMP	no	no	very slight inhibition	no effect
UMP	no	no	very slight inhibition	no effect
IMP	no	no	very slight inhibition	no effect
AMP	no	no	strong inhibition	inhibition
GDP	yes	yes[b]	inhibition	inhibition
CDP	yes	yes[b]	inhibition	inhibition
UDP	yes	yes[b]	inhibition	inhibition
IDP	yes	yes[b]	inhibition	inhibition
GTP	no	no	inhibition	enhancement
CTP	no	no	inhibition	enhancement
UTP	no	no	inhibition	enhancement
ITP	no	no	inhibition	enhancement
ATP	no	no	inhibition	enhancement

[a] See Guccione *et al.* (1971) and Packham *et al.* (1972, 1974).
[b] Shape change and weak aggregation with 830 μM.

inhibited ADP-induced shape change. It inhibited the conversion of [^{14}C]ADP to [^{14}C]ATP in either the absence or presence of externally added ATP. It is important to note that AMP is not converted to adenosine in these suspensions of washed platelets and in most experiments the AMP was treated with adenosine deaminase to remove any traces of adenosine (Packham *et al.* 1972). All of the nucleoside diphosphates induced shape change with suspensions of washed rabbit or human platelets and caused some degree of platelet aggregation, particularly when the sensitivity of the platelets was enhanced by the presence of adrenaline. In high concentrations all of the nucleoside diphosphates inhibited ADP-induced aggregation and the conversion of [^{14}C]ADP to [^{14}C]ATP. The nucleoside triphosphates all enhanced the conversion of [^{14}C]ADP to [^{14}C]ATP but only ATP was effective at low concentrations. The addition of the nucleoside triphosphates to suspensions of washed rabbit platelets inhibited ADP-induced platelet aggregation but ATP produced the most marked inhibition. Higher concentrations of the other nucleoside triphosphates were required for inhibition.

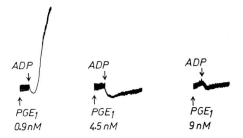

FIG. 1. Effect of PGE$_1$ on ADP-induced aggregation and shape change of washed rabbit platelets. PGE$_1$ at the concentrations indicated was added 15 seconds before ADP (4.5 μM). Aggregation is indicated by an upward deflection of the curve (increase in light transmission). Change in platelet shape from disks to a more rounded form with pseudopods causes a small downward deflection of the aggregation curve and loss of the oscillations of light transmission.

The effect of inhibitors of ADP-induced platelet aggregation on nucleoside-diphosphate kinase activity

The addition of prostaglandin E$_1$ to a suspension of washed rabbit platelets inhibited ADP-induced aggregation and shape change (Fig. 1). Table 3 shows the effect of these concentrations of PGE$_1$ on the conversion of [^{14}C]ADP to [^{14}C]ATP and [^{14}C]AMP by washed rabbit platelets. The concentration of PGE$_1$ which produced maximum inhibition of ADP-induced shape change and aggregation was the concentration which produced the maximum inhibition of the conversion of [^{14}C]ADP to [^{14}C]ATP. If an external phosphoryl group donor were made available for the nucleosidediphosphate kinase, PGE$_1$ did not inhibit the conversion of [^{14}C]ADP to [^{14}C]ATP (Table 3). PGE$_1$ did not inhibit the slight conversion of [^{14}C]ADP to [^{14}C]AMP in these suspensions of washed platelets.

Hydroxylamine has been reported by Iizuka & Kikugawa (1972) to inhibit platelet aggregation. Concentrations of hydroxylamine which inhibit the conversion of [^{14}C]ADP to [^{14}C]ATP (Table 4) also blocked ADP-induced shape change (Fig. 2). The effect of hydroxylamine appears to be similar to that of prostaglandin E$_1$ in that hydroxylamine did not inhibit the conversion of [^{14}C]ADP to [^{14}C]ATP in the presence of ATP in the suspending fluid (Table 4). Hydroxylamine did not inhibit the conversion of [^{14}C]ADP to [^{14}C]AMP in these suspensions of washed platelets.

Dibutyryl cyclic AMP at final concentrations between 0.45mM and 4.5 mM did not have any effect on the conversion of [^{14}C]ADP to [^{14}C]ATP by washed rabbit platelets (Table 5). However, at a concentration of 450 μM, dibutyryl cyclic AMP inhibited ADP-induced platelet aggregation and at 4500 μM it inhibited the ADP-induced platelet shape change (Fig. 3).

TABLE 3

Effect of PGE_1 on conversion of $[^{14}C]ADP$ to $[^{14}C]ATP$ and $[^{14}C]AMP$ by suspensions of washed rabbit platelets and the influence of external ATP on these reactions

Expt	Addition		% of label as $[^{14}C]ATP$, $[^{14}C]ADP$ or $[^{14}C]AMP$ after incubation with platelets				
			0.5 min	1 min	2 min	5 min	10 min
1	Control solution	ATP	0.1	1.4	3.0	9.8	—
		ADP	99.8	98.4	94.6	87.5	—
		AMP	0.1	0.2	2.4	2.7	—
	PGE_1 9nM	ATP	0	0	0.4	1.9	—
		ADP	100	100	98.8	94.6	—
		AMP	0	0	1.4	3.5	—
	PGE_1 4.5nM	ATP	0	0	0.6	2.3	—
		ADP	100	100	98.8	94.2	—
		AMP	0	1.0	0.6	3.5	—
	PGE_1 0.9nM	ATP	0	0.1	1.1	4.4	—
		ADP	100	99.3	97.7	91.8	—
		AMP	0	0.6	1.2	3.8	—
2	Control solution + Tyrode	ATP	—	2.0	4.6	10.1	16.5
	Control solution + ATP 80 μM	ATP	—	15.4	28.4	56.4	73.2
	PGE_1 8 μM + Tyrode	ATP	—	0.9	1.0	1.9	2.9
	PGE_1 8 μM + ATP 80 μM	ATP	—	12.3	23.0	45.0	70.0

In experiment 1, the $[^{14}C]ADP$ (4.5 μM) was added 15 seconds after the PGE_1 or control solution (solvent used to dissolve PGE_1). In experiment 2, the PGE_1 or control solution was incubated with the platelet suspension for 10 minutes at 37 °C before the addition of ATP or Tyrode solution, followed by $[^{14}C]ADP$ (3.35 μM) 15 seconds later. About 0.3% of the $[^{14}C]ADP$ ran in the ATP spot on chromatograms of $[^{14}C]ADP$ that had not been exposed to platelets. This percentage has been subtracted from the $[^{14}C]ATP$ values.

EGTA and EDTA are known to inhibit ADP-induced platelet aggregation but they do not inhibit the ADP-induced shape change if they are added immediately before the ADP. We examined the effect of EDTA and EGTA on the conversion of $[^{14}C]ADP$ to $[^{14}C]ATP$ by washed rabbit platelets. Fig. 4 shows that EDTA inhibited the conversion of $[^{14}C]ADP$ to $[^{14}C]ATP$ and that this effect was not influenced by the addition of unlabelled ATP to the suspending fluid. In contrast, Fig. 5 shows that although EGTA inhibited the conversion of $[^{14}C]ADP$ to $[^{14}C]ATP$, this inhibitory effect was overcome if ATP were added to the suspending fluid. Since the shape change occurs during the first few seconds following the addition of ADP, studies were done

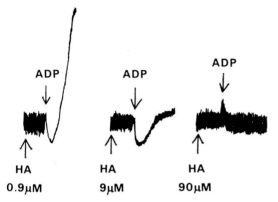

FIG. 2. Effect of hydroxylamine on ADP-induced aggregation and shape change of washed rabbit platelets. Hydroxylamine at the concentrations indicated was added 15 seconds before ADP (4.5 μM). (See caption of Fig. 1 for explanation of changes in light transmission.)

to determine whether there was detectable conversion of [^{14}C]ADP to [^{14}C]-ATP in the presence of EDTA or EGTA during the first minute (Table 6). Samples were taken 30 seconds and 60 seconds after the addition of [^{14}C]ADP to the platelet suspension and assayed for [^{14}C]ATP formation. In every experiment there was more [^{14}C]ATP at 30 seconds and 60 seconds in the suspending fluid containing platelets than in the suspending medium to which [^{14}C]ADP was added. Although the amount of conversion in the presence of the chelating agents was less than in their absence, it is clear that the chelating agents did not completely block the conversion of [^{14}C]ADP to [^{14}C]ATP during the first minute.

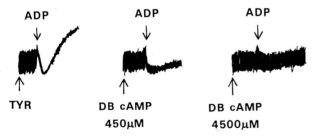

FIG. 3. Effect of dibutyryl cyclic AMP (DB cAMP) on ADP-induced aggregation and shape change of washed rabbit platelets. Dibutyryl cyclic AMP at the concentrations shown was added 15 seconds before ADP (4.5 μM). A control experiment in which Tyrode solution (TYR) was added is shown at the left. (See caption of Fig. 1 for explanation of changes in light transmission.)

TABLE 4

Effect of hydroxylamine on conversion of [^{14}C]ADP to [^{14}C]ATP and [^{14}C]AMP by suspensions of washed rabbit platelets and the influence of external ATP on these reactions

Expt	Addition		% of label as [^{14}C]ATP, [^{14}C]ADP or [^{14}C]AMP after incubation with platelets			
			0.5 min	1 min	2 min	5 min
1	Tyrode	ATP	2.3	3.9	5.0	12.6
		ADP	96.4	93.4	91.1	82.8
		AMP	1.7	2.7	4.9	5.0
	Hydroxylamine 90μM	ATP	2.2	1.4	0.7	3.0
		ADP	95.6	96.3	95.0	89.4
		AMP	2.2	2.3	4.3	7.6
	Hydroxylamine 45μM	ATP	1.1	1.5	1.9	2.2
		ADP	96.3	95.7	94.4	89.3
		AMP	2.6	2.8	3.7	8.5
	Hydroxylamine 9μM	ATP	1.2	1.6	3.2	4.7
		ADP	97.1	96.1	93.8	88.5
		AMP	1.7	2.3	3.0	6.8
	Hydroxylamine 0.9μM	ATP	2.0	3.2	4.0	8.3
		ADP	95.7	93.4	89.5	85.0
		AMP	2.3	3.4	6.5	6.7
2	Tyrode + Tyrode	ATP	0	0.5	2.0	7.5
	Tyrode + ATP 8μM	ATP	1.9	3.3	7.7	25.5
	Hydroxylamine 45μM	ATP	0	0	0	0
	Hydroxylamine 45μM + ATP 8μM	ATP	1.0	3.7	12.6	26.8

In experiment 1, the [^{14}C]ADP (4.5μM) was added 15 seconds after the hydroxylamine or Tyrode solution. In experiment 2, ATP (or Tyrode) was added 15 seconds after the hydroxylamine (or Tyrode) followed by [^{14}C]ADP (4.2μM) 15 seconds later.

About 0.6% of the [^{14}C]ADP ran in the ATP spot on chromatograms of [^{14}C]ADP that had not been exposed to platelets. This percentage has been subtracted from the [^{14}C]ATP values.

TABLE 5

Conversion of [^{14}C]ADP to [^{14}C]ATP by suspensions of washed rabbit platelets in the presence of dibutyryl cyclic AMP

Addition to platelet suspension	% of label as [^{14}C]ATP at 5 min			
	Expt 1	Expt 2	Expt 3	Expt 4
Tyrode	4.9	12.9	7.5	13.6
Dibutyryl cyclic AMP				
0.45mM	4.6	10.6	7.7	11.5
0.9mM	4.8	9.8	6	12.2
4.5mM	4.0	–	–	9.7

Dibutyryl cyclic AMP or Tyrode solution was added to the platelet suspensions 15 seconds before [^{14}C]ADP (4.5μM).

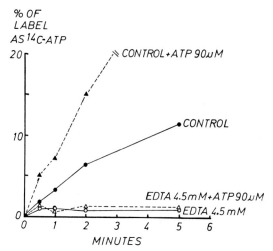

FIG. 4. Effect of EDTA on the conversion of [^{14}C]ADP to [^{14}C]ATP by washed rabbit platelets in the presence and absence of external ATP. EDTA or Tyrode solution (control) was added 30 seconds before [^{14}C]ADP; ATP (or Tyrode solution) was added 15 seconds before [^{14}C]ADP.

TABLE 6

Effect of EDTA or EGTA on conversion of [^{14}C]ADP to [^{14}C]ATP by washed rabbit platelets

Addition to platelet suspension	% of label as [^{14}C]ATP (mean ± s.e.)	
	30 seconds	60 seconds
Tyrode	1.9 ± 0.28	2.9 ± 0.42
EDTA 4.7mM	1.2 ± 0.20	1.4 ± 0.31
Tyrode	2.3 ± 0.31	3.6 ± 0.37
EGTA 4.7 mM	1.6 ± 0.50	2.2 ± 0.42

EDTA, EGTA or Tyrode solution was added 30 seconds before [^{14}C]ADP. Concentrations of [^{14}C]ADP between 1 and 5μM were used. Results shown are the mean values of 9 experiments with EDTA and 6 experiments with EGTA. About 0.4% of the [^{14}C]ADP ran in the ATP spot on chromatograms of [^{14}C]ADP that had not been exposed to platelets. This percentage was subtracted before the mean values for [^{14}C]ATP were calculated. Paired difference analysis indicated that in the presence of EDTA or EGTA the amount of [^{14}C]ADP converted to [^{14}C]ATP at 30 seconds and 60 seconds was significantly greater than zero. $P < 0.005$.

The addition of acetylsalicylic acid to suspensions of washed rabbit platelets had no effect on the conversion of 3.4 μM [^{14}C]ADP to [^{14}C]ATP (percentage [^{14}C]ATP at five minutes: control, 10.6; ASA 1mM, 9.8; ASA 5mM, 9.7).

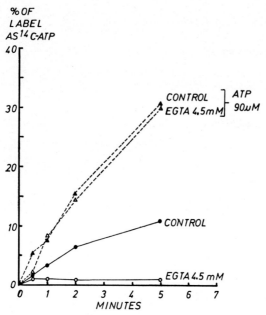

FIG. 5. Effect of EGTA on the conversion of [^{14}C]ADP to [^{14}C]ATP by washed rabbit platelets in the presence and absence of external ATP. Additions were made as described for Fig. 4.

Measurement of ATP and ADP in the suspending fluid

Table 7 shows the results of experiments in which the ATP and ADP in the supernatant were measured 10 minutes after the addition of ADP to a suspension of washed rabbit platelets. The total amount of ADP plus ATP in the supernatant of the platelet suspensions to which ADP had been added was similar to the total amount of ADP plus ATP in suspending medium without platelets to which ADP was added. The amount of ATP appearing in the supernatant following the addition of ADP, expressed as the percentage of ADP converted to ATP, was similar to that measured in the experiments with [^{14}C]ADP. Table 7 also shows that the amount of ATP in the supernatant of a platelet suspension without added ADP was usually less than 0.1 μM. The addition of aspirin to a suspension of washed rabbit platelets had no effect on the amount of ATP appearing in the suspending fluid after the addition of ADP (Table 7).

Table 8 shows that the addition of prostaglandin E$_1$ to a suspension of washed rabbit platelets before the addition of ADP inhibited the amount of ATP appearing in the supernatant fluid. In conjunction with one of these

TABLE 7

Concentration of ADP and ATP in supernatant of a suspension of washed rabbit platelets 10 minutes after addition of ADP

Expt	Solution analysed	Additions	Supernatant or suspending fluid		% of added ADP converted to ATP
			ATP + ADP (μM)	ATP (μM)	
1	Suspending medium	ADP	7.90	0.06	
	Supernatant from platelet suspension	TYR[a]	0.08	0.04	
		ADP	9.3	2.8	35.4
2	Suspending medium	ADP	11.7	0.1	
	Supernatant from platelet suspension	TYR	0.2	0.1	
		ADP	11.8	0.6	5.1
3	Suspending medium	ADP	18.0	0.1	
	Supernatant from platelet suspension	TYR	0.21	0.07	
		ADP	15.0	1.90	10.6
4	Suspending medium	ADP	11.0	0.2	
	Supernatant from platelet suspension	TYR	0.3	0.2	
		ADP	10.3	2.1	19.1
5	Suspending medium	TYR + ADP	37.0	0.06	
	Supernatant from platelet suspension	TYR + TYR	—	0.06	
		ASA[b] + TYR	—	0.06	
		TYR + ADP	—	3.5	9.5
		ASA[b] + ADP	—	3.4	9.2

[a] TYR, Tyrode solution.
[b] ASA (acetylsalicylic acid) concn, 0.5mM.

experiments, the amount of [^{14}C]ADP converted to [^{14}C]ATP was measured at 10 minutes; the percentage converted to [^{14}C]ATP was 12% and the percentage converted in the presence of 9μM PGE_1 was 2.4%. These values approximate those found with the firefly assay.

TABLE 8

Effect of PGE$_1$ on the concentration of ADP and ATP in supernatant of suspensions of washed rabbit platelets 10 minutes after addition of ADP

Expt	Solution analysed	Additions	Supernatant or suspending fluid		% of added ADP converted to ATP
			ATP + ADP (μM)	ATP (μM)	
1	Suspending medium	ADP	16.2	0.1	
	Supernatant from platelet suspension[c]	PGE$_1$[a]+TYR	0.1	0.07	
		TYR+ADP	15.0	1.90	11.7
		PGE$_1$[a]+ADP	15.1	0.40	2.5
2	Suspending medium	ADP	40	0.1	
	Supernatant from platelet suspension	PGE$_1$[b]+TYR	—	0.1	
		TYR+ADP	—	6.2	15.5
		PGE$_1$[b]+ADP	—	0.41	1.2
3	Suspending medium	ADP	37	0.1	
	Supernatant from platelet suspension	PGE$_1$[a]+TYR	—	0.1	
		TYR + ADP	—	3.3	8.9
		PGE$_1$[a]+ADP	—	0.23	0.6

[a] 8.5μM.
[b] 0.85μM.
[c] With the same suspension of washed rabbit platelets, the percentage of 3.35μM[14C]ADP converted to [14C]ATP was 12% with Tyrode solution and 2.4% with 9μM PGE$_1$ in 10 minutes.

Source of ATP in the suspending fluid

Although the findings indicated that ATP *per se* probably was not lost or released from the platelets, further experiments were done to investigate this possibility. To determine whether cytoplasmic constituents were lost after the addition of ADP under the conditions of these experiments, washed rabbit platelets were labelled with ^{51}Cr and the accumulation of radioactivity in the suspending fluid was measured. Suspensions of washed ^{51}Cr-labelled rabbit platelets warmed for five minutes before the addition of ADP did not show any increased accumulation of radioactivity in the suspending fluid in comparison to the control (Table 9). Furthermore, after 30 minutes at 37 °C there

TABLE 9

Loss of ^{51}Cr from prelabelled washed rabbit platelets at 37 °C[a]

Addition	Supernatant ^{51}Cr as % of platelet ^{51}Cr (mean $\pm$ S.E.)		
	5 min	15 min	30 min
Tyrode	2.6 $\pm$ 0.2	2.8 $\pm$ 0.3	3.1 $\pm$ 0.3
ADP 0.9μM	2.5 $\pm$ 0.2	3.0 $\pm$ 0.3	3.3 $\pm$ 0.4
ADP 9μM	2.9 $\pm$ 0.3	2.8 $\pm$ 0.3	3.2 $\pm$ 0.3

[a] Mean values from four experiments. The labelled platelets were incubated at 37 °C for the times indicated before the addition of ADP. Samples were centrifuged 5 minutes after the addition of ADP and the amount of ^{51}Cr in the supernatant was determined.

was no significant difference between the values for ^{51}Cr in the suspending fluid for the ADP-stimulated platelets or the control platelets.

The possibility of loss of cytoplasmic constituents was also examined by incubating suspensions of washed rabbit platelets with [^{14}C]adenosine to label the ATP and ADP in the metabolic pool. In these experiments, the specific activity of the [^{14}C]ATP was such that if the ATP appearing in the suspending fluid had come from the cytoplasm, it would have been detectable as [^{14}C]ATP. Table 10 shows that there was no apparent increase in [^{14}C]ATP in the supernatant of these prelabelled washed rabbit platelets after the addition of ADP.

To investigate the possibility that the terminal phosphoryl group of platelet ATP was being transferred to added ADP, washed rabbit platelets were labelled by incubation with [^{32}P]orthophosphate to produce [^{32}P]ATP in the metabolic

TABLE 10

Loss of [^{14}C]ATP from washed rabbit platelets preincubated with [^{14}C] adenosine

Expt	Addition	Supernatant [^{14}C]ATP as % of platelet [^{14}C]ATP at 10 min	Estimated concentration of ATP in supernatant at 10 min[a] (μM)
1	Tyrode	0.39	0.096
	ADP 9μM	0.32	0.079
	ADP 90μM	0.37	0.091
2	Tyrode	0.77	0.19
	ADP 9μM	0.73	0.18
	ADP 90μM	0.42	0.11

[a] Calculated from the supernatant [^{14}C]ATP and based on 62 nmol ATP per 7 $\times$ 10^8 rabbit platelets (Ardlie et al. 1970) and the assumption that only 40% of the total platelet ATP is in the metabolic pool which can be labelled readily by preincubation of the platelets with [^{14}C]adenosine.

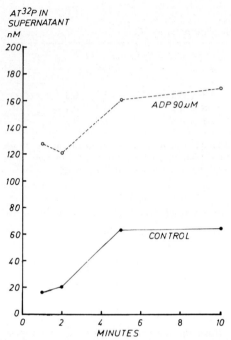

FIG. 6. ADP-induced appearance of [^{32}P]ATP in suspending fluid of washed rabbit platelets prelabelled by incubation with [^{32}P]orthophosphate. The calculation of molarity of ATP in the supernatant is based on the [^{32}P]ATP in the supernatant fluid and on 62 nmol ATP per 7×10^8 rabbit platelets (Ardlie *et al.* 1970) and the assumption that only 40% of the total ATP is in the metabolic pool which can be labelled readily with ^{32}P.

pool. Over the time interval studied, there was a greater amount of [^{32}P]ATP in the supernatant of the platelet suspension to which ADP had been added than in the controls (Fig. 6). The results from another experiment of this type are summarized in Table 11. In this experiment, ADP caused an increase in [^{32}P]ATP in the supernatant and this increase was not inhibited by acetyl-salicylic acid. There appeared to be some inhibition by prostaglandin E$_1$ of the ADP-induced appearance of [^{32}P]ATP in the suspending fluid.

Suspensions of washed human platelets

We have found that human platelets exhibit more ecto-ATPase activity than rabbit platelets; this makes it difficult to demonstrate their nucleoside-diphosphate kinase activity because [^{14}C]ATP formed from [^{14}C]ADP is dephosphorylated more rapidly (J. F. Mustard & D. W. Perry, unpublished observations).

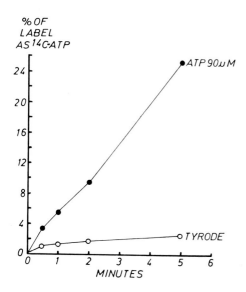

FIG. 7. Conversion of 10μM [¹⁴C]ADP to [¹⁴C]ATP by washed human platelets in the presence and absence of external ATP. ATP (or Tyrode solution) was added 15 seconds before [¹⁴C]ADP.

Fig. 7 shows that there is some conversion of [¹⁴C]ADP to [¹⁴C]ATP by a suspension of washed human platelets and that the addition of external ATP leads to extensive conversion, as is seen with rabbit platelets. Table 12 shows a comparison between the results of the firefly assay method of examining the conversion of ADP to ATP and the [¹⁴C]ADP method. Approximately the

TABLE 11

ADP-induced appearance of [³²P]ATP in suspensions of ³²P-labelled washed rabbit platelets

Additions	Supernatant [³²P]ATP as % of platelet [³²P]ATP at 10 min	Estimated concentration of ATP in supernatant at 10 min[a] (μM)
Tyrode	0.95	0.24
ADP 80μM	2.37	0.60
Tyrode + ASA[b] 1mM	1.06	0.26
ADP 80μM + ASA 1mM	3.15	0.78
Tyrode + PGE₁ 8μM	1.15	0.28
ADP 80μM + PGE₁ 8μM	1.77	0.44

[a] Calculated from the supernatant [³²P]ATP and based on 62 nmol of ATP per 7×10^8 rabbit platelets (Ardlie *et al.* 1970) and the assumption that only 40% of the total platelet ATP is in the metabolic pool which can be labelled readily with ³²P.
[b] ASA, acetylsalicylic acid.

TABLE 12

Conversion of ADP to ATP by washed human platelets

Expt	Assay method	Concentration of added ADP (μM)	% of ADP converted to ATP in 10 min
1	Firefly	12	2
2	Firefly	16	0.6
3	[^{14}C]ADP	10	2.2
4	[^{14}C]ADP	5	2
5	[^{14}C]ADP	5	6
6	[^{14}C]ADP	5	2
7	[^{14}C]ADP	3.6	1

same amount of ADP was found to be converted to ATP in 10 minutes by the two methods of assay.

DISCUSSION

When [^{14}C]ADP is added to a suspension of washed rabbit platelets it is partially converted to [^{14}C]ATP. We have established previously that this is caused by a nucleosidediphosphate kinase and is not due to adenylate kinase. Since Haslam & Mills (1967) and Mills *et al.* (1968) have reported that platelet damage causes loss of the latter enzyme, it is evident that platelets prepared by the technique used in the present study are undamaged as judged by the criterion of adenylate kinase loss.

In earlier studies (Guccione *et al.* 1971) and in the present studies, we observed a slight formation of [^{14}C]AMP during the much greater formation of [^{14}C]-ATP following addition of [^{14}C]ADP. We attribute this to an ADPase on the platelet surface. Further evidence that [^{14}C]AMP formation is not due to adenylate kinase is that both PGE$_1$ and hydroxylamine inhibit the formation of [^{14}C]ATP from [^{14}C]ADP but do not inhibit the formation of [^{14}C]AMP from [^{14}C]ADP.

The addition of an external phosphoryl group donor in the form of ATP greatly accelerated the conversion of [^{14}C]ADP to [^{14}C]ATP. However, the conversion to [^{14}C]ATP seen when [^{14}C]ADP was added to the suspension of washed platelets without added ATP cannot be attributed to ATP in the suspending medium for several reasons:

1. We established previously that when ADP is added to washed rabbit or human platelets suspended in Tyrode solution containing 0.35% albumin there

is no detectable release of ATP, ADP or 5-hydroxytryptamine from the amine storage granules (Packham *et al.* 1973; Mustard *et al.* 1975);

2. We could not show loss of cytoplasmic contents by prelabelling platelet adenine nucleotides by incubating platelets with [^{14}C]adenosine and examining the suspending fluid for [^{14}C]ATP and [^{14}C]ADP after addition of ADP;

3. We have not found that addition of ADP to suspensions of washed rabbit platelets causes loss of lactate dehydrogenase from the platelets into the suspending fluid (Joist *et al.* 1974). Since this cytoplasmic enzyme is not lost, it is concluded that lysis does not occur;

4. In the experiments reported in this paper, platelets prelabelled with ^{51}Cr did not lose labelled material into this suspension following the addition of ADP. ^{51}Cr labels cytoplasmic components. Therefore the observation that ^{51}Cr is not lost indicates that the platelets retain their cytoplasmic contents, which would include ADP and ATP.

5. Acetylsalicylic acid, which inhibits ADP-induced release from human platelet granules in citrated plasma, had no effect on the conversion of [^{14}C]-ADP to [^{14}C]ATP by suspensions of washed rabbit platelets.

Thus neither the rabbit platelet granules nor cytoplasm contribute ATP *per se* to the suspending medium after ADP addition. Furthermore, the ATP level in the suspending fluid is usually less than 0.1 μM whereas the amount of added ATP required to produce detectable acceleration of the conversion of [^{14}C]ADP to [^{14}C]ATP is 50 times greater. Thus the weight of the evidence indicates that the source of the phosphoryl group for the conversion of [^{14}C]ADP to [^{14}C]ATP has to be the platelets, possibly the platelet membrane.

We previously established that the enzyme must be on the surface of the platelets (Guccione *et al.* 1971). We have been able to demonstrate nucleosidediphosphate kinase activity in platelet membranes isolated by the method of Marcus *et al.* (1966) (D. W. Perry & J. F. Mustard, unpublished observations). In contrast, Nachman & Ferris (1974) reported that their human platelet membrane preparations did not exhibit nucleosidediphosphate kinase activity, although it is not clear that they added the phosphoryl group donor that would be required to demonstrate conversion of [^{14}C]ADP to [^{14}C]ATP.

The experiments in which the ATP and ADP concentrations in the suspending fluid were measured before and after the addition of ADP to a suspension of washed platelets are also in keeping with the concept that the platelet membrane nucleosidediphosphate kinase can transfer a phosphoryl group from the membrane to ADP in the suspending fluid. In these experiments the amount of ATP in the suspending fluid increased without there being any increase in the total ADP and ATP concentration. Thus, ADP in the suspending fluid must have been converted to ATP by the transfer of a phosphoryl group from the platelets via the membrane nucleosidediphosphate kinase.

The effects of the other nucleoside diphosphates and triphosphates on the platelets are compatible with the concept that nucleosidediphosphate kinase is the receptor for ADP which is involved in the ADP-induced platelet shape change and aggregation. The high molar concentrations of CDP, GDP, UDP and IDP required to induce platelet shape change and aggregation could be due to considerably lower affinity of the enzyme for these compounds, compared with its affinity for ADP (Packham *et al.* 1974). Some nucleosidediphosphate kinases from other cells show a higher affinity for ADP than for the other nucleoside diphosphates (Glaze & Wadkins 1967). The results with ATP and the other nucleoside triphosphates are in agreement with this concept, since in the presence of a phosphoryl group donor in the suspending medium, donation of a phosphoryl group from the platelets should be inhibited and therefore ADP-induced platelet shape change and aggregation should be inhibited. The fact that the nucleoside triphosphates other than ATP are less effective as phosphoryl group donors is also in keeping with the observation that the other nucleoside triphosphates are less effective inhibitors of ADP-induced shape change and aggregation than is ATP.

The results with the inhibitors of nucleosidediphosphate kinase activity also are compatible with the hypothesis that the nucleosidediphosphate kinase on the surface of rabbit platelets is the receptor for ADP and that it is the inter-action of ADP with this enzyme which induces platelet shape change and platelet aggregation. Compounds which inhibit the conversion of [^{14}C]ADP to [^{14}C]ATP in the absence of an external source of ATP all inhibit ADP-induced platelet aggregation. The compounds of this type which we have studied are AMP, *p*-chloromercuribenzene sulphonate (PCMBS) (Guccione *et al.* 1971), EGTA, EDTA, prostaglandin E_1, hydroxylamine, and nucleoside diphosphates other than ADP. In the presence of external ATP, only AMP, the other nucleoside diphosphates, PCMBS, and EDTA are inhibitory. In the case of AMP and the nucleoside diphosphates other than ADP it seems most likely that they compete with ADP for a site on the enzyme. AMP and other nucleo-side monophosphates have been shown to inhibit the nucleosidediphosphate kinase of red blood cells (Mourad & Parks 1966) but not the mitochondrial enzyme (Goffeau *et al.* 1967). At the concentrations used in these experiments, AMP was the only nucleoside monophosphate which inhibited the activity of the platelet enzyme. Reagents which block SH groups have been shown to inhibit both erythrocytic and mitochondrial nucleosidediphosphate kinase (Agarwal & Parks 1971; Goffeau *et al.* 1968).

Among the compounds which inhibit the donation of a phosphoryl group from the platelet to external ADP are EGTA, PGE_1 and hydroxylamine. At the concentrations tested, however, these compounds do not inhibit the activity of the enzyme since [^{14}C]ADP is converted to [^{14}C]ATP in the presence of these inhibitors providing there is an external source of ATP.

The failure of dibutyryl cyclic AMP to inhibit the conversion of [^{14}C]ADP to [^{14}C]ATP makes it questionable that the inhibition of nucleosidediphosphate kinase activity by prostaglandin E$_1$ is due to the increased platelet cyclic AMP levels. If it were, one would have expected dibutyryl cyclic AMP at concentrations which completely inhibit ADP-induced platelet shape change and aggregation to have shown some effect on nucleosidediphosphate kinase activity. As suggested by Salzman (1972), it may be that prostaglandin E$_1$, by stimulating adenylate cyclase, diverts ATP to form cyclic AMP so that ATP is not available to the nucleosidediphosphate kinase.

Although EDTA and EGTA inhibit the nucleosidediphosphate kinase and ADP-induced platelet aggregation they do not inhibit ADP-induced platelet shape change when they are added to a platelet suspension immediately before ADP. If platelets are incubated with EDTA at 37 °C they gradually lose their ability to change shape upon the addition of ADP (J. F. Mustard & D. W. Perry, unpublished observations). This evidence would seem to indicate that the nucleosidediphosphate kinase activity is not involved in the ADP-induced shape change. However, examination of the changes during the first minute showed that neither EGTA nor EDTA completely inhibited the conversion of [^{14}C]ADP to [^{14}C]ATP by the platelets. Thus it is possible that the shape change produced by ADP in the presence of EDTA and EDGA could be due to the slight interaction of ADP with the enzyme which occurs in the presence of EDTA and EGTA.

The compounds which inhibited ADP-induced platelet shape change produced almost complete inhibition of the conversion of [^{14}C]ADP to [^{14}C]ATP during the first minute after the addition of [^{14}C]ADP (these include AMP, PGE$_1$ and hydroxylamine). This may indicate that to prevent ADP-induced shape change there must be virtually complete inhibition of the phosphoryl group transfer during the first few seconds after ADP addition.

Under suitable conditions of temperature, stirring, and divalent cation concentration, platelet aggregation occurs after the initial shape change. Although the platelet aggregates eventually de-aggregate, the platelets are refractory to aggregation by the same concentration of ADP that was used to induce the first aggregation response (Born & Cross 1963). The timing of the events is such, however, that the platelets continue to convert [^{14}C]ADP to [^{14}C]ATP during this period. This may indicate that once the initial response to ADP in terms of the transfer of the phosphoryl group and shape change has occurred, further phosphoryl group transfers make the platelets refractory to further additions of ADP.

The transfer to external ADP of the phosphoryl group presumably diverts it from a reaction which is essential to maintain the platelets in their normal disk shape.

Among the possibilities are:

1. An effect on the production of platelet cyclic AMP and thereby on platelet calcium and the platelet contractile protein (Gerrard *et al.* 1974).

2. An effect on the turnover of the phosphate groups of the phosphatidyl inositols, resulting in changes in the transfer of ions, particularly calcium, across the platelet membrane (this has been suggested for phosphatidyl inositols in other cells (Hendrickson & Reinertsen 1971)). It is known that ADP causes increased turnover of the phosphate groups of phosphatidic acid and some of the phosphatidyl inositols during platelet shape change and aggregation (Lloyd *et al.* 1973).

3. A diversion of ATP from sites in the membrane where it is used to maintain the membrane contractile protein in a contracted state.

Although it has not been studied in as much detail, nucleosidediphosphate kinase is also present on the surface of human or pig platelets. Study of the enzyme on the surface of human platelets is more difficult than with rabbit platelets because of the greater amount of ecto-ATPase activity which appears to be associated with the human platelet membrane.

ACKNOWLEDGEMENTS

The technical assistance of Mrs C. Fagerstroem and Miss S. J. Turner is gratefully acknowledged. These studies were supported by Medical Research Council of Canada grants MT 1309 and MT 2629.

References

AGARWAL, R. P. & PARKS, R. E., JR (1971) Erythrocytic nucleoside diphosphokinase. V. Some properties and behavior of the pI 7.3 isozyme. *J. Biol. Chem. 246*, 2258-2264

ARDLIE, N. G., PACKHAM, M. A. & MUSTARD, J. F. (1970) Adenosine diphosphate-induced platelet aggregation in suspensions of washed rabbit platelets. *Br. J. Haematol. 19*, 7-17

ARDLIE, N. G., PERRY, D. W., PACKHAM, M. A. & MUSTARD, J. F. (1971) Influence of apyrase on the stability of suspensions of washed rabbit platelets. *Proc. Soc. Exp. Biol. Med. 136*, 1021-1023

BOOYSE, F. M. & RAFELSON, M. E., JR (1969) Studies on human platelets. III. A contractile protein model for platelet aggregation. *Blood 33*, 100-103

BORN, G. V. R. (1965) Uptake of adenosine and of adenosine diphosphate by human blood platelets. *Nature (Lond.) 206*, 1121-1122

BORN, G. V. R. & CROSS, M. J. (1963) The aggregation of blood platelets. *J. Physiol. (Lond.)* *168*, 178-195

BOULLIN, D. J., GREEN, A. R. & PRICE, K. S. (1972) The mechanism of adenosine diphosphate induced platelet aggregation: binding to platelet receptors and inhibition of binding and aggregation by prostaglandin E_1. *J. Physiol. (Lond.)* *221*, 415-426

CAZENAVE, J.-P., PACKHAM, M. A. & MUSTARD, J. F. (1973) Adherence of platelets to a collagen-coated surface: development of a quantitative method. *J. Lab. Clin. Med.* *82*, 978-990

CHAMBERS, D. A., SALZMAN, E. W. & NERI, L. L. (1967) Characterization of 'Ecto-ATPase' of human blood platelets. *Arch. Biochem. Biophys.* *119*, 173-178

CHAMBERS, D. A., SALZMAN, E. W. & NERI, L. L. (1968) Platelet nucleotide metabolism and platelet aggregation. *Exp. Biol. Med.* *3*, 62-70

FEINBERG, H., BELAMARICH, F. & BORN, G. V. R. (1973) Transphosphorylation in human and rabbit platelet suspensions. *Fed. Proc.* *32*, 220abs

GAARDER, A., JONSEN, J., LALAND, S., HELLEM, A. J. & OWREN, P. A. (1961) Adenosine diphosphate in red cells as a factor in the adhesiveness of human blood platelets. *Nature (Lond.)* *192*, 531-532

GERRARD, J. M., WHITE, J. G. & RAO, G. H. R. (1974) Effects of the ionophore A 23187 on blood platelets. II. Influence on ultrastructure. *Am. J. Pathol.* *77*, 151-159

GLAZE, R. P. & WADKINS, C. L. (1967) Properties of a nucleoside diphosphokinase from liver mitochondria and its relationship to the adenosine triphosphate-adenosine diphosphate exchange reaction. *J. Biol. Chem.* *242*, 2139-2150

GOFFEAU, A., PEDERSEN, P. L. & LEHNINGER, A. L. (1967) The kinetics and inhibition of the adenosine diphosphate-adenosine triphosphate exchange catalyzed by a purified mitochondrial nucleoside diphosphokinase. *J. Biol. Chem.* *242*, 1845-1853

GOFFEAU, A. PEDERSEN, P. L. & LEHNINGER, A. L. (1968) Reactivity of thiol groups in active and inactive forms of a mitochondrial nucleoside diphosphokinase. *J. Biol. Chem.* *243*, 1685-1691

GUCCIONE, M. A., PACKHAM, M. A., KINLOUGH-RATHBONE, R. L. & MUSTARD, J. F. (1971) Reactions of ^{14}C-ADP and ^{14}C-ATP with washed platelets from rabbits. *Blood 37*, 542-555

HAMPTON, J. R. & MITCHELL, J. R. A. (1966) An estimate of the number of adenosine diphosphate binding sites on human platelets. *Nature (Lond.)* *211*, 245-246

HASLAM, R. J. & MILLS, D. C. B. (1967) The adenylate kinase of human plasma, erythrocytes and platelets in relation to the degradation of adenosine diphosphate in plasma. *Biochem. J.* *103*, 773-784

HENDRICKSON, H. S. & REINERTSEN, J. L. (1971) Phosphoinositide interconversions: A model for control of Na^+ and K^+ permeability in the nerve axon membrane. *Biochem. Biophys. Res. Commun.* *44*, 1258-1266

IIZUKA, K. & KIKUGAWA, K. (1972) Platelet aggregation inhibitors. I. Hydroxylamine: a potent inhibitor of platelet aggregation *Chem. Pharm. Bull. (Tokyo)* *20*, 614-616

JENKINS, C. S. P., PACKHAM, M. A., KINLOUGH-RATHBONE, R. L. & MUSTARD, J. F. (1971) Interactions of polylysine with platelets. *Blood 37*, 395-412

JOIST, H. J., DOLEZEL, G., LLOYD, J. V., KINLOUGH-RATHBONE, R. L. & MUSTARD, J. F. (1974) Platelet factor-3 availability and the platelet release reaction. *J. Lab. Clin. Med.* *84*, 474-482

KALBHEN, D. A. & KOCH, H. J. (1967) Methodische Untersuchungen zur quantitativen Mikrobestimmung von ATP in biologischem Material mit dem Firefly-Enzymsystem. *Z. Klin. Chem. 5*, 299-304

KINLOUGH-RATHBONE, R. L., PACKHAM, M. A. & MUSTARD, J. F. (1970) The effect of prostaglandin E_1 on platelet function in vitro and in vivo. *Br. J. Haematol.* *19*, 559-571

LLOYD, J. V., NISHIZAWA, E. E., HALDAR, J. & MUSTARD, J. F. (1972) Changes in ^{32}P-labelling of platelet phospholipids in response to ADP. *Br. J. Haematol.* *23*, 571-585

LLOYD, J. V., NISHIZAWA, E. E. & MUSTARD, J. F. (1973) Effect of ADP-induced shape change on incorporation of ^{32}P into platelet phosphatidic acid and mono-, di- and triphosphatidyl inositol. *Br. J. Haematol. 25*, 77-99

MARCUS, A. J., ZUCKER-FRANKLIN, D., SAFIER, L. B. & ULLMAN, H. L. (1966) Studies on human platelet granules and membranes. *J. Clin. Invest. 45*, 14-28

MILLS, D. C. B., ROBB, I. A. & ROBERTS, G. C. K. (1968) The release of nucleotides, 5-hydroxytryptamine and enzymes from human blood platelets during aggregation. *J. Physiol. (Lond.) 195*, 715-729

MOLNAR, J. & LORAND, L. (1961) Studies on apyrases. *Arch. Biochem. Biophys. 93*, 353-363

MOURAD, N. & PARKS, R. E., Jr (1966) Erythrocytic nucleoside diphosphokinase. 1. Isolation and kinetics. *J. Biol. Chem. 241*, 271-278

MOURAD, N. & PERT, J. H. (1967) An enzymatic method to determine damage in human platelets. *Proc. Soc. Exp. Biol. Med. 125*, 643-645

MUSTARD, J. F., PERRY, D. W., ARDLIE, N. G. & PACKHAM, M. A. (1972) Preparation of suspensions of washed platelets from humans. *Br. J. Haematol. 22*, 193-204

MUSTARD, J. F., PERRY, D. W., KINLOUGH-RATHBONE, R. L. & PACKHAM, M. A. (1975) Factors responsible for ADP-induced release reaction of human platelets. *Am. J. Physiol. 228*, 1757-1765

NACHMAN, R. L. & FERRIS, B. (1974) Binding of adenosine diphosphate by isolated membranes from human platelets. *J. Biol. Chem. 249*, 704-710

PACKHAM, M. A., ARDLIE, N. G. & MUSTARD, J. F. (1969) The effect of adenine compounds on platelet aggregation. *Am. J. Physiol. 217*, 1009-1017

PACKHAM, M. A., GUCCIONE, M. A., PERRY, D. W., KINLOUGH-RATHBONE, R. L. & MUSTARD, J. F. (1972) AMP inhibition of reactions of ADP with washed platelets from humans and rabbits. *Am. J. Physiol. 223*, 419-424

PACKHAM, M. A., GUCCIONE, M. A., CHANG, P.-L. & MUSTARD, J. F. (1973) Platelet aggregation and release: effects of low concentrations of thrombin or collagen. *Am. J. Physiol. 225*, 38-47

PACKHAM, M. A., GUCCIONE, M. A., PERRY, D. W. & MUSTARD, J. F. (1974) Interactions of nucleoside di- and triphosphates with rabbit platelets. *Am. J. Physiol. 227*, 1143-1148

REIMERS, H. J., PACKHAM, M. A., KINLOUGH-RATHBONE, R. L. & MUSTARD, J. F. (1973) Effect of repeated treatment of rabbit platelets with low concentrations of thrombin on their function, metabolism and survival. *Br. J. Haematol. 25*, 675-689

SALZMAN, E. W. (1972) Cyclic AMP and platelet function. *N. Engl. J. Med. 286*, 358-363

SALZMAN, E. W., ASHFORD, T. P., CHAMBERS, D. A. & NERI, L. L. (1969) Platelet incorporation of labelled adenosine and adenosine diphosphate. *Thromb. Diath. Haemorrh. 22*, 304-315

SPAET, T. H. & LEJNIEKS, I. (1966) Studies on the mechanism whereby platelets are clumped by adenosine diphosphate. *Thromb. Diath. Haemorrh. 15*, 36-51

Discussion

Haslam: If your hypothesis turns out to be correct, it will be the first authenticated case of an agonist acting according to rate theory rather than occupation theory. That could be extremely important in pharmacology.

I also became interested in the effects of hydroxylamine on platelet aggregation, mainly because of the ability of this compound to react with acyl phosphates. Thus, if high-energy phosphate is transferred from ATP to ADP through the platelet membrane, this could involve an intermediate glutamyl-γ-phosphate residue in a membrane protein. However, the concentrations of hydroxylamine required to react with glutamyl-γ-phosphate (approximately 1M) are much higher than are required to inhibit ADP-induced platelet aggregation. Moreover, after confirming the effects of hydroxylamine on ADP-induced aggregation described by Iizuka & Kikugawa (1972), I found that it also blocked the aggregating action of 5-hydroxytryptamine (5HT), which suggests a non-specific mechanism of action. I also investigated the effect of hydroxylamine on the inhibition by ADP of the increase in platelet cyclic AMP produced by PGE_1 (unpublished results). This effect of ADP is probably mediated by the same receptor as is responsible for inducing aggregation. I found that hydroxylamine had no effect on this reaction under conditions in which it completely inhibited aggregation. Because of these observations I suggest that the action of hydroxylamine has no specific connection with the ADP receptor. Perhaps hydroxylamine affects platelet energy metabolism.

Mustard: This suggestion about an inhibition of metabolism may be valid. With washed rabbit platelets, conversion of [^{14}C]ADP to [^{14}C]ATP is inhibited in the presence of 2-deoxyglucose and antimycin (J. F. Mustard, D. W. Perry, R. L. Kinlough-Rathbone & M. A. Packham, unpublished work).

Feinberg: We did some similar experiments (Feinberg *et al.* 1973). We used the same system of washed rabbit platelets incubated with [^{14}C]ADP or [^{3}H]ADP and studied the distribution of radioactivity among ATP, ADP, AMP and in some cases IMP and the nucleosides found in the neutralized perchloric acid extract of the platelet suspension. In general we also found that about 10% of the radioactivity was from purine-labelled ATP after five minutes of incubation at 37 °C. We found that radioactivity in AMP increased as well—an indication that, in part, the redistribution stemmed from adenylate kinase activity; however, there was much more redistribution to ATP than to AMP. We also showed a small redistribution of radioactivity to ATP from labelled ADP added to the suspension medium after the platelets had been removed, indicating an elution of enzymic activity from the platelets. As mentioned by Professor Mustard, these results argue for the possibility that the platelets transfer a phosphoryl group from their surface to exogenous ADP—a process which may destabilize the membrane.

If platelets are involved as a phosphorylated intermediate in an ADP–ATP exchange reaction it ought to be possible to phosphorylate the platelet with [γ-^{32}P]ATP. We incubated platelets with [α-^{32}P]ATP or [γ-^{32}P]ATP to determine if ATP *per se* binds to the platelet. Only [γ-^{32}P]ATP radioactivity was taken up by platelets; hence uptake of radioactivity from [γ-^{32}P]ATP involves either a phosphorylation of a site on the platelet or a prior hydrolysis of ATP and uptake of inorganic ^{32}P. We then compared the uptake of inorganic ^{32}P and ^{32}P from [γ-^{32}P]ATP and found the latter to occur at higher rates. Finally we added non-isotopic inorganic PO_4 along with $[\gamma\text{-}^{32}P]ATP$, on the basis that uptake would be much reduced if it depended on prior hydrolysis. We found little decrease in the rate of uptake of ^{32}P. We concluded that $[\gamma\text{-}^{32}P]ATP$ phosphorylates platelet membrane sites—presumably the same sites that transfer phosphoryl groups to ADP.

Mustard: In our early experiments (Packham *et al.* 1969) we showed that suspensions of washed rabbit platelets did not convert $[^{14}C]ADP$ to $[^{14}C]$adenosine. Hence there was no likelihood of uptake of labelled material by the platelets nor of formation of $[^{14}C]ATP$ within the platelets. In preliminary experiments we had found no difference in the formation of $[^{14}C]ATP$ from $[^{14}C]ADP$ when the platelets were separated before addition of the supernatant to perchloric acid, compared with direct addition of the platelet suspension to perchloric acid. It should be noted that we routinely add non-radioactive ATP, ADP and AMP with the perchloric acid to prevent changes in the ^{14}C-labelled compounds. In 1971 (Guccione *et al.*) we showed that the formation of $[^{14}C]AMP$ from $[^{14}C]ADP$ could not be attributed to adenylate kinase (myokinase) activity.

In that study we examined the question of adenylate kinase in some detail. With suspensions of washed rabbit platelets prepared by the method of Ardlie *et al.* (1970), we could not demonstrate detectable adenylate kinase activity in the platelet suspensions.

Packham: These experiments involved the addition of $[^{14}C]AMP$ and unlabelled ATP to the platelet suspensions. In some cases the platelets were also exposed to 0.1 unit/ml of thrombin. No formation of $[^{14}C]ADP$ was detected (Guccione *et al.* 1971).

Mustard: One of the interesting findings with both prostaglandin E_1 and hydroxylamine is that the $[^{14}C]AMP$ still appears but $[^{14}C]ATP$ is not formed. If $[^{14}C]AMP$ formation were due to adenylate kinase activity both $[^{14}C]ATP$ and $[^{14}C]AMP$ should be formed. Thus there must be another enzyme associated with the platelets which causes the formation of the $[^{14}C]AMP$.

Crawford: The most prominent enzyme in our surface membrane subfraction is a phosphodiesterase and we now routinely use this as our surface membrane marker enzyme. The enzyme splits bis-(*p*-nitrophenyl) phosphate extremely well and is 6–8-fold enriched in the fraction with respect to homogenate activity. However, we have had considerable difficulty in our search for its physiological substrate. There are, as you know, a number of nucleotide phosphohydrolases present in the membrane and phospholipid phosphodiesterases too. One feature, however, is that the activity towards the synthetic substrate is competitively inhibited by ATP, so the enzyme might be another source of AMP within your membrane system.

Haslam: Does this phosphodiesterase hydrolyse cyclic nucleotides?

Crawford: No, it does not, although I should say we have only tried cyclic AMP. Nor does it seem to operate against nucleoside disphosphates.

Mills: Dr Mustard, is there any evidence that the reaction of ADP with a nucleosidediphosphate kinase initiates the shape change and aggregation, or are the activation of this enzyme and the trans-membrane phosphorylation the result of a conformational change in the platelet membrane induced by ADP?

Mustard: That is a perfectly valid question of a type that one can ask of many phenomena. The only thing we can say is that compounds which inhibit the shape change completely inhibit the enzyme and, conversely, compounds that completely inhibit the enzyme (such as AMP) also inhibit the shape change.

Mills: In your hands and in your system, how good is *p*-chloromercuri-benzene sulphonate an inhibitor of the shape change? In human platelets in plasma the shape change induced by ADP is unaffected by 3–5mM-PCMBS.

Mustard: Without plasma proteins present the concentrations of PCMBS required are much less.

Mills: According to Ellman (1959) there is only 0.133 mmole of free SH per litre of plasma.

Packham: In our original experiments with PCMBS, we were not examining the phenomenon in terms of shape change and the concentrations that inhibit shape change (Guccione *et al.* 1971). The results of our recent experiments indicate that PCMBS is not an effective inhibitor of the ADP-induced shape change, nor does it completely block the nucleosidediphosphate kinase reaction (J. F. Mustard, D. W. Perry & M. A. Packham, unpublished work). PCMBS is not as effective an inhibitor as prostaglandin E_1.

Nachman: What do you know about this enzyme in its soluble form? What is its molecular weight, and how does its rate kinetics compare to its state on the membrane?

Packham: The difficulty would be to quantify how much enzyme is in the soluble form and how much is on the membrane; one cannot compare rates unless one has known amounts.

Nachman: Have you tried freeze–thawing the platelets and determining whether it all comes off, or only half comes off?

Packham: We have not done freeze–thaw experiments. We can detect some nucleosidediphosphate kinase activity in the supernatant medium and also in the supernatant of thrombin-treated platelets. With the latter preparation, we removed the released ATP and ADP by dialysis and then examined the enzyme activity by adding non-radioactive ATP as well as [^{14}C]ADP (Guccione *et al.* 1971).

Born: If your biological effect depends on the removal of a transferrable phosphate group from somewhere on the platelet surface, for example from a serine or histamine, would it be reasonable to assume that adding a phosphatase should have the same effect? The large molecules of a phosphatase might not have access to this substrate. However, it would be interesting to try this; and it might also answer the question whether the ATP that is formed in your reaction has an effect. What about other aggregating agents, like 5HT? Here you are adding something which cannot act as an acceptor for phosphate. You might get over this difficulty by postulating that the first thing 5HT does after reacting with its receptor is to cause a conformational change in which ADP is formed locally from ATP, thereby allowing the nucleosidediphosphate kinase reaction to start. That is conceivable if one imagines, for example, that the transport of 5HT starts immediately and that it is associated with the breakdown of membrane ATP to ADP. In that way your system could get going. But this sort of hypothesis could not explain the initiation of aggregation by other agents, including adrenaline or thrombin.

Mustard: I can't answer either point specifically, but if one is going to argue that the transfer of a phosphoryl group, presumably from ATP, is a key step, then logically anything else that initiated this should produce a similar effect.

Born: Let us suppose there is another acceptor system: something else apart from water which accepts phosphate.

Holmsen: I find it hard to see any connection between the nucleosidediphosphate kinase activity and aggregation, since the enzymic reaction goes on long after the aggregation has reached its maximum, which occurs within half a minute. However, can I urge you not to *stir* when you incubate your platelet suspensions with ADP and determine the production of ATP. Under these conditions refractoriness towards ADP should develop, which takes several minutes to reach a maximum (Rozenberg & Holmsen 1968). Have you any thoughts on whether there may be any connection between the duration and activity of nucleosidediphosphate kinase and the refractory state?

Mustard: The experiments are done with platelets suspended in Tyrode's solution without apyrase. These platelets will be refractory to further additions of ADP, unless the ADP is removed. However, the nucleosidediphosphate kinase is still active. Perhaps, after the initial response, the platelets remain refractory as long as the enzyme is converting ADP to ATP.

Born: Of course, it could be a question of relative rates; for example, it could be that rephosphorylation of membrane proteins from inside the platelets is comparatively slow.

Mustard: If one removes the external source of ADP, the platelets return to their disk shape and will again respond to ADP. Of course, nucleosidediphosphate kinase activity cannot be demonstrated unless ADP is present.

Stimulus-response coupling in the thrombin-platelet interaction

THOMAS C. DETWILER, BERNICE M. MARTIN and RICHARD D. FEINMAN

Department of Biochemistry, State University of New York, Downstate Medical Center, Brooklyn, New York

Abstract Recently developed methods for measuring secretion of Ca^{2+} or ATP and activation of phosphorylase have been used to investigate (*i*) the enzymic role of thrombin in platelet stimulation and (*ii*) the coupling of the receptor signal to platelet responses.

To resolve the apparent discrepancy between a requirement for catalytically active thrombin and the lack of thrombin 'turnover' expected for a catalytic mechanism, we compared the proteinase specificity, the pH dependence and the effects of a competitive inhibitor for platelets and other substrates. All proteinases that were active were specific for the hydrolysis of basic amino acid peptides but there was no requirement for structural homology with thrombin. With low levels of thrombin, the rate of stimulation had the same pH dependence as the hydrolysis of synthetic substrates, but at high levels of thrombin the reaction was independent of pH, indicating a change in the rate-determining step. A competitive inhibitor also affected rate, as expected for a proteinase reaction. However, the extent of the platelet reaction was also dependent on pH and on a competitive inhibitor. A proposed mechanism includes formation of a thrombin–receptor complex followed by a *reversible* reaction with no dissociation of thrombin from the modified receptor. The extent of the platelet responses is determined by the equilibrium concentration of the complex of thrombin and modified receptor. Thus, the proposed model combines aspects of an enzyme reaction and an agonist–receptor equilibrium.

The roles of intracellular messengers in coupling stimulation to responses were investigated by observing the effects of various drugs on secretion of ATP or activation of phosphorylase. The divalent cation ionophore A23187 induced secretion identical to that induced by thrombin. Elevation of intracellular cyclic AMP blocked secretion induced by thrombin but had no effect on A23187-induced secretion. Inhibition of prostaglandin synthesis had no effect on either reaction, while cytochalasin B accelerated the secretory process induced by either agent. Thrombin and A23187 caused phosphorylase activation; cyclic AMP blocked the thrombin activation but not the A23187 activation. A model is proposed in which the thrombin–membrane reaction is followed by a pH-independent, cyclic AMP-blocked step that is rate-determining at high thrombin concentrations.

77

This is followed by a faster reaction, probably involving an intracellular Ca^{2+} flux, that is the first step common to the thrombin and A23187 reaction.

The essential feature of platelet function is their response to various stimuli. We have studied the stimulation of platelets by thrombin in the framework of two general questions. What is the mechanism of the interaction of thrombin with the platelet membrane? How is the 'signal' transmitted to the various responses?

Thrombin is a proteolytic enzyme of the active serine class (E.C. 3.4.21.5) (Magnusson 1971). The mechanism of its reaction with platelets has been presumed to be proteolysis of a membrane protein, but such a thrombin-sensitive receptor has not been conclusively identified. In an attempt to better characterize the reaction, we studied its kinetics, using secretion of Ca^{2+} or ATP to follow the reaction (Detwiler & Feinman 1973*a*, *b*). A surprising aspect of these studies was that the amount secreted depended on the thrombin concentration, suggesting that thrombin does not turn over as expected for an enzyme. We therefore evaluated the enzymic aspect of the thrombin–platelet reaction and we propose a mechanism analogous to the reaction of trypsin with soybean trypsin inhibitor.

There is little known about how the thrombin stimulus triggers the many observed platelet responses. There are several well-known intracellular regulatory agents, or 'second messengers', such as Ca^{2+}, cyclic AMP and prostaglandins, and there is circumstantial or indirect evidence that each of these may be involved in platelet function. However, their precise roles in platelets are not known. In an attempt to identify and order the key events and processes in the complex sequence of events leading from stimulation by thrombin to the final responses, we have studied the effects of various drugs on thrombin-induced secretion, a key functional response, and the activation of phosphorylase, a primary metabolic response.

In this paper we (1) summarize our previous kinetic studies of the thrombin–platelet reaction, (2) describe studies of the enzymic role of thrombin, (3) consider the processes involved in stimulus–secretion coupling and (4) propose a model for the initiation of secretion by thrombin and the activation of phosphorylase.

METHODS

The work described here was performed with human platelets that were washed and suspended in a Tris-NaCl-citrate isotonic buffer. Most of the experiments were based on the continuous recording of the secretion of either Ca^{2+} or ATP, as previously described (Detwiler & Feinman 1973a, b). Released Ca^{2+} was measured spectrophotometrically using the metallochromic indicator murexide with a dual wavelength spectrophotometer. This instrument allows one to measure very small spectral changes in turbid and optically dense solutions without interference from changes in light scattering or total absorbance. Released ATP was measured with a firefly luminescent assay.

Phosphorylase was assayed by a sensitive coupled enzyme fluorometric assay (Chaiken et al. 1975). Details of the procedures and of reagents used have been published (Detwiler & Feinman 1973a, b; Friedman & Detwiler 1975; Martin et al. 1975).

RESULTS AND DISCUSSION

Kinetics of the thrombin–platelet reaction

Time-progress curves for the continuous recording of the secretion of Ca^{2+} and ATP are shown in Fig. 1. The calcium curve has the characteristics of the appearance of product in a series first-order reaction (Frost & Pearson 1961) and this curve could be fitted by analogue computer simulation of this simple mechanism. Thus, as a minimal mechanism the process may be considered as in reaction 1, where P is platelet, P* represents some intermediate state of the

$$P \xrightarrow{k_1} P* \xrightarrow{k_2} \text{secretion (ATP or } Ca^{2+}) \quad (1)$$

platelet, k_1 is the observed rate constant for the first step and k_2 is the rate constant for the second step. This type of reaction is subject to rather straight-forward analysis. The inflection point in the curve is the point of maximum P* and will depend on the relative rates of the two reaction steps. We have shown the rate of the second step to be constant under most conditions, so the time to the inflection, t_i, can be used to determine the rate of the first step. The exact mathematical relationship is complex (Detwiler & Feinman 1973a), but for the purpose of this paper it is sufficient that a longer t_i indicates a slower formation of P*. We also measure yield, the total amount of Ca^{2+} released, calculated from added standards.

The concentration dependence of the kinetics showed that k_2 was platelet- and thrombin-independent, but that the apparent first-order rate constant, k_1 (app), was dependent on thrombin concentration; the fact that this constant saturated at high concentrations of thrombin (Fig. 2) led us to expand this model to include a prior equilibrium (Detwiler & Feinman 1973a), which may

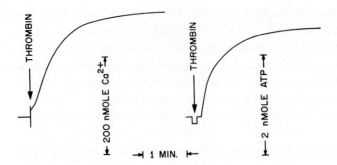

FIG. 1. Time-progress curves for the secretion of Ca^{2+} and ATP. Ca^{2+} secretion was measured spectrophotometrically as described by Detwiler & Feinman (1973*a*); this tracing is from an experiment with 10^{-8}M thrombin, a saturating amount. ATP secretion was measured by the firefly extract luminescence procedure as described by Detwiler & Feinman (1973*b*). This tracing is from an experiment with 4×10^{-8}M thrombin since the phosphate buffer required for this assay increases the K_m of the thrombin–platelet reaction (Martin *et al.* 1975).

be considered analogous to ES complex formation in classical enzyme kinetics.

$$nT + P \underset{}{\overset{\overbrace{\qquad\qquad}^{k_1\,(\text{app})}}{\underset{K}{\rightleftharpoons}}} T_nP \overset{k_1}{\rightarrow} T_nP^* \overset{k_2}{\rightarrow} \text{secretion} \qquad (2)$$

ATP secretion curves (Fig. 1) are qualitatively similar to Ca^{2+} release curves except for the distinct delay before any reaction. We concluded that most Ca^{2+} was released with a nearly identical time course to ATP, while a small but significant fraction of released Ca^{2+} *preceded* the release of ATP.

A significant feature of both these reactions is that the yield, or total amount secreted, is dependent on thrombin concentration (Fig. 2) and we proposed that the enzyme becomes bound in the course of the reaction. This raised the crucial question whether thrombin does, in fact, function as an enzyme.

Enzymic role of thrombin in platelet stimulation

In evaluating the enzymic role of thrombin in platelet stimulation it is useful to compare the thrombin reaction with that of other proteinases. While it is known that certain other proteinases can cause functional changes in platelets (Davey & Lüscher 1967), there have been no detailed and quantitative comparative studies. We therefore compared the reactions of thrombin, trypsin, chymotrypsin, plasmin, papain and phenylmethylsulphonyl-thrombin (PMS-thrombin). The first four enzymes are serine proteinases with considerable structural homology but different peptide specificities, while papain is an

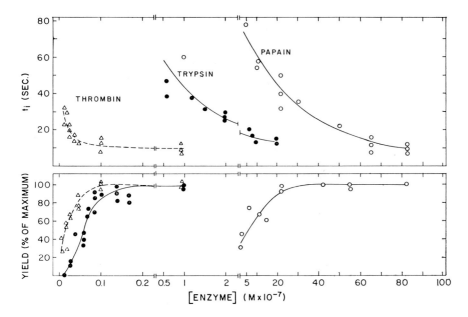

Fig. 2. Effect of enzyme concentration on the proteinase-induced secretion of Ca^{2+}. Yield is the amount of Ca^{2+} released and t_i is the time to the inflection point in the time-progress curve (see Fig. 1); a long t_i reflects a slow thrombin reaction.

SH-proteinase with no structural similarity to thrombin but a similar peptide specificity (Blow 1971; Glazer 1971; Keil 1971; Magnusson 1971). PMS-thrombin is an active-site-blocked enzyme. These enzymes thus permit evaluation of the contributions of peptide specificity and protein structure. Plasmin (2×10^{-7}M), chymotrypsin (8×10^{-7}M) and PMS-thrombin (3×10^{-7}M) did not induce secretion, while trypsin and papain caused secretion of both Ca^{2+} and ATP with a time-course that was identical to that induced by thrombin when saturating levels of enzymes were used. There were, however, three significant differences between the reactions of these enzymes. (*i*) The concentrations required varied by three orders of magnitude (Fig. 2). (*ii*) While rate and yield had the same concentration dependence with thrombin, they were greatly different with trypsin (Fig. 2). (*iii*) With low levels of enzyme, the reactions of trypsin and papain had long initial lags so that they could not be fitted by the series first-order mechanism that characterizes thrombin reactions.

Thrombin and papain have unrelated structures, with specificity for the hydrolysis of basic amino acid peptides their only common property. Trypsin (active with platelets) also has specificity for basic amino acid peptides, whereas chymotrypsin (*not* reactive with platelets) has a high degree of structural homology with thrombin but no reactivity with peptides of basic amino acids. It thus appears that the ability to hydrolyse basic amino acid peptides is the main requirement for reactivity with platelets. The unreactivity of plasmin, which shows a preference for lysyl side chains, and the high reactivity of thrombin, which has a preference for arginyl side chains, suggest that an arginine peptide is the susceptible peptide of the thrombin receptor. However, specificity for protein and membrane substrates undoubtedly depends on more than the side groups immediately next to the peptide bond hydrolysed.

If the stimulation of platelets by thrombin does involve proteolysis, variation of pH or the addition of a competitive inhibitor should have predictable effects. The pH dependence of the rate of thrombin stimulation (Fig. 3) is, in fact, nearly identical to that for hydrolysis of other substrates by serine proteinases. This pH dependence is apparently *not* due to effects of pH on the platelet, since the dependence on pH with papain (Martin *et al.* 1975) parallels the different pH dependence for the hydrolysis of synthetic substrates by this enzyme. Thus, changing pH has the expected effect for a mechanism involving proteolysis by these enzymes. It is significant that the pH effect could be overcome at high thrombin concentration; this demonstrates a change in the rate-determining step from pH dependent at low thrombin to pH independent at high thrombin levels. Thus, the model in reaction (1) should include an additional step. The effect of a competitive inhibitor of thrombin on the rate of stimulation (Fig. 4) was also consistent with a reaction involving the enzyme active site. There was, however, a very surprising result with the pH and competitive inhibitor experiments; yield, as well as rate, was affected. We had previously attributed the thrombin dependence of yield to 'burst' kinetics, with an initial fast reaction followed by very slow enzyme turnover so that thrombin was essentially irreversibly bound. If this were true, a competitive inhibitor could slow the rate but should have no effect on yield, since eventually all thrombin would be bound.

The evidence for a catalytic role of thrombin in platelet stimulation may be summarized as (*i*) active-site-blocked thrombin is not effective, (*ii*) the reactivity of different proteinases is related to similar peptide specificity and not to structural similarity, (*iii*) the pH dependence is the same as for hydrolysis of synthetic substrates, and (*iv*) a competitive inhibitor inhibits rate as expected for a proteolytic reaction. The most immediate problem is understanding how thrombin concentration, pH and the competitive inhibitor affect yield. Direct measurements indicate that thrombin is bound to platelets (Detwiler & Feinman 1973a; Tollefsen *et al.* 1974), but it is not yet clear whether the binding is only to functional receptors or to other sites (that is, the platelet could act as an irreversible antithrombin in competition with the receptor). If there are non-

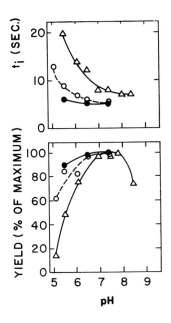

FIG. 3. Effect of pH on thrombin-induced secretion of Ca^{2+}. The kinetic parameter t_i is the time to the inflection in curves such as Fig. 1; a long t_i reflects a slow rate of thrombin stimulation. Yield is expressed as the amount of Ca^{2+} released as a percentage of that released at pH 7.4. △—△, 5×10^{-8}M thrombin; ○- - -○, 3×10^{-7}M thrombin; ●—●, 2×10^{-6}M thrombin.

receptor binding sites, anything that slowed the reaction with the receptor would decrease the amount of reaction before the thrombin was completely removed. The observation that active-site-inhibited thrombin competes with ^{125}I-labelled thrombin for binding but not for stimulation (Tollefsen *et al.* 1974) suggests that the major part of the thrombin binding is, in fact, to sites other than the active receptors. However, this is an equilibrium binding, so that all receptors should eventually be 'hit', and the question is whether the equilibrium is sufficiently slow to allow for essentially no turnover.

Since there is at present little basis for deciding whether such competing 'antithrombins' are present, we have tentatively interpreted our data with the assumption that only active receptors are involved. We propose a scheme that can account for all of our results and most other published results on the interaction of thrombin and platelets. This proposal, which is an elaboration of the model described by reaction (2), is shown in reaction (3), where R is a

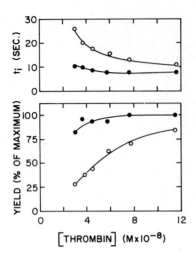

FIG. 4. Effect of a competitive inhibitor on thrombin-induced secretion of ATP. Yield is the amount of ATP released as a percentage of the amount released with 10^{-7}M thrombin and no inhibitor. ●—●, no inhibitor; ○—○, 0.05 mM p-(p'-nitrophenoxypropoxy) benzamidine benzene sulphonate (NPPBA).

membrane receptor and k_{cat} is the rate constant for the catalytic step. The

$$T + R \underset{k_{-cat}}{\overset{K}{\rightleftharpoons}} TR \overset{k_{cat}}{\rightleftharpoons} TR^{\circ}$$

$$P \overset{k_1}{\rightarrow} P^* \overset{k_2}{\rightarrow} \text{secretion}$$

(3)

thrombin–receptor reaction is distinct from the thrombin-independent platelet steps; the broken line connecting these two processes does not imply a separate kinetic step but is intended only to show the dependence of the intracellular processes on the membrane reaction. The novel feature of this model is that the catalytic step is reversible, with yield determined by the equilibrium concentration of TR°. Thus, the model is described in terms of both an enzyme reaction and the classical occupation theory of hormone action (Furchgott 1972). The rate of formation of TR° and the equilibrium concentration of TR° would both be affected by a competitive inhibitor or by a change in k_{cat} (as with changes in pH). The molecular analogy of this model is the reaction of trypsin with soybean trypsin inhibitor (Laskowski & Sealock 1971), which involves the reversible formation of a stable covalent enzyme–inhibitor complex.

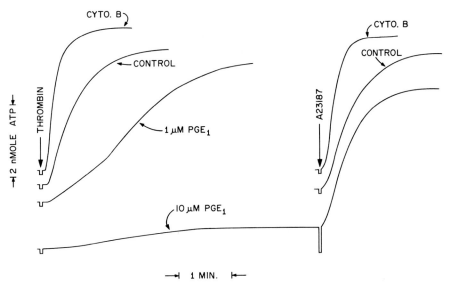

FIG. 5. Effects of drugs on thrombin- and A23187-induced secretion of ATP. Drugs were added as ethanol solutions one minute before starting the reactions with 3×10^{-8}M thrombin or 1μM A23187. Cyto. B, 10μM cytochalasin B.

A similar interaction has been proposed for the thrombin–antithrombin III reaction (Rosenberg & Damus 1973).

While this model is speculative, it is consistent with experimental observations, it defines the problem in a new way, and it suggests specific experimental approaches. One aspect significant to other studies is that a proteolytic product need not exist.

Stimulus–response coupling

While there is little known about how the stimulus, presumably a membrane reaction, is transmitted to the various platelet responses, it is likely that some of the 'second messengers' known to function in cellular regulatory processes in other tissues are involved. In an attempt to identify the processes involved and to place them in their proper sequence we have used various drugs to modify thrombin-induced secretion of ATP. These experiments were planned and analysed in terms of the scheme in reaction (3).

Calcium ions. There is considerable circumstantial evidence for a key role of calcium ions in some platelet responses, and we have shown that the divalent cation ionophore A23187, which discharges divalent cation gradients, induces secretion of ATP. The ionophore-induced secretion (Fig. 5) has a time course

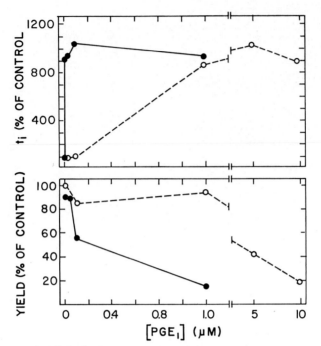

FIG. 6. Effect of PGE$_1$ on the thrombin-induced secretion of ATP. Thrombin concentration was 3×10^{-8}M. ●—●, all reactions included 250 μM theophylline; ○- - -○, no theophylline. Drugs were added 1 minute before thrombin.

and yield very similar to that induced by thrombin except for a shorter lag phase (Feinman & Detwiler 1974). We proposed that A23187 by-passed the thrombin reaction and directly affected some regulatory mechanism to trigger the normal secretory process. Further work has confirmed this, making A23187 a valuable tool for studying the stimulus–response coupling mechanism. The evidence that the secretory processes induced by thrombin and A23187 are the same is: (*i*) the rate constants for secretion (k_2 in reaction 3) are identical, (*ii*) yields of ATP are identical, (*iii*) the activation energies are identical (Friedman & Detwiler 1975), and (*iv*) drugs that affect the secretory process have the same effect whether secretion is induced by thrombin or A23187 (see below). The mechanism of A23187 action is presumed to involve its known ability to transfer cations across membranes (Pressman 1973) and from knowledge of regulatory mechanisms in other tissues it seems likely that the essential cation is Ca^{2+}. (The role of Ca^{2+} is discussed further under Summary and Conclusions, pp. 88–90.)

Cyclic AMP. Since cyclic AMP is known to regulate many cell processes and is known to affect platelet function, we studied the effects of elevation of intracellular cyclic AMP levels on thrombin- and A23187-induced secretion. Intracellular cyclic AMP was increased with PGE_1 (an adenylate cyclase activator), with theophylline (a phosphodiesterase inhibitor) and with dibutyryl cyclic AMP. Since the effects of these agents were qualitatively the same and since prostaglandin E_1 and theophylline were synergistic (see Fig. 6), their effects are almost certainly through an increase in intracellular cyclic AMP. An example of the effects is shown in Fig. 5 for PGE_1 and is quantified in Fig. 6. With thrombin-induced secretion, low levels increase the lag (slow the formation of P* in reaction 3) while higher levels also inhibit yield. We have never seen an effect on A23187-induced secretion, in contrast to the report of White et al. (1974) that cyclic AMP inhibited A23187-induced secretion.

It is possible to determine which step in the formation of P* is inhibited by comparing the inhibition when the rate-determining step is either formation of TR° (e.g. with very low enzyme concentrations) or the k_1 step (as with higher levels of enzyme in Fig. 5). This is difficult, however, because with low levels of thrombin the yield is also low, so that when the formation of TR° is solely the rate-determining step there is not enough reaction to measure. We therefore made use of the unusual feature of the trypsin reaction shown in Fig. 2; yield is saturated at a much lower trypsin level than is rate, so that rate can be markedly slowed without a decrease in yield. With high trypsin levels (when the k_1 step was rate-determining), cyclic AMP increased the lag, but with low trypsin (when the formation of TR° was rate-determining), the long lag was not further increased by elevating cyclic AMP. Thus, cyclic AMP apparently inhibits the k_1 step in reaction 3.

Prostaglandins. Prostaglandins are known to be rapidly synthesized after platelet stimulation (Smith et al. 1974); the process is inhibited by aspirin and indomethacin. We found no effect of these inhibitors on thrombin- or A23187-induced secretion of ATP, confirming a previous report by Smith & Willis (1971) and indicating that prostaglandins are not 'second messengers' in this process.

Microfilaments and microtubules. Platelets contain microfilaments and microtubules, structures that have been implicated in secretory processes in other cells (Allison 1973). To investigate whether microfilaments are involved in platelet secretion we tested the effect of cytochalasin B, which disrupts microfilament systems, on the secretion of ATP (Fig. 5). Low levels of cyto-chalasin B accelerated the exponential phase (the k_2 step of reaction 3) of secretion induced by either thrombin or A23187, but had no effect on the lag phase (formation of P* in reaction 3). Similar experiments with drugs specific for microtubules showed no effects on secretion unless very high concentrations of drugs were used.

Inhibitors of energy metabolism. Holmsen *et al.* (1969) considered a dependence on energy derived from glycolysis or oxidative phosphorylation to be one of the identifying features of the platelet 'release reaction', so we attempted to determine which part of the overall process required energy. However, prolonged incubation with deoxyglucose and addition of antimycin A had no effect on yield or on any of the kinetic parameters. Interpretation of these results is complicated by the fact that there is no specific and potent inhibitor of glycolysis, but they suggest that any requirement for ATP must be very small. We believe it important to note that there is no *a priori* requirement that secretion be an energy-driven process.

Phosphorylase activation

Secretion is a key functional response of platelets to stimulation, but there are other morphological and metabolic responses and it is important to establish whether all responses are induced by the same mechanism. Activation of glycogen phosphorylase (E.C. 2.4.1.1), which plays a major regulatory role in energy metabolism, is one of the quickest metabolic responses (Detwiler 1972) and is therefore ideal for comparing the induction of a functional response (secretion) with a primary metabolic response. Regulation of phosphorylase was therefore studied in intact platelets and in platelet extracts (Chaiken *et al.* 1975). Phosphorylase in intact platelets was activated quickly by either thrombin or A23187; elevation of cyclic AMP blocked activation by thrombin but not by A23187. Thus, the activation of phosphorylase seems to proceed through essentially the same processes as does the induction of secretion. In addition to blocking stimulation by thrombin, at higher levels cyclic AMP caused activation of phosphorylase in the absence of thrombin or A23187.

SUMMARY AND CONCLUSIONS

Until a thrombin receptor is isolated, there is no proof that such a receptor actually exists; it is possible that anything that 'destabilizes' the membrane, such as proteolytic attack, could induce the observed platelet responses. However, the proteinase specificity suggests that this is not the case and we have interpreted our data on the assumption of a specific thrombin receptor; we consider stimulus–response coupling in the thrombin–platelet reaction as shown in Fig. 7. We propose that thrombin reacts with a specific membrane

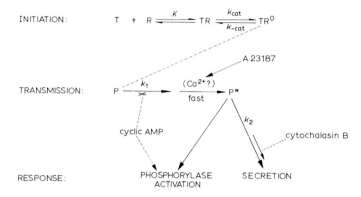

FIG. 7. Model for stimulus–response coupling in platelets. The thrombin–receptor reaction is as proposed in reaction (3), with the equilibrium concentration of TR° determining the amount, but not the rate, of conversion of P to P*. Two steps are shown between P and P* to account for the observations that the process is faster with A23187 than with thrombin and that only the thrombin reaction is inhibited by cyclic AMP. The fast step may involve an intracellular Ca^{2+} flux (see text). Cyclic AMP has been shown, as indicated, to both block stimulation by thrombin and activate phosphorylase in the absence of stimulation (Chaiken *et al.* 1975).

receptor by a reaction analogous with the reaction of trypsin with soybean trypsin inhibitor. The magnitude of the stimulus is viewed as a function of the equilibrium [TR°], the complex of thrombin and modified receptor. The subsequent platelet changes, whereby the initial 'signal' is transmitted to various responses, cannot yet be analysed in terms of chemical reactions and they are connected to the receptor reaction by a dotted line that does not imply any mechanism or even a distinct kinetic step.

There is some 'activated' state of the stimulated platelet, P*, that appears to be a common intermediate for either secretion or activation of phosphorylase. The conversion of P to P* is shown as at least a two-step process. While this is not demanded by the data it is the simplest mechanism consistent with our data. The k_1 step is the pH-independent step and the rate-determining step at high concentrations of thrombin. This step is by-passed by A23187, so that ionophore-induced secretion has a shorter lag and is not inhibited by cyclic AMP. A significant aspect of this scheme is that cyclic AMP blocks stimulation, or transmission of the signal, but does not block the actual responses.

The formation of P* may involve a Ca^{2+} flux, consistent with the observed role of A23187. Although there is no direct evidence for such a key role for Ca^{2+}, there is considerable circumstantial and indirect evidence. The arguments in favour of an involvement of Ca^{2+} follow. (1) Some responses (e.g. secretion, activation of phosphorylase) are known to be Ca^{2+} dependent in other tissues

(Stormorken 1969; Brostrom *et al.* 1971). (2) Several of the responses of platelets may involve actomyosin, known to be regulated by Ca^{2+} in skeletal muscle. While similar regulatory mechanisms may not be present in smooth muscle or non-muscle cells, effects of Ca^{2+} on platelet actomyosin ATPase activity have been reported (Cohen *et al.* 1973; Hanson *et al.* 1973; Malik *et al.* 1975). There is, however, no definitive evidence that regulation of platelet contractility is an essential part of platelet responses. (3) After stimulation by thrombin, an extracellular Ca^{2+} flux precedes the secretion of ATP (Detwiler & Feinman 1973*b*). (4) Intracellular calcium pools have been observed and at least one of these is discharged within seconds of thrombin stimulation (Sato *et al.* 1975). (5) The divalent cation ionophore induces some, and possibly all, platelet responses (Feinman & Detwiler 1974; White *et al.* 1974).

It is, of course, clear that none of these is direct evidence for a regulatory role of Ca^{2+} and taken together they are only circumstantial. Until definitive evidence is obtained that responses are *preceded* by an increase in *intracellular* Ca^{2+} and that some response is regulated by changes in Ca^{2+}, the role of Ca^{2+} in stimulus–response coupling should be considered an hypothesis. If Ca^{2+} is involved, it must be from an intracellular source (Feinman & Detwiler 1974).

Prostaglandin synthesis is a serious omission in the scheme in Fig. 7. Since inhibitors of prostaglandin synthesis do not affect thrombin–secretion coupling, prostaglandins apparently do not serve as second messengers in this process, but it would be very helpful to know how prostaglandin synthesis fits in with the other responses. Specifically, does cyclic AMP block thrombin-induced prostaglandin synthesis and does A23187 induce prostaglandin synthesis?

ACKNOWLEDGEMENTS

We are grateful to Drs J. W. Fenton, II, and T. J. Ryan, Division of Laboratories and Research, New York State Department of Health, Albany, USA, for their generous gifts of highly purified human thrombin and plasmin and the thrombin inhibitor and for stimulating discussions.

This work was supported by grants HL 10099 and HL 16355 from the United States Public Health Service.

References

ALLISON, A. C. (1973) in *Locomotion of Tissue Cells (Ciba Found. Symp. 14)*, pp. 109-143, Associated Scientific Publishers, Amsterdam

BLOW, D. M. (1971) in *The Enzymes* (Boyer, P. D., ed.), vol. 3, pp. 185-205, Academic Press, New York

BROSTROM, C. O., HUNKELER, F. L. & KREBS, E. G. (1971) The regulation of skeletal muscle phosphorylase kinase by Ca^{2+}. *J. Biol. Chem. 246*, 1961-1967

CHAIKEN, R., PAGANO, D. & DETWILER, T. C. (1975) Regulation of platelet phosphorylase. *Fed. Proc. 34*, 242 (abs.)

COHEN, I., KAMINSKI, E. & DE VRIES, A. (1973) Actin-linked regulation of the human platelet contractile system. *FEBS (Fed. Eur. Biochem. Soc.) Lett. 34*, 315-317

DAVEY, M. G. & LÜSCHER, E. F. (1967) Action of thrombin and other coagulant and proteolytic enzymes on blood platelets. *Nature (Lond.) 216*, 857-858

DETWILER, T. C. (1972) Control of energy metabolism in platelets. The effects of thrombin and cyanide on glycolysis. *Biochim. Biophys. Acta 256*, 163-174

DETWILER, T. C. & FEINMAN, R. D. (1973a) Kinetics of the thrombin-induced release of calcium (II) by platelets. *Biochemistry 12*, 282-289

DETWILER, T. C. & FEINMAN, R. D. (1973b) Kinetics of the thrombin-induced release of adenosine triphosphate by platelets. Comparison with release of calcium. *Biochemistry 12*, 2462-2468

FEINMAN, R. D. & DETWILER, T. C. (1974) Platelet secretion induced by divalent cation ionophores. *Nature (Lond.) 249*, 172-173

FRIEDMAN, F. & DETWILER, T. C. (1975) Stimulus-secretion coupling in platelets. Effects of drugs on secretion of ATP. *Biochemistry 14*, 1315-1320

FROST, A. A. & PEARSON, R. D. (1961) *Kinetics and Mechanism*, 2nd edn, pp. 166-169, Wiley, New York

FURCHGOTT, R. F. (1972) in *Handbook of Experimental Pharmacology New Series* (Blaschko, H. & Muscholl, E., eds.), vol. 33, pp. 284-335, Springer-Verlag, New York

GLAZER, A. N. (1971) in *The Enzymes* (Boyer, P. D., ed.), vol. 3, pp. 502-545, Academic Press, New York

HANSON, J. P., REPKE, D. I., KATZ, A. M. & ALEDORT, L. M. (1973) Calcium ion control of platelet thrombosthenin ATPase activity. *Biochim. Biophys. Acta 314*, 382-389

HOLMSEN, H., DAY, H. J. & STORMORKEN, H. (1969) The blood platelet release reaction. *Scand. J. Haematol.* Suppl. 8

KEIL, B. (1971) in *The Enzymes* (Boyer, P. D., ed.), vol. 3, pp. 249-273, Academic Press, New York

LASKOWSKI, M., JR & SEALOCK, R. W. (1971) in *The Enzymes* (Boyer, P. D., ed.), vol. 3, pp. 376-457, Academic Press, New York

MAGNUSSON, S. (1971) in *The Enzymes* (Boyer, P. D., ed.), vol. 3, pp. 278-320, Academic Press, New York

MALIK, M. N., ROSENBERG, S., DETWILER, T. C. & STRACHER, A. (1975) Role of Ca^{2+} in the allosteric regulation of platelet actomyosin. *Biochem. Biophys. Res. Commun. 61*, 1071-1075

MARTIN, B. M., FEINMAN, R. D. & DETWILER, T. C. (1975) Platelet stimulation by thrombin and other proteases. *Biochemistry 14*, 1308-1314

PRESSMAN, B. C. (1973) Properties of ionophores with broad range of cation selectivity. *Fed. Proc. 32*, 1698-1703

ROSENBERG, R. D. & DAMUS, P. S. (1973) The purification and mechanism of action of human antithrombin-heparin cofactor. *J. Biol. Chem. 248*, 6490-6505

SATO, T., HERMAN, L., CHANDLER, J., STRACHER, A. & DETWILER, T. C. (1975) Localization of a thrombin-sensitive calcium pool in platelets. *J. Histochem. Cytochem. 23*, 103-106

SMITH, J. B. & WILLIS, A. L. (1971) Aspirin selectively inhibits prostaglandin production in human platelets. *Nature New Biol. 231*, 235-237

SMITH, J. B., SILVER, M. J., INGERMAN, C. & KOCSIS, J. J. (1974) in *Platelets and Thrombosis* (Sherry, S. & Scriabine, A., eds.), pp. 81-90, University Park Press, Baltimore

STORMORKEN, H. (1969) The release reaction of secretion. *Scand. J. Haematol.* Suppl. 9

TOLLEFSEN, D. M., FEAGLER, J. R. & MAJERUS, P. W. (1974) The binding of thrombin to the surface of human platelets. *J. Biol. Chem. 249*, 2646-2651

WHITE, J. G., RAO, G. H. R. & GERRARD, J. M. (1974) Effects of the ionophore A23187 on blood platelets. I. Influence on aggregation and secretion. *Am. J. Pathol. 77*, 135-149

Discussion

Nachman: I would like to pursue your idea about a complex between thrombin and a modified receptor (TR°). You are suggesting that it is analogous to the soybean trypsin inhibitor complex. In this system the inhibitor itself undergoes proteolysis. Is this part of your model—does the TR° step include the concept of a proteolytic cleavage?

Detwiler: In its most general form it can, but it doesn't need to. We think it probably does, but that is not the essence of the model.

Nachman: Most other inhibitor systems that have been studied carefully enough lead one to think that the definition of inhibitor function is consonant with, if not dependent on, a previous proteolytic cleavage.

Detwiler: This is what we are now concerned with. Proteolytic cleavage would explain why we see aspects of a catalytic mechanism; it would explain why the competitive inhibitor and pH affect the rate of stimulation in the way expected for an enzyme reaction. But the essential feature of our model is an equilibrium between native and modified receptor. The receptor must differ from a true substrate, such as fibrinogen, in that any proteolysis would be reversible.

Sneddon: We have done experiments using trypsin in low concentrations in the presence of EDTA to initiate the platelet release reaction (see Sneddon & Williams 1973). In the presence of EDTA trypsin produces no release of 5-hydroxytryptamine (5HT) or adenine nucleotides. However, if we add trypsin inhibitor, wash the platelet suspension to remove the EDTA, then add Ca^{2+}, both 5HT and adenine nucleotides, but not cytoplasmic enzymes, are released. Similar experiments have been reported by Mürer (1972).

If the experiment is repeated, but instead of adding Ca^{2+} within seconds of the washing step we continue to incubate the platelet suspension at 36 °C, we have found that these trypsin-treated platelets lose their Ca^{2+} sensitivity. This suggested to us that trypsin caused proteolytic cleavage of the platelet membrane, and that the membrane is capable of repair after removal of the trypsin. This 'repair' is prevented by cooling the platelets to 0-4 °C, but not by inhibitors of protein synthesis.

Detwiler: We have been trying to design analogous experiments with thrombin instead of trypsin. Our scheme predicts that if one could do the thrombin–platelet reaction in a condition in which the transmission of the signal is blocked, this should be reversed by simply putting in either a competitive inhibitor or something which will pull off the thrombin. This is I think analogous to your experiment with trypsin?

Sneddon: That is our acute experiment, and you are suggesting that when we add calcium and soybean trypsin inhibitor simultaneously we are pulling the enzyme off its receptor with the inhibitor?

Detwiler: We would predict that result. We have never been able to design a really stringent test of the concept, but that is the critical test of the scheme we propose: that the enzyme–receptor reaction is reversible. The only way to see that is to block the response while you do the experiment.

Sneddon: I have tried this with thrombin in rat or rabbit platelets. The high concentrations of EDTA (Sneddon 1972; Sneddon & Williams 1973) needed to block the thrombin release reaction are sufficient to reduce subsequent responses to calcium. Thus, although the block is not complete, you can reduce thrombin-triggered release with EDTA; however when you inhibit the thrombin with heparin and then add Ca^{2+}, the Ca^{2+}-induced release reaction is smaller than anticipated.

Detwiler: Have you tried adding hirudin instead of heparin?

Sneddon: No.

Smith: Of course, when you start to talk about the use of EDTA and calcium ions to dissociate the initiation and extrusion phases of the release reaction, you are bringing in the additional problem of species differences. I don't know about rat platelets, but I do know that pig and rabbit platelets show a much greater dependence on extracellular calcium ions for release than do human platelets (Mürer 1972).

Feinberg: Dr G. LeBreton and I have evidence for an increase in the calcium ion concentration within platelets in response to ADP (LeBreton & Feinberg 1974). We incubated human platelets in plasma with dimethyl sulphoxide (5 %) and the calcium ion indicator murexide (0.5 mM). We resuspended the platelets in murexide–DMSO-free plasma and were able to show that the murexide pertained to the platelet. The addition of 10^{-5}M-ADP resulted in a spectral shift characteristic for Ca–murexide formation. In parallel experiments it was shown that ^{45}Ca was not taken up after the addition of ADP, and so we interpreted the spectral shift as an indication of a redistribution of intraplatelet calcium ion. Inhibition of granule release after treatment with aspirin did not abolish the formation of Ca–murexide—an indication that granule calcium was not the source of the redistributed calcium.

Haslam: Your suggested scheme is fascinating, Dr Detwiler. However, we find that PGE_1 does inhibit the release reaction induced by the ionophore A23187, at least for a while (R. J. Haslam & M. D. McClenaghan, unpublished work), which seems to conflict with your data. Eventually, the inhibition by PGE_1 is at least partly overcome by the ionophore, perhaps because the ADP that is released increasingly inhibits the formation of cyclic AMP induced by the PGE_1. We have studied the effects of cytochalasin B on the release reaction induced by collagen (Haslam *et al.* 1975) and in preliminary experiments we have used thrombin as the release stimulus with similar results. With low concentrations of cytochalasin B (0.1 μg/ml; i.e. 0.2 μM in suspensions of washed platelets) there was a marked potentiation not only of the rate of release of 5HT but also of the extent of release. I wonder if this last finding can be accommodated by your scheme.

Detwiler: We found no effect of cytochalasin on the extent of reaction.

Haslam: To obtain a marked potentiation by cytochalasin B of the extent of release we have, of course, to use a weak collagen or thrombin stimulus.

Detwiler: Yes; we routinely evaluate these drugs by using just a saturating level of thrombin; if we see any effect we vary the thrombin concentration from very low to very high to further analyse it.

Haslam: What I am asking is whether an increase in the extent of release is consistent with an action of cytochalasin B at the point you suggest. Is the extent of release totally dependent in your scheme on the amount of TR°?

Detwiler: In the simplest case, it is inconsistent with our scheme.

Adelstein: What concentration of cytochalasin B were you using in these experiments? And what do you feel cytochalasin B is doing under these conditions?

Detwiler: We get a maximum effect at 10μM and the effect is essentially instantaneous. In most cases we can go substantially lower, to 1μM, and still see an effect on the rate of secretion. I don't know what it does, but others have speculated that if secretory granules are held in place in a cell by microfilaments that restrict intracellular movement, movement of secretory granules to the membrane would be facilitated by disruption of microfilaments. That is speculation and there is no real evidence. There are generally two effects of cytochalasin B: it either inhibits or stimulates, although it is probably not as simple as that.

Haslam: In our experiments with collagen (Haslam *et al.* 1975) we found that cytochalasin B either inhibited or stimulated the release reaction, depending on its concentration; it may act similarly in other systems. With suspensions of washed platelets, concentrations of about 1 μg/ml (2μM) inhibited release; lower concentrations potentiated. In the presence of plasma the concentrations required for both effects were markedly increased.

Mills: Is this effect specific to cytochalasin B?

Detwiler: That is the only one I have used, so I don't know.

Haslam: We have also only used cytochalasin B in studies on the release reaction.

Crawford: Cytochalasin B might act in another way as well, if one subscribes to the view that cell microfilaments may also be associated with the interior wall of the surface membrane. Some of the experiments on the effect of cyto-chalasin on the phenomenon of 'capping' in lymphocytes (that is, the movement of surface antigens to one pole of the cell as a result of combination with added specific antibody) suggest that any change in the character of microfilaments could increase the potential for lateral diffusibility of the membrane proteins, thus perhaps allowing different types of hydrophobic interactions to occur. This may change the permeability properties of the membrane simply as a result of loss of the constraint exercised by the associated microfilaments.

Lüscher: If proteolytic cleavage of a substrate on the platelet surface is the essential primary event in thrombin-mediated platelet activation, it must be assumed that the thrombin–receptor complex in fact is an enzyme–substrate complex. If platelets are treated with thrombin at low temperature, under conditions where the membranes are largely immobilized, secondary reactions will not be observed, although proteolytic cleavage has occurred. When hirudin is added in order to block the remaining thrombin, these secondary reactions will take place upon rewarming, in spite of the fact that no active enzyme is present. It could perhaps be argued that the thrombin–receptor complex is still stable under these conditions: however, in view of the generally transient combination of an enzyme with its substrate, this seems rather unlikely. It must be pointed out that the active thrombin-binding site is quite different from the 'high affinity' site which also binds thrombin (Phillips 1974), although it is not involved at all in platelet activation.

Detwiler: This is related to the trypsin experiments described by Dr Sneddon. How long after adding hirudin do you wait before you warm the cells? Do you wait long enough to reverse the membrane reaction?

Lüscher: We wait for 3–4 minutes.

Detwiler: The second question is how far the transmission of the signal has gone before you add hirudin. If you add thrombin and only two or three seconds later add hirudin, secretion proceeds normally (Detwiler & Feinman 1973) because the reaction has been started and can go on without thrombin. These are the kinds of experiments that we hope to do to test our hypothesis, but they are difficult to design because one doesn't know, as in the experiment you described, how far the transmission of the signal had gone before one stops and warms the platelets. If it has gone beyond the initial thrombin–receptor reaction, anything else you do to the thrombin or the receptor will make no difference.

Lüscher: It is indeed difficult to say just how unreactive the platelet membrane is at temperatures from 4 °C to 10 °C.

There would be one other way of distinguishing between the proteolytic and complex formation theories of thrombin action. By adding subthreshold amounts of thrombin several times it should be possible to claeve most of the glycoprotein substrate. Such platelets should—according to the proteolytic theory—no longer be reactive whereas, according to your hypothesis, they should still react normally upon the addition of a critical amount of thrombin.

Detwiler: We have done that. We were looking for two things. One was to determine whether the platelets would become refractory after incubating them with a small amount of thrombin. Our results were not consistent but if there is any refractoriness, it is hard to show it. Secondly, the simplest explanation for many of our results (to explain for instance why, when you slow the rate of the thrombin reaction, you also decrease the yield), was that when you stimulate slowly, the effect is less than if you stimulate rapidly. To test this we added small amounts of thrombin repeatedly instead of the same total amount at one time. In every case the effect was cumulative; a repeated very small addition gave the same ultimate response as one large addition. In fact, it was only after a month of these experiments that we were forced to think through the whole problem and make the equilibrium proposal.

Mustard: We have evidence that platelets do become unresponsive to thrombin after thrombin treatment (Reimers *et al.* 1973; Kinlough-Rathbone *et al.* 1975). Washed rabbit platelets were treated with thrombin to cause release of their amine storage granule contents and the platelets were recovered. These platelets respond normally to ADP in terms of shape change and aggregation. They also change shape in response to collagen and show shape change and aggregation responses to the ionophore A23187. They contain no detectable releasable material and if they are reinfused into the circulation of rabbits they survive normally. When thrombin is added to these degranulated platelets no shape change or aggregation occurs. It appears that the ability of the platelets to respond to thrombin has been destroyed.

Lüscher: This brings up an interesting question. If platelets are not allowed to aggregate, for example in a system which contains no calcium, then the so-called contact effect is absent (cf. Massini & Lüscher 1972), which, for instance with ADP in the presence of calcium and fibrinogen, is required for release. Perhaps such 'non-contacted' platelets represent a special case.

Mustard: We have found that close platelet contact does not always cause the release reaction. For example, polylysine does not cause release from washed rabbit platelets although it certainly causes them to adhere to each other (Jenkins *et al.* 1971). In citrated human platelet-rich plasma, polylysine does cause a release reaction (Packham & Guccione 1973). If one suspends washed *human* platelets in a system containing both Ca^{2+} and Mg^{2+}, the release reaction does not occur during ADP-induced aggregation, or upon the addition of polylysine. If one takes human blood into hirudin and prepares platelet-rich plasma, release does not occur on the addition of ADP. If one adds citrate to the hirudin platelet-rich plasma or to heparin platelet-rich plasma and then adds ADP, the release reaction takes place. If citrate is added to a suspension of washed human platelets in a medium containing calcium and magnesium, the release reaction occurs. Furthermore, if washed human platelets are suspended in a medium containing magnesium but *no* added calcium, aggregation and release occur on the addition of ADP. Therefore the release reaction that appears to be related to close cell contact can be observed only in a citrate system or in a system containing magnesium but no calcium (Mustard *et al.* 1975). Simple contact between platelets, induced by ADP or by polylysine, does not induce the release reaction.

Smith: Did the suspension of washed human platelets contain fibrinogen when you were adding citrate and then ADP?

Mustard: Yes; in the washed human platelet system, fibrinogen is necessary in the suspending fluid for ADP-induced aggregation. In the rabbit system it is not necessary.

Holmsen: Mürer (1972) has subdivided the thrombin-induced release reaction experimentally into an initiation and an extrusion step. He showed that Ca^{2+} inhibited the initiation phase, but enhanced or had no effect on the extrusion step. Do you know which of these steps might be inhibited by Ca^{2+} during (secondary) aggregation?

Mustard: It is inhibiting something, certainly, because if one prepares a suspension of washed human platelets in a medium containing magnesium only, and adds increasing amounts of calcium, and tests the response to ADP, a point is reached where the release reaction no longer occurs.

Haslam: Mürer is talking about induction by thrombin, not by ADP.

Mustard: This has not been tested with thrombin.

Holmsen: We have done some preliminary experiments on the effect of extracellular Ca^{2+} on the overall release reaction induced by thrombin at 37 °C. (Note that Mürer [1972] produced the 'initiation step' by exposing platelets to thrombin at 0 °C, then removed thrombin by washing or by using hirudin, and finally warmed the incubation mixture to 37 °C in order to produce the 'extrusion step'.) Platelets were washed with EDTA-containing solutions as described elsewhere (Holmsen & Day 1970), and Ca^{2+} was added in concentrations up to 3 mM above the endogenous EDTA concentration before thrombin was introduced. Ca^{2+} indeed inhibited the release of both adenine nucleosides and acid hydrolases, and the inhibition increased with increasing time of exposure and concentration of Ca^{2+}. We also found that these platelets lost metabolic ATP progressively during incubation with Ca^{2+}. Perhaps the inhibition was related to Ca^{2+}-induced depletion of ATP? However, no effect of Ca^{2+} on the release reaction was observed with platelets isolated by gel filtration in a medium containing no EDTA or Ca^{2+} (Lages *et al.* 1975).

Nachman: When the rabbit platelets have been degranulated with thrombin and then reinfused into the circulation, and show all the expected reactions except to thrombin, do they have fibrinogen on them?

Mustard: One would expect so, but we haven't examined this.

Holmsen: I have a comment on terminology. Some years ago we suggested (Holmsen *et al.* 1969) a subdivision of the release reaction into three consecutive steps: induction, transmission and extrusion. During induction the release inducer interacts with the outer surface of the platelet (receptors), by which a 'signal' or 'messenger substance' is liberated from the membrane. The 'signal' then propagates to a locus in the cell where it catalyses processes directly involved in movement of the granules and the plasma membrane toward each other. (A 'signal' could be a substance, such as calcium.) This propagation was referred to as transmission, and the processes connected with granule/membrane movements were parts of the extrusion process. I see that you, Dr Detwiler, have restricted the induction step to include the interaction between extracellular inducer and the receptor only, while your term 'transmission' includes the processes involved in *liberation* of the messenger substances, in addition to the propagation. I think this is a more concise subdivision of the secretory process than we made. So, with reference to Fig. 7 (p. 89) in your paper, we could now define the two first steps in the process:

Induction (initiation) = interaction between inducer and receptor resulting in inducer-modified receptor complex.

Transmission = with the receptor in the modified state, 'the signal' is liberated and propagates to a locus in the cell where it triggers reactions causing granules and membranes to move together.

Secondly, in your paper, you suggested that the ionophore-induced secretion *by-passed* a cyclic AMP-sensitive step, which then would explain why an increase in cyclic AMP does not inhibit this form of secretion, although it inhibits secretion induced by thrombin. I wonder whether the by-pass mechanism is applicable, in light of the enhancing effect of cyclic AMP on calcium uptake in calcium-storing vesicles, that has been shown in several tissues (Rabinowitz *et al.* 1965; Mohinder & Pritchard 1973; Dhalla *et al.* 1973). In accordance with this, we suggested (Day & Holmsen 1971) that cyclic AMP may inhibit the release reaction by stimulating the uptake of calcium into intracellular vesicles, thereby lowering the concentration of Ca^{2+} in the cytoplasm with a resulting inhibition of contractile systems. The ionophore makes Ca^{2+} available by rendering the vesicle membrane permeable to Ca^{2+}. The calcium that is pumped back in again will immediately leak out since the membrane is permeable. This is *not* a by-pass mechanism, rather an introduction of an alternative way of making calcium available, which cannot be counteracted by the cyclic AMP-sensitive calcium pump. (It could actually be likened to the impossible task of pumping liquid into a vessel where the physical walls have been removed or perforated.) How would this action of cyclic AMP fit with your hypothesis?

Detwiler: That's an excellent idea. With an action of cyclic AMP as you describe, we could consider the transmission step in Fig. 7 of my paper to be as shown in Fig. 1 below. This would explain the failure of PGE_1 to inhibit

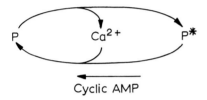

Fig. 1 (Detwiler). Transmission step (revised) in stimulus–response coupling in platelets.

ionophore-induced secretion, and it would be consistent with our observation that inhibition by cyclic AMP depended on the thrombin concentration; that is, the effect of cyclic AMP could be overcome by a strong enough 'stimulus' (Friedman & Detwiler 1975). On this aspect of cyclic AMP inhibition, we have said that '... it is as if cAMP regulates the *amplitude* of the transmission of a thrombin dependent signal' (Friedman & Detwiler 1975). We couldn't think of a mechanism, but the one shown above seems fully consistent with the observed phenomena. However, I would still say that the ionophore by-passes the thrombin–receptor reaction.

References

Day, H. J. & Holmsen, H. (1971) Concepts of the platelet release reaction. *Ser. Haematol. 4*, 3-27

Detwiler, T. C. & Feinman, R. D. (1973) Kinetics of the thrombin-induced release of calcium (II) by platelets. *Biochemistry 12*, 282-289

Dhalla, N. S., Sulakhe, P. V. & McNamara (1973) Studies on the relationship between adenylate cyclase activity and calcium transport by cardiac sarcotubular membranes. *Biochim. Biophys. Acta 323*, 276-284

Friedman, F. & Detwiler, T. C. (1975) Stimulus-secretion coupling in platelets. Effects of drugs on secretion of ATP. *Biochemistry 14*, 1315-1320

Haslam, R. J., Davidson, M. M. L. & McClenaghan, M. D. (1975) Cytochalasin B, the blood platelet release reaction and cyclic GMP. *Nature (Lond.) 253*, 455-457

HOLMSEN, H. & DAY, H. J. (1970) The selectivity of the thrombin-induced platelet release reaction: subcellular localization of released and retained substances. *J. Lab. Clin. Med.* *85*, 840-855

HOLMSEN, H., DAY, H. J. & STORMORKEN, H. (1969) The blood platelet release reaction. *Scand. J. Haematol.* Suppl. 8, 1-26

JENKINS, C. S. P., PACKHAM, M. A., KINLOUGH-RATHBONE, R. L. & MUSTARD, J. F. (1971) Interactions of polylysine with platelets. *Blood 37*, 395-412

KINLOUGH-RATHBONE, R. L., CHAHIL, A. & MUSTARD, J. F. (1975) Effect of A23,187 on thrombin-degranulated washed rabbit platelets. *Fed. Proc. 34*, 855 (abstr.)

LAGES, B., SCRUTTON, M. C. & HOLMSEN, H. (1975) Studies on gel-filtered human platelets: isolation and characterization in a medium containing no added Ca^{2+}, Mg^{2+} or K^+. *J. Lab. Clin. Med. 85*, 811-825

LEBRETON, G. & FEINBERG, H. (1974) ADP-induced changes in intraplatelet Ca^{2+} ion concentration. *Pharmacologist 16*, 313

MASSINI, P. & LÜSCHER, E. F. (1972) On the mechanism by which cell contact induces the release reaction of blood platelets; the effect of cationic polymers. *Thromb. Diath. Haemorrh. 27*, 121-133

MOHINDER, S. N. & PRITCHARD, E. T. (1973) Calcium binding by a plasma membrane fraction isolated from rat submandibular glands. *Biochim. Biophys. Acta 323*, 391-395

MÜRER, E. H. (1972) Factors influencing the initiation and the extrusion phase of the platelet release reaction. *Biochim. Biophys. Acta 261*, 435-443

MUSTARD, J. F., PERRY, D. W., KINLOUGH-RATHBONE, R. L. & PACKHAM, M. A. (1975) Factors responsible for ADP-induced release reaction of human platelets. *Am. J. Physiol. 228*, 1757-1765

PACKHAM, M. A. & GUCCIONE, M. A. (1973) Reactions of polylysine with platelets in plasma and in suspensions of washed platelets. *IVth International Congress on Thrombosis and Haemostasis*, Vienna, abstr. 143, p. 177

PHILLIPS, D. R. (1974) Thrombin interaction with human platelets. Potentiation of thrombin-induced aggregation and release by inactivated thrombin. *Thromb. Diath. Haemorrh. 32*, 207-215

RABINOWITZ, M., DESALLES, L., MEISSLER, J. & LORAN, L. (1965) Distribution of adenyl cyclase activity in rabbit skeletal muscle fractions. *Biochim. Biophys. Acta 97*, 29-35

REIMERS, H. J., PACKHAM, M. A., KINLOUGH-RATHBONE, R. L. & MUSTARD, J. F. (1973) Effect of repeated treatment of rabbit platelets with low concentrations of thrombin on their function, metabolism and survival. *Br. J. Haematol. 25*, 675-689

SNEDDON, J. M. (1972) Divalent cations and the blood platelet release reaction. *Nature New Biol. 236*, 103-104

SNEDDON, J. M. & WILLIAMS, K. I. (1973) Effects of cations on the blood platelet release reaction. *J. Physiol. (Lond.) 235*, 625-637

The interaction of platelet actin, myosin and myosin light chain kinase

ROBERT S. ADELSTEIN, MARY ANNE CONTI, JAMES L. DANIEL and
WILLIAM ANDERSON, Jr

*Section on Molecular Cardiology, Cardiology Branch, National Heart and Lung Institute,
Bethesda, Md.*

Abstract   Human blood platelets contain two proteins very similar in structure
and function to the contractile proteins of muscle: actin and myosin. Platelet
actin has a similar molecular weight (43 000 daltons) and amino acid composition
to muscle actin. It polymerizes into long filaments which can form 'arrowheads'
with skeletal muscle and platelet myosin subfragment-1 (S-1) as viewed in the
electron microscope. These 'arrowheads' are dissociated by Mg-ATP. Platelet
actin activates the ATPase activity of muscle heavy meromyosin to approximately
the same extent as muscle actin.

Platelet myosin (molecular weight 460 000), like muscle myosin, is composed
of heavy chains (200 000 daltons) and light chains (20 000 and 16 000 daltons).
The light chains resemble those found in other cytoplasmic (non-muscle) myosins
and smooth muscle myosin in charge (at pH 8.4) and size and differ from the
light chains of skeletal muscle and cardiac myosin.

Human platelets contain a kinase that transfers the terminal phosphate from
γ-labelled $AT^{32}P$ to the 20 000 dalton light chain of platelet myosin. When platelet myosin is phosphorylated, its actin-activated ATPase activity is markedly increased. Moreover, if phosphorylated myosin is dephosphorylated with *E. coli*
alkaline phosphatase, its actin-activated ATPase activity is decreased. These
findings indicate that the phosphorylation–dephosphorylation of platelet myosin
is a major controlling factor in platelet actin–myosin interaction. The ability of
platelet myosin kinase to phosphorylate myosin from fibroblast and smooth
muscle cells suggests that myosin phosphorylation may play a functional role
in other cells.

Human blood platelets contain proteins similar in structure and function to the
muscle proteins actin and myosin (Bettex-Galland & Lüscher 1965; Booyse
et al. 1971; Adelstein & Conti 1972; Booyse *et al.* 1973). Indeed, it is now
known that cytoplasmic actin and myosin are present in a large variety of
non-muscle cells from human and other vertebrate and non-vertebrate systems
(for a review on the subject of cytoplasmic actin and myosin, see Pollard &
Weihing 1974).

Our laboratory has been studying platelet myosin, actin and a recently isolated enzyme, platelet myosin light chain kinase, in order to understand the interaction of these proteins in platelets. The purpose of these studies is to discover the role these proteins play in specialized cell functions such as the platelet 'release reaction' and clot retraction as well as their possible role in functions common to all cells, such as motility and cell division.

In this paper we briefly review the structural and chemical properties of platelet actin and myosin. We shall then discuss the following properties of these proteins: (1) the phosphorylation of platelet myosin by a recently purified endogenous kinase, (2) the use of this platelet kinase to phosphorylate other cytoplasmic and smooth muscle myosins, (3) the effect of phosphorylation on the interaction of platelet actin and myosin.

PLATELET ACTIN

A number of methods for purifying platelet actin have been described (Adelstein & Conti 1972; Booyse *et al.* 1973). Human platelet actin has a molecular weight (43 000 daltons) and an amino acid composition similar to muscle actin. This includes the presence of 1 mole per molecule of the unusual amino acid N^{τ}-methyl histidine. Recent studies in the laboratory of Dr Marshall Elzinga (unpublished) on the cyanogen bromide fragments of platelet actin indicate identical amino acid sequences for some of the platelet actin and rabbit skeletal muscle actin peptides (Elzinga *et al.* 1973). There are a few discrete amino acid replacements which might reflect either a species difference or a difference between cytoplasmic and muscle actin.

Recently, Lazarides & Weber (1974) showed that non-muscle and muscle actin have similar antigenic determinants. They prepared antibodies to mouse fibroblast actin eluted from sodium dodecyl sulphate–polyacrylamide gels and found that these antibodies cross-reacted with chicken muscle actin.

Studies on the function of platelet actin are less complete. We have shown that human platelet actin activates rabbit skeletal muscle heavy meromyosin (HMM) to approximately the same extent as rabbit muscle actin. The activation measured at low ionic strength and 37 °C was from 0.1 to 1.5 μmoles P_i/mg protein per min. Skeletal muscle troponin-tropomyosin conferred Ca^{2+} sensitivity on this system (Adelstein & Conti 1972). Lower activation levels reported by others for cytoplasmic actins (Pollard & Weihing 1974) may reflect partial denaturation of the protein.

The process of polymerization, transforming platelet G-actin (globular) to F-actin (fibrous) in the presence of 0.1 M-KCl and 2 mM-MgCl$_2$, is known to

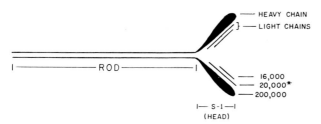

FIG. 1. Schematic representation of the platelet myosin molecule. *Indicates the phosphor-ylated light chain. The products of proteolytic cleavage (rod, S-1) are indicated (Adelstein *et al.* 1971). Diagram based on that for muscle myosin (Lowey *et al.* 1969).

occur but has not been as well studied as in the case of muscle actin (Oosawa & Kasai 1971). We have noted a marked pH dependence for this process in the platelet protein, the optimum being pH 7.5. Polymerized platelet actin is capable of forming 'arrowheads' with platelet myosin subfragment-1 (S-1), as well as skeletal muscle myosin S-1, as viewed in the electron microscope. These 'arrowheads' can be dissociated by Mg-ATP (Adelstein *et al.* 1971).

In a recent study on actin isolated from neutrophilic polymorphonuclear leucocytes, Boxer *et al.* (1974) reported that actin from leucocytes with sub-normal locomotion and ingestion capabilities failed to polymerize under con-ditions that fully polymerized normal leucocyte actin.

The existence of a second form of platelet actin has been described by Probst & Lüscher (1972) and Abramowitz *et al.* (1975). This second form of actin, similar in amino acid content to the primary form described above, remains depolymerized under conditions leading to the polymerization of ordinary platelet actin. It has been postulated that this actin may play a role in deter-mining cell shape, that unlike the usual form of actin it does not interact with platelet myosin, but that it may undergo polymerization–depolymerization inside the platelet.

PLATELET MYOSIN

Platelet myosin has a molecular weight of approximately 460 000 and is composed of two heavy chains (200 000 daltons) and two different light chains (20 000 and 16 000 daltons). We have isolated the intact molecule as well as the proteolytic fragments S-1 and rod (see Fig. 1). As is the case for skeletal muscle myosin, the platelet myosin S-1 fragment retains the ATPase activity as well as the ability to bind reversibly to actin. The rod portion retains the ability to form bare thick filaments at low ionic strength (Adelstein *et al.* 1971).

The two light chains of platelet myosin are similar in molecular weight to the light chains of other cytoplasmic (e.g., fibroblast) and smooth muscle myosins. They also resemble these light chains in charge, as evidenced by their electrophoretic mobility, in polyacrylamide-urea gels (pH 8.4). On the other hand, the platelet light chains differ in these parameters from the light chains of skeletal and cardiac muscle myosin (Adelstein & Conti 1974).

Although platelet myosin and smooth muscle myosin have similar light chains, Willingham *et al.* (1974) have immunological evidence for differences in the heavy chains. Antibodies to fibroblast myosin cross-react with the isolated rod portion of the platelet myosin molecule (for the isolation of platelet rod, see Adelstein *et al.* 1971). These particular antibodies fail to cross-react with smooth muscle myosin, indicating a difference in the rod portion of platelet and smooth muscle myosin.

In summary, platelet myosin resembles other cytoplasmic myosins as well as smooth muscle myosin in containing a similar (possibly identical) complement of light chains. These light chains differ from those of skeletal and cardiac muscle myosin. At least part of the rod portion of the heavy chains of platelet and fibroblast myosin differs from that of smooth muscle myosin.

Recent experiments with antibodies to non-muscle myosin indicate a potential method for localizing myosin in platelet cells. Using antibodies to fibroblast myosin, Willingham *et al.* (1974) showed that a part of the fibroblast myosin is localized on the outside of the fibroblast cell membrane. Weber & Groeschel-Stewart (1974) prepared antibodies to chicken gizzard myosin which they used to locate cytoplasmic myosin inside fibroblast cells from human, mouse and chicken sources. It is of interest that when Willingham *et al.* (1974) made antibodies to smooth muscle myosin (mouse uterus) they failed to cross-react with mouse fibroblast myosin, although they did cross-react with chicken gizzard myosin. Before firm conclusions can be drawn about myosin localization it must definitely be established: (*a*) that the myosin being utilized in antibody production is pure by a number of criteria and (*b*) that the antibodies produced not only cross-react with a cellular component *in situ*, but also cross-react with myosin isolated from the cell.

Table 1 summarizes the enzymic activity of platelet myosin at high ionic strength and compares it to that of smooth, skeletal and cardiac myosin. As is the case with the light chains, the ATPase activity of platelet myosin resembles that of smooth muscle more than cardiac and skeletal muscle myosin. This is also true for the actin-activated ATPase activity measured in the presence of Mg^{2+} at low ionic strength. This last parameter is thought to be the most physiologically relevant of the *in vitro* enzymic measurements, and we shall return to it below in discussing the effect of platelet myosin phosphorylation.

TABLE 1

ATPase specific activity of platelet and muscle myosin

| | ATPase specific activity ($\mu mol\ P_i/mg$ protein per min[a]) | |
	K[+]-EDTA	Ca[2+]
Non-muscle		
Human platelet	1.4	0.7
Muscle		
Horse smooth[b]	1.37	0.8
Rabbit skeletal (white)	4.2	0.36
Human cardiac	2.0	0.3

[a] Assay conditions: 20 mM-Tris·HCl (pH 7.2), 2 mM-EDTA or 10 mM-CaCl$_2$; 0.5 M-KCl, 2 mM-ATP, 0.25 mg/ml myosin, 37 °C.
[b] Yamaguchi *et al.* (1970). The rest of the values are from this laboratory.

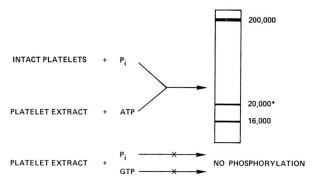

FIG. 2. Schematic representation of platelet myosin phosphorylation. A 7.5% polyacrylamide-sodium dodecyl sulphate gel showing the relative mobility or the myosin chains is on the right. *Indicates phosphorylated chain.

PHOSPHORYLATION

In an effort to understand the factors controlling actin–myosin interaction in the platelet as well as other non-muscle cells, we began a study on platelet protein phosphorylation. Since kinases are often bound to their substrate, our initial studies involved the addition of γ-labelled AT^{32}P to a high salt (0.5 M-KCl) extract of lysed platelets at pH 7.5 (see Fig. 2).

The only protein phosphorylated in this extract is myosin, specifically the 20 000 dalton light chain (Adelstein *et al.* 1973). This corresponds to the findings of Perrie *et al.* (1973) who phosphorylated the 18 500 dalton light chain of rabbit skeletal muscle myosin using an exogenous kinase. As mentioned above, this light chain differs both in size and charge from the phosphorylated platelet light chain.

The original experiments on myosin phosphorylation in a platelet extract revealed that ^{32}P could be utilized from γ-labelled $AT^{32}P$ (and not $GT^{32}P$ or $^{32}P_i$) to form a stable covalent (ester type) bond (see Fig. 2). Subsequently, we found that if fresh intact platelets are incubated in the presence of $^{32}P_i$, small but significant quantities of $^{32}P_i$ are incorporated into the 20 000 dalton light chain of the purified myosin. This suggests that ^{32}P is first incorporated into the platelet pool of ATP and is then used to phosphorylate the myosin light chain. We are now repeating this $^{32}P_i$ incubation in the presence of ADP, thrombin and dibutyryl cyclic AMP to see if these reagents, known to affect platelet aggregation, have any effect on the incorporation of $^{32}P_i$ into platelet myosin.

PLATELET MYOSIN LIGHT CHAIN KINASE

The enzyme was purified from human platelets by an initial extraction at low ionic strength to separate it from myosin, and subsequent column chromatography on DEAE-Sephadex, Biogel P-200 and hydroxyapatite (for details of purification, see Daniel *et al.* 1974 and Adelstein *et al.* 1975). This procedure resulted in an approximately 500-fold purification of the kinase. The enzyme was not purified to homogeneity since approximately seven bands were seen on polyacrylamide gel electrophoresis (done in the absence of SDS in order to preserve the native enzyme structure), only one of which possessed enzymic activity after elution from the gel.

The properties of the purified enzyme are summarized in Table 2. It is similar to the skeletal muscle kinase purified by Pires *et al.* (1974) in size and apparent independence of cyclic AMP for its phosphorylating activity. Unlike the skeletal muscle enzyme, the platelet kinase has no Ca^{2+} requirement but does require Mg^{2+} for its activity.

SUBSTRATES

The substrate specificity of the platelet kinase is quite interesting, particularly since it follows the structural and functional similarities of the myosins outlined above (Table 2). The platelet kinase phosphorylates the 20 000 dalton light chain of mouse fibroblast and chicken gizzard myosin. The platelet kinase is inhibited by rabbit and human skeletal muscle myosin and cannot phosphorylate human cardiac myosin. The inhibition by skeletal muscle myosin suggests a

TABLE 2

Properties of platelet myosin kinase

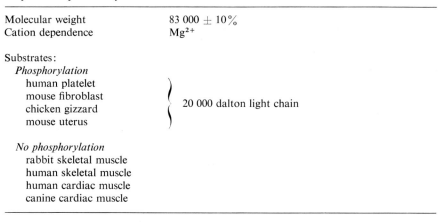

Molecular weight	83 000 ± 10%
Cation dependence	Mg²⁺

Substrates:
Phosphorylation
  human platelet
  mouse fibroblast
  chicken gizzard
  mouse uterus

    20 000 dalton light chain

No phosphorylation
  rabbit skeletal muscle
  human skeletal muscle
  human cardiac muscle
  canine cardiac muscle

basic similarity in the site to which the enzyme can bind without being able to transfer the phosphate group. The finding that the platelet kinase can phosphorylate another cytoplasmic myosin (i.e., fibroblast) suggests that the process of phosphorylation may extend to myosins in cells other than platelets. Indeed, we have used the platelet enzyme as a probe in an effort to uncover the presence of non-muscle myosin in human rhabdomyosarcoma cells.

At present, we are investigating the hypothesis that tumour cells contain significant amounts of cytoplasmic myosin which functions in cell division. We chose the malignant skeletal muscle tumour rhabdomyosarcoma to see if these cells contain normal skeletal muscle myosin as well as cytoplasmic myosin. Our working hypothesis is that cytoplasmic myosin, which is involved in cell division, would be present in unusually large amounts in neoplastic rhabdomyosarcoma cells. Since some of these cells continue to show evidence of myofibrils, we would also expect to isolate skeletal muscle myosin. We hoped to differentiate muscle and cytoplasmic myosin by the ability of the latter to be phosphorylated by platelet kinase as well as by the size and charge of the light chains.

Myosin prepared from the excised tumour of a 4-year-old girl was found to contain a mixture of human skeletal and cytoplasmic myosin (see Fig. 3). Because cytoplasmic myosin only partially dissociates from actin under conditions which completely dissociate skeletal muscle actomyosin (i.e., the presence of Mg-ATP), the two myosins could be separated by chromatography on Sepharose 4B. Incubation of cytoplasmic myosin with platelet myosin kinase and [γ-³²P]ATP resulted in phosphorylation of the 20 000 dalton light chain, whereas the enzyme had no effect on the normal human skeletal muscle myosin

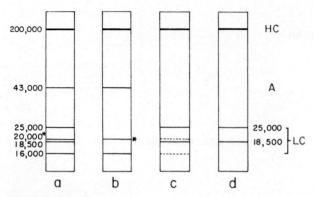

FIG. 3. Schematic representation of 7.5% polyacrylamide-sodium dodecyl sulphate gels of rhabdomyosarcoma and human skeletal myosin. (*a*) rhabdomyosarcoma myosin before Sepharose chromatography, (*b*) cytoplasmic myosin purified from *a* by Sepharose chromatography, (*c*) human skeletal myosin with trace cytoplasmic myosin, purified from *a*, (*d*) control sample of human skeletal myosin. HC, heavy chain; A, actin; LC, light chains. *Phosphorylated light chain.

(see Fig. 3). Further studies will be necessary to ascertain that the tumour cells are the source of both myosins. Dr Donald Henson and Rachel Levinson (National Cancer Institute) are using antibodies to both human skeletal and fibroblast myosin to study the localization of myosin in sections made from the same tumour. Of relevance is our finding that a pure line of human rhabdomyosarcoma cells (A204), grown *in vitro* and showing no evidence of myofibrillar formation, contain light chains of cytoplasmic myosin (i.e., 20 000 and 16 000 dalton) and not human skeletal muscle myosin (25 000 and 18 500).

THE ROLE OF PHOSPHORYLATION

The effect of phosphorylating platelet myosin is to increase the actin-activated ATPase activity measured in the presence of Mg^{2+} at low ionic strength (see Table 3) (Adelstein *et al.* 1975). Phosphorylation has no effect on the myosin ATPase activity measured in the presence of K^+-EDTA at high ionic strength. Table 3 shows that myosin, before phosphorylation, can be activated to some extent but the resulting specific activity is one-fifth the specific activity of actin-activated phosphorylated myosin. We do not yet know if this low level of activation is an inherent property of the myosin or reflects partial phosphorylation of the myosin during the purification procedure.

Although a platelet phosphatase which dephosphorylates platelet myosin has yet to be isolated, we have succeeded in partially dephosphorylating

TABLE 3

The effect of phosphorylation on ATPase specific activity

	ATPase specific activity (μmol P_i/mg protein per min)		
	Actin-activated[a]		Myosin alone[b]
	– Actin	+ Actin	K+-EDTA
Control myosin	0.002	0.020	0.57
Phosphorylated myosin	0.009	0.100	0.61

[a] Assay conditions: 10 mM-Tris·HCl (pH 7.2), 1.4 mM-MgCl$_2$, 1 mM-ATP, 30 mM-KCl, 0.13 mg/ml myosin, 1.2 mg/ml actin, 37 °C.
[b] Assay conditions: 20 mM-Tris·HCl (pH 7.2), 2 mM-EDTA, 0.5 M-KCl; 2 mM-ATP, 0.25 mg/ml myosin 37 °C. (For details of assay, see Adelstein et al. 1971. For details of phosphorylation, see Adelstein et al. 1975.)

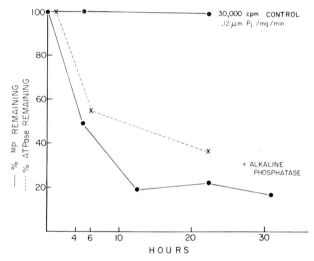

FIG. 4. Release of ^{32}P from phosphorylated myosin incubated with alkaline phosphatase. ^{32}P-labelled phosphorylated myosin was incubated with alkaline phosphatase and samples removed at the times indicated for (●) determination of ^{32}P remaining and (×) actin-activated ATPase specific activity remaining. The upper line (control) shows that counts were not lost from a control sample incubated under the same condition without alkaline phosphatase. The phosphorylated myosin contained 30 000 c.p.m./0.05 mg of protein and an actin-activated ATPase specific activity of 0.12 μmol P_i/mg myosin per min.

platelet myosin using *E. coli* alkaline phosphatase (Adelstein *et al.* 1974; Conti & Adelstein 1975). Fig. 4 illustrates a time course for the release of ^{32}P from previously phosphorylated platelet myosin in the presence of alkaline phosphatase. The actin-activated ATPase activity for the appropriate time is plotted on the same graph. Dephosphorylation is accompanied by a decrease in the actin-activated myosin ATPase activity but, like phosphorylation, it has no effect on the K^+-EDTA and Ca^{2+}-activated myosin ATPase activity measured at high ionic strength.

These studies suggest that phosphorylation acts as a switch that turns on myosin so that it can interact, in a physiologically meaningful way, with actin. Since interaction with actin (detected by an increase in the actin-activated ATPase activity) does not result in dephosphorylation, the switch evidently remains on until a phosphatase turns it off by dephosphorylating myosin. The ability of the platelet enzyme to phosphorylate other non-muscle myosins, such as fibroblast myosin and chicken gizzard myosin, suggests that this process may play a role in the numerous other non-muscle cells in which myosin and actin have been detected, as well as in smooth muscle.

Phosphorylation does not appear to confer Ca^{2+} sensitivity on the platelet actin–myosin system. This means that phosphorylated myosin is activated by actin both in the presence and absence of Ca^{2+}. In muscle, the troponin–tropomyosin complex confers Ca^{2+} sensitivity. It is possible that this fine tuning of the switch is also conferred by troponin–tropomyosin in the platelets (Cohen *et al.* 1973). The identification of platelet tropomyosin has been described by Cohen & Cohen (1972). Positive identification of platelet and other cytoplasmic troponins has yet to be accomplished.

Both general and specialized cell functions may be affected by the interaction of actin with phosphorylated myosin. Specialized cell functions in the platelet include the process of clot retraction and platelet aggregation. In secretory cells, specialized functions involve the release of substances such as hormones and neurotransmitters (Puszkin & Kochwa 1974). General cellular processes that might be affected by this interaction include cell division, as discussed above in the case of rhabdomyosarcoma cells, and cell migration, which is of particular importance in blood cells, as well as embryonic cells, particularly during the earliest stages of development. The challenge of these speculations awaits the proof of further experimentation.

SUMMARY

(1) Human blood platelets contain myosin which is similar in structure and function to smooth muscle myosin and to cytoplasmic myosins from other non-muscle sources.

(2) Platelet myosin light chain kinase can phosphorylate the 20 000 dalton light chain of platelet myosin, fibroblast myosin and chicken gizzard myosin.

(3) The effect of phosphorylation is to increase the actin-activated ATPase activity of platelet myosin.

(4) Phosphorylation might play a similar role in controlling actin–myosin interaction in other cells found to contain these proteins.

ACKNOWLEDGEMENTS

The authors gratefully acknowledge the help of Dr Donald Henson and Rachel Levinson for growing the A204 rhabdomyosarcoma cells and Dr John Ziegler for the rhabdomyosarcoma surgical specimens. We also thank Mrs Kathy Knudsen for typing the manuscript.

References

ABRAMOWITZ, J. W., STRACHER, A. & DETWILER, T. C. (1975) A second form of actin. *Arch. Biochem. Biophys.* 167, 230-237

ADELSTEIN, R. S. & CONTI, M. A. (1972) The characterization of contractile proteins from platelets and fibroblasts. *Cold Spring Harbor Symp. Quant. Biol.* 37, 599-606

ADELSTEIN, R. S. & CONTI, M. A. (1974) Myosin and myosin-like molecules in cells other than muscle. In *Exploratory Concepts in Muscular Dystrophy* (Proceedings of an International Conference, Carefree, Arizona, October, 1973) (Milhorat, A. T., ed.), *Excerpta Medica ICS 333*, 70-78

ADELSTEIN, R. S., POLLARD, T. D. & KUEHL, W. M. (1971) Isolation and characterization of myosin and two myosin fragments from human blood platelets. *Proc. Natl. Acad. Sci. U.S.A.* 68, 2703-2707

ADELSTEIN, R. S., CONTI, M. A. & ANDERSON, W., JR (1973) Phosphorylation of human platelet myosin. *Proc. Natl. Acad. Sci. U.S.A.* 70, 3115-3119

ADELSTEIN, R. S., DANIEL, J. L., CONTI, M. A. & ANDERSON, W., JR (1975) Platelet myosin phosphorylation: studies on the kinase, substrate and effect of phosphorylation. *Proc. Fed. of Europ. Biochem. Socs., 9th Meeting*, Budapest, vol. 31, pp. 177-186, North-Holland, Amsterdam

BETTEX-GALLAND, M. & LÜSCHER, E. F. (1965) in *Advances in Protein Chemistry*, vol. 20 (Anfinsen, C. B. *et al.*, eds.), pp. 1-34, Academic Press, New York

BOOYSE, F. M., HOVEKE, T. P., ZSCHOCKE, D. & RAFELSON, M. E., Jr (1971) Human platelet myosin. *J. Biol. Chem.* 246, 4291-4297

BOOYSE, F. M., HOVEKE, T. P. & RAFELSON, M. E., Jr (1973) Human platelet actin, isolation and properties. *J. Biol. Chem.* 248, 4083-4091

BOXER, L. A., HEDLEY-WHYTE, E. T. & STOSSEL, T. P. (1974) Neutrophil actin dysfunction and abnormal neutrophil behavior. *N. Engl. J. Med.* 291, 1093-1099

COHEN, I. & COHEN, C. (1972) A tropomyosin-like protein from human platelets. *J. Mol. Biol.* 68, 383-387

COHEN, I., KAMINSKI, E. & DE VRIES, A. (1973) Actin-linked regulation of the human platelet contractile system. *FEBS Lett.* 34, 315-317

CONTI, M. A. & ADELSTEIN, R. S. (1975) Platelet myosin phosphorylation controls actin activation of myosin ATPase activity. *Fed. Proc.* 34, 540a

DANIEL, J., CONTI, M. A. & ADELSTEIN, R. S. (1974) Platelet myosin phosphorylation: studies on the kinase and phosphorylated light chain. *Fed. Proc.* 33, 2009a

ELZINGA, M. E., COLLINS, J. H., KUEHL, W. M. & ADELSTEIN, R. S. (1973) Complete amino acid sequence of actin of rabbit skeletal muscle. *Proc. Natl. Acad. Sci. U.S.A.* 70, 2687-2691

LAZARIDES, E. & WEBER, K. (1974) Actin antibody: the specific visualization of actin filaments in non-muscle cells. *Proc. Natl. Acad. Sci. U.S.A.* 71, 2268-2272

Lowey, S., Slayter, H. S., Weeds, A. G. & Baker, H. (1969) Substructure of the myosin molecule. *J. Mol. Biol. 42*, 1-29

Oosawa, F. & Kasai, M. (1971) in *Subunits in Biological Systems*, part A (Timasheff, S. N. & Fasman, G. D., eds.) (*Biological Macromolecules Series*, vol. 5), pp. 261-320, Marcel Dekker, New York

Perrie, W. T., Smillie, L. B. & Perry, S. V. (1973) A phosphorylated light chain component of myosin from skeletal muscle. *Biochem. J. 135*, 151-164

Pires, E., Perry, S. V. & Thomas, M. A. W. (1974) Myosin light chain kinase, a new enzyme from striated muscle. *FEBS Lett. 41*, 292-296

Pollard, T. D. & Weihing, R. R. (1974) Actin and myosin and cell movement. In *CRC Critical Reviews of Biochemistry*, vol. 2, pp. 1-65, CRC Press, Inc., Cleveland, Ohio

Probst, E. & Lüscher, E. F. (1972) Studies on thrombosthenin A, the actin-like moiety of the contractile protein from blood platelets. I. Isolation, characterization, and evidence for two forms of thrombosthenin A. *Biochim. Biophys. Acta 278*, 577-584

Puszkin, S. & Kochwa, S. (1974) Regulation of neurotransmitter release by a complex of actin with relaxing protein isolated from rat brain synaptosomes. *J. Biol. Chem. 249*, 7711-7714

Weber, K. & Groeschel-Stewart, U. (1974) Antibody to myosin: the specific visualization of myosin-containing filaments in non-muscle cells. *Proc. Natl. Acad. Sci. U.S.A. 71*, 4561-4564

Willingham, M. C., Ostlund, R. E. & Pastan, I. (1974) Myosin is a component of the cell surface of cultured cells. *Proc. Natl. Acad. Sci. U.S.A. 71*, 4144-4148

Yamaguchi, M., Miyazawa, Y. & Sekine, T. (1970) Preparation and properties of smooth muscle myosin from horse esophagus. *Biochim. Biophys. Acta 216*, 411-421

Discussion

Nachman: You discussed the antigenic relationships between the various actomyosins. Becker and I, using actomyosin from a human pregnant uterus, made an antibody in rabbits (Becker & Nachman 1973). This antibody to smooth muscle actomyosin stains human megakaryocytes and platelets. An antibody to crude thrombosthenin, which contains tropomyosin, actin and all the myosin fragments, stains human uterus. By immunodiffusion there is partial identity between thrombosthenin and uterine actomyosin. So in the human system there is clear-cut evidence of an antigenic relationship between platelet actomyosin and uterine actomyosin.

Adelstein: Two laboratories working with non-muscle myosin have found that antibodies to these myosins fail to cross-react with smooth muscle myosin. Willingham *et al.* (1974) found that antibodies to mouse fibroblast myosin failed to cross-react with mouse uterus myosin, and Pollard found that antibodies to human platelet myosin did not cross-react with human uterus myosin (T. D. Pollard, personal communication).

On the other hand, antibodies to mouse fibroblast myosin do cross-react with human platelet myosin, specifically with the rod portion of the molecule (M. C. Willingham & R. S. Adelstein, unpublished work).

These findings do not exclude the possibility that cytoplasmic (non-muscle) myosin may have some antigenic sites in common with smooth muscle myosin which would result in a population of antibodies that would cross-react with both myosins. I would simply like to point out that one must always be careful about the purity of the antigen—in this case, the myosin.

Cohen: Dr Adelstein described some of the similarities and differences among myosins from platelets and muscle cells. We have also studied the properties of platelet myosin, particularly of platelet light meromyosin (LMM), obtained by splitting the myosin molecule with trypsin. We find an axial periodicity of 14.5 nm (145Å) in tactoids of platelet LMM, which is similar to the periodicity of LMM from smooth and skeletal muscle. This may indicate a fundamental similarity in the structure of these molecules, at least in respect of their assembly.

The most striking difference between muscle and platelet systems lies in the tropomyosin molecule. Platelet tropomyosin is smaller than other, muscle tropomyosins. This two-chain α-helical molecule has a subunit molecular weight of 30 000 and forms paracrystals with an axial period of 34.5 nm, which is close to the length of the molecule (Cohen & Cohen 1972). It is therefore smaller in size than the 40 nm long tropomyosins from muscle. Tropomyosin may be involved in the regulation of contraction which we have demonstrated to be of the actin-linked type in platelets (Cohen *et al.* 1973). Fine *et al.* (1973) have shown characteristics for tropomyosin from brain tissue similar to those of platelet tropomyosin. This may imply distinctive structural and spatial relationships in the contractile elements of non-muscular systems, as compared with muscle systems.

Dr Adelstein, you discussed the function of phosphorylation in the platelet system and mentioned that the actin activation of myosin is increased by phosphorylation. Compared to that of skeletal muscle myosin, the actin activation of platelet myosin is rather weak. Pollard (1975) has shown that the actin activation of platelet myosin is increased by the presence of a co-factor, which he has not yet completely identified. Could this co-factor be related to a protein kinase?

Adelstein: At present, since the co-factor has not been purified, it is not possible to determine whether it might be a kinase. However, the following points should be made: (*a*) Pollard's co-factor was isolated from *rabbit skeletal muscle* and added to platelet myosin; (*b*) the actin-activated ATPase activity found in the presence of the co-factor is the same order of magnitude as that found by us for phosphorylated myosin (T. D. Pollard, personal communication). Until the co-factor is at least partially purified it is not possible to know whether it is a kinase or not.

Haslam: Perhaps it is not surprising that cyclic AMP did not activate the phosphorylation of the myosin light chains, Dr Adelstein. As you found an increase in actin-activated ATPase after phosphorylation and some evidence that ADP increases the phosphorylation of platelet myosin, it is likely that, if anything, increased phosphorylation would be associated with decreased cyclic AMP levels. This raises the question of whether myosin light chain kinase is activated by cyclic GMP, which does increase in response to ADP (see my paper, Fig. 7, p. 135).

Adelstein: We have tried cyclic GMP and not found any effect, but the experiment needs to be repeated. Our original thought was that cyclic AMP actually *decreased* the kinase activity, but we have not yet substantiated this. Our experiment using ^{32}P and ADP, which causes aggregation, has only been done once and must be repeated.

Crawford: Do you always, in your myosin activation experiments, titrate to maximal response? In other words, do you establish the most favourable combining ratio for the actin and myosin?

Adelstein: Yes; we have had to do that.

Crawford: It occurs to me that some of the activation of the myosin by actin may depend upon a number of factors which are difficult to control experiment-ally—for example, variability in the length and polarity of the actin polymer and whether or not it is present as the two-stranded helical structure you get in muscle or as a single-stranded Mg^{2+} polymer, of the kind seen in *Physarum* and *Dictyostelium* (Hatano & Oosawa 1966; Woolley 1972). There may even be lateral association of the polymeric units. All these factors could influence the combining properties of the two polymers and I would think it would be extremely difficult to define such interactions in quantitative terms.

Adelstein: We are using rabbit skeletal muscle actin which has been poly-merized in the presence of 30 mM-KCl, 2 mM-MgCl$_2$, 7 mM-Tris·HCl (pH 7.5) and 2.5 mM-DTT. We use a 10–15-fold excess of actin (mg/mg) over platelet myosin. Platelet actin polymerized under these conditions appears to activate platelet myosin to the same extent (R. S. Adelstein & M. A. Conti, unpublished results).

Detwiler: We have been interested in these systems for some time, and one problem relates to the preparation of the platelet actin. I wonder what your normal yield of polymerizable actin is and whether you are dealing with a very small fraction of the total actin of the cell, or a substantial part of it. I am not specifically referring to the second form of actin that we described (Abramowitz *et al.* 1975), but if you go through the conventional procedures for preparing actin, you obtain only a small amount of material. I am worried by discussions of actin-activated myosin ATPase when platelet actin is used; it might be just some small part of the total actin that is capable of this activity.

Adelstein: In the experiments on the actin-activated ATPase activity we purify platelet myosin free of platelet actin and in most cases we add back rabbit skeletal muscle actin. We have also added back platelet actin but the procedure we employ for isolating platelet actin makes use of the ability of actin to polymerize at high ionic strength (Adelstein & Conti 1972).

We have never quantified how much platelet actin can be polymerized but we do know that unlike rabbit skeletal muscle actin, the polymerization of platelet actin is very sensitive to pH. Platelet actin, shown to be polymerized at pH 7.5 by both flow birefringence and increased viscosity, was depolymerized by simply raising the pH to 8.3. Polymerization was restored by lowering the pH to 7.5 (Adelstein & Conti 1972).

Lüscher: The yields of purified actin isolated from crude platelet actomyosin are certainly deplorably low. However, once actin is in the fibrillar F form, it can be depolymerized and repolymerized with a 95 % yield.

Crawford: There are also difficulties with conventional acetone powder preparations of whole platelets. The extractability of the actin from the powder is quite low and you certainly leave some actin behind, probably a considerable proportion. I suspect, since in our own cell fractionation studies that I referred to earlier (p. 42) the cytosol actin seems not to combine with skeletal muscle myosin, that the low ionic strength extraction of acetone powder probably favours the extraction of this non-combinable actin. This may be G-actin or perhaps an effete monomer which is no longer polymerizable under any conditions. Perhaps, in fact, we leave the contractile-competent platelet actin in the acetone powder debris, protected from extraction by its association with the particulate elements of the cell.

Lüscher: It remains most intriguing that there is no electron microscopical evidence for the presence of pre-formed cytoplasmic actin microfibrils in a resting platelet. These become immediately discernible upon stimulation. In what form is the actin present in resting platelets?

Adelstein: Without knowing for sure, I would favour the existence of small polymers which would polymerize into long fibrous polymers under the right stimulus.

Lüscher: Thus one is faced with the interesting situation that in the platelet, unlike for example striated muscle, there is no evidence for a morphologically defined contractile structure which can as such be stimulated into activity. In order to have contractile activity, it is necessary to assemble such a system first.

Adelstein: A current problem in studies of smooth muscle, similar to one that exists in non-muscle contractile systems, is the positive identification of troponin. Troponin is a complex of proteins that together with tropomyosin confers calcium sensitivity on skeletal muscle actomyosin; that is to say, actin-activation of the myosin ATPase activity will occur only in the presence of Ca^{2+}. In a recent article Bremel (1974) suggests that troponin may not be present in smooth muscle and that calcium sensitivity may be conferred by myosin, similar to the findings of Lehman *et al.* (1972) in molluscs.

Cohen: I agree with you about the likelihood of the existence of small oligomers of actin in the intact cell. These would grow into long filaments when the cell is stimulated by some as yet unknown mechanism. You might have tropomyosin bound to these small actin oligomers, as only seven actin molecules are needed to provide a site of attachment for one tropomyosin molecule. Seven actin molecules would make quite a small oligomer.

Detwiler: May I pose a general question related to platelet contractile proteins? Dr Lüscher initially pointed out the very large amount of actomyosin in platelets and in the literature one frequently encounters statements about the function of this protein (cf. Bettex-Galland & Lüscher 1965). But to my mind there is no real evidence for any function of platelet contractile proteins. Can anyone tell me what the possible functions of these proteins are, and defend these suggestions with some evidence?

Lüscher: Of course one could argue that the relatively large amount of contractile protein in platelets is simply due to the fact that the megakaryocyte is an extremely mobile cell and that therefore the platelet cannot help containing a lot of actomyosin! There is also, of course, another answer to your question. Microscopical observation of spontaneous haemostasis shows that first a relatively fragile platelet mass is formed, which is barely able to resist the eroding forces of the streaming blood. This loose aggregate suddenly becomes solid and impermeable. This striking phenomenon certainly is not due to the formation of fibrin but rather to active contraction of the aggregate. In fact, *in vitro*, platelet aggregates will contract at 37 °C within two to three minutes, which corresponds roughly to a normal bleeding time. I think this consolidation of a haemostatic plug, or of a platelet thrombus, is a most important manifestation of contractility.

Furthermore, long spikes form early during the shape change, and later can be retracted completely. Extrusion as well as the withdrawal of these pseudopods certainly are again manifestations of contractility.

Detwiler: You are saying that these are phenomena that are easily attributed to a contractile protein. Intuitively it seems that that would be a nice function of the contractile protein, but there is really no *evidence* that it is the contractile protein doing that.

Lüscher: I really have difficulties in offering any other explanation for the active contraction of a platelet aggregate or for clot retraction.

Born: One way to analyse the retraction of the spikes is to isolate them; we have been trying to do this but it is very difficult. Dr Lüscher is right. These cells can pack together almost as tightly as is theoretically possible for them (Born & Hume 1967); the intercellular space becomes very small indeed, and there must be some mechanism for deforming these cells so that they can pack in this way. But what evidence is there about this mechanism?

Feinberg: How would Dr Detwiler explain all the observed movements— spike formation and so on—without contractile proteins?

Detwiler: I couldn't, but a biophysicist could talk about the extrusion of water from a gel and things of that sort which do not necessarily involve contractile protein. The point is that lack of an obvious alternative explanation is not proof of anything.

Cohen: I don't think we have syneresis here. We do have a contractile phenomenon, as Budtz-Olsen (1951) has shown by comparing the kinetics of syneresis and clot retraction. So it is not just water coming out.

Haslam: What we would like to have is a specific inhibitor of the action of thrombosthenin, so that we could then identify unequivocally all the processes in which thrombosthenin is involved. I don't know of any such compound. Thiol reagents, which are usually non-specific, do react with thrombosthenin and do block these processes. What sort of progress has been made towards synthesizing a useful specific irreversible inhibitor of myosin ATPase? Yount *et al.* (1972) described irreversible inhibition by a purine disulphide analogue of ATP, but this sort of compound would not be able to penetrate the platelet membrane because of its negative charge.

Cohen: I would suggest the use of cytochalasin B. This fungal drug inhibits contraction by disorganizing microfilaments. It also inhibits shape change, and I believe that shape change is a manifestation of contraction.

Haslam: There are problems here. The evidence that cytochalasin B is a sufficiently specific inhibitor of contractile processes is unconvincing. Cytochalasin B is also an extremely potent inhibitor of the transport of sugars and nucleosides across cell membranes and may therefore interfere with cell metabolism. Even the concentrations of cytochalasin B which potentiate the release reaction (i.e. less than 2 μM with washed platelets) can inhibit membrane transport. One could explain this by postulating that there is some connection between the insertion of microfilaments into the membrane and the transport mechanism, so that both are disrupted at the same time. However, at the moment we really do not know enough about how cytochalasin B acts to be able to draw any firm conclusions.

Cohen: J. G. White (1971) has shown that cytochalasin B inhibits shape change, but primary aggregation is unaffected and occurs between disk-shaped platelets.

Haslam: In our hands (Haslam *et al.* 1975) this inhibitory effect of cyto-chalasin B on platelet shape change was seen only with high concentrations (e.g. 40 μM in platelet-rich plasma). When you have an inhibitory action of cytochalasin B the possibility of its being metabolic in origin requires in-vestigation.

Cohen: You can reverse the effect of cytochalasin B; you can wash it out and the platelets regain their normal function.

Haslam: The metabolic effects of an inhibition of membrane transport processes may also be reversible.

Lüscher: I would fully subscribe to your doubts, Dr Haslam, because, for instance, cytochalasin B is unable to inhibit the so-called 'superprecipitation' of actomyosin, generally considered to mimic contraction under *in vitro* conditions.

Mustard: I am a bit confused; Dr Detwiler asked a question, to which he received a partial answer, which suggested that when platelets change their shape and form spikes the contractile protein is involved in the shape change. I find that somewhat inconsistent. If the contractile protein restores the platelet disk shape, is it also causing the shape change?

Born: We are using 'contractile protein' in too loose a sense here. There is evidence now for both the sliding mechanism of striated muscle and proteins which contract through a change in conformation.

Lüscher: One has to keep in mind that besides contractile protein which is dispersed in the cytoplasm, the platelet contains preformed contractile material, sometimes termed submembranous fibrils (Zucker-Franklin 1970), just beneath the cell membrane. Since it is likely that calcium first becomes available in the vicinity of the membrane, be it by influx or from storage organelles localized along the microtubules, it is conceivable that these submembranous fibrils will be the first to contract. The formation of the long spikes is then perhaps explained as resulting from the compression of the platelet's cell body. Next, the cytoplasmic contractile system will become organized and activated.

It is only then that contraction of the pseudopods will start. Thus, it is the time-sequence of activation of different compartments of contractile material which determines the course of the morphological manifestations of contractility.

Mustard: To make that explanation acceptable you would have to postulate that the membrane system is not able to contract uniformly; it would have to contract in a differential manner, with parts that contract and parts that do not contract.

Cohen: This is how locomotion happens in amoebae, where cyclic changes occur with parts of the cell in a contracted state and parts in a relaxed state (Taylor *et al.* 1973).

References

ABRAMOWITZ, J. W., STRACHER, A. & DETWILER, T. C. (1975) A second form of actin: platelet microfilaments depolymerized by ATP and divalent cations. *Arch. Biochem. Biophys. 167*, 230-237

ADELSTEIN, R. S. & CONTI, M. A. (1972) The characterization of contractile proteins from platelets and fibroblasts. *Cold Spring Harbor Symp. Quant. Biol. 37*, 599-606

BECKER, C. G. & NACHMAN, R. L. (1973) Contractile proteins of endothelial cells; platelets and smooth muscle. *Am. J. Pathol. 71*, 1-18

BETTEX-GALLAND, M. & LÜSCHER, E. F. (1965) Thrombosthenin, the contractile protein from blood platelets and its relationship to other contractile proteins. *Adv. Protein Chem. 20*, 1-35

BORN, G. V. R. & HUME, M. (1967) Effects of the number and sizes of platelet aggregates on the optical density of plasma. *Nature (Lond.) 215*, 1027-1029

BREMEL, R. D. (1974) Myosin-linked calcium regulation in vertebrate smooth muscle. *Nature (Lond.) 252*, 405-406

BUDTZ-OLSEN, O. E. (1951) The mechanism of clot retraction. In *Clot Retraction*, pp. 64-67, Thomas, Springfield, Ill.

COHEN, I. & COHEN, C. (1972) A tropomyosin-like protein from human platelets. *J. Mol. Biol. 68*, 383-387

COHEN, I., KAMINSKI, E. & DE VRIES, A. (1973) Actin-linked regulation of the human platelet contractile system. *FEBS Lett. 34*, 315-317

FINE, R. E., BLITS, A. L., HITCHCOCK, S. E. & KAMINER, B. (1973) Tropomyosin in brain and growing neurones. *Nature (Lond.) 245*, 182-186

HASLAM, R. J., DAVIDSON, M. M. L. & McCLENAGHAN, M. D. (1975) Cytochalasin B, the blood platelet release reaction and cyclic GMP. *Nature (Lond.) 253*, 455-457

HATANO, S. & OOSAWA, F. (1966) Isolation and characterisation of plasmodium actin. *Biochim. Biophys. Acta 127*, 488

LEHMAN, W., KENDRICK-JONES, J. & SZENT-GYORGYI, A. G. (1972) Myosin-linked regulatory systems: comparative studies. *Cold Spring Harbor Symp. Quant. Biol. 37*, 319-330

POLLARD, T. D. (1975) Functional implications of the biochemical and structural properties of cytoplasmic contractile proteins. In *Molecules and Cell Movement* (Inoue, S. & Stephens, R. E., eds.), pp. 259-285, Raven Press, New York

TAYLOR, D. L., CONDEELIS, J. S., MOORE, P. L. & ALLEN, R. D. (1973) The contractile basis of amoeboid movement. I. The chemical control of motility in isolated cytoplasm. *J. Cell Biol. 59*, 378-394

WHITE, J. G. (1971) Platelet microtubules and microfilaments: effects of cytochalasin B on structure and function. In *Platelet Aggregation* (Caen, J., ed.), pp. 15-52, Masson, Paris

WILLINGHAM, M. C., OSTLUND, R. E. & PASTAN, I. (1974) Myosin is a component of the cell surface of cultured cells. *Proc. Natl. Acad. Sci. U.S.A. 71*, 4144-4148

WOOLLEY, D. E. (1972) An actin-like protein from amoebae of *Dictyostelium discoideum*. *Arch. Biochem. Biophys. 150*, 519-530

YOUNT, R. G., FRYE, J. S. & O'KEEF, K. R. (1972) Inhibition of heavy meromyosin by purine disulfide analogs of ATP. *Cold Spring Harbor Symp. Quant. Biol. 37*, 113-119

ZUCKER-FRANKLIN, D. (1970) The submembranous fibrils of human blood platelets. *J. Cell Biol. 47*, 293-299

Roles of cyclic nucleotides in platelet function

RICHARD J. HASLAM

Department of Pathology, McMaster University, Hamilton, Ontario

Abstract A reinvestigation of the effects of inducers of platelet aggregation on platelet cyclic AMP levels using a variety of methods has confirmed that no measurable changes occur. Nevertheless, aggregating agents have diverse effects on the unstimulated adenylate cyclase activity measurable in intact platelets in the presence of inhibitors of cyclic AMP phosphodiesterase; ADP inhibits and adrenaline stimulates this activity, while noradrenaline, 5-hydroxytryptamine and vasopressin have no significant net effects. These findings suggest that the functional pool of cyclic AMP is a small fraction of the total present in the resting platelet.

Differing effects of aggregating agents on the prostaglandin E_1 (PGE_1)-stimulated adenylate cyclase activity of intact platelets can also be demonstrated. ADP causes a non-competitive inhibition of this activity (K_i about 1 μM), while vasopressin has no inhibitory action. This suggests that a specific inhibitory interaction may occur within the platelet membrane between the ADP receptor mechanism and adenylate cyclase. The relationship between platelet cyclic AMP levels and the inhibition by PGE_1 of ADP-induced aggregation has been explored in detail. The inhibition of adenylate cyclase by ADP markedly reduces the inhibitory activity of PGE_1. Inhibition of aggregation was much more closely related to the cyclic AMP level about 15 s before measurement of the inhibition than to the level at the time of addition of ADP or at the time of measurement of inhibition. As significant aggregation occurs at elevated cyclic AMP levels, a fall in cyclic AMP concentration cannot be required to initiate aggregation.

The role of cyclic GMP in platelet function is less clear. Increases in platelet cyclic GMP (2 to 4-fold) are observed in response to either ADP or collagen in human heparinized platelet-rich plasma and appear to be associated with both platelet aggregation and the initiation of the release reaction. On the other hand, studies in dog platelets have shown that both aggregation and the release reaction induced by cholinergic agonists can occur in the absence of measurable increases in cyclic GMP, though the potentiation of the release reaction by extracellular Ca^{2+} ions is closely correlated with the elevation of cyclic GMP levels. The results suggest that cyclic GMP may have a regulatory role in platelet function secondary to that of Ca^{2+} ions, but cannot alone mediate either aggregation or release.

The blood platelet has several advantages as a model system for the analysis of the biochemical changes associated with pharmacological effects. Thus, platelets are readily obtained free from other cells and respond to a wide range of agonists. They show two principal types of reactions: shape change with aggregation, which has many features in common with the contraction of smooth muscle (White 1968; Haslam & Rosson 1972), and the release of granule constituents, which is analogous to secretion by exocytosis in other cells (Stormorken 1969). Substantial evidence has accumulated that a number of agents, including prostaglandin E_1 (PGE_1), adenosine, methylxanthines, papaverine and pyrimidopyrimidines, inhibit these processes by increasing the intracellular concentration of cyclic AMP (Salzman 1972; Haslam 1973). This view has not, however, been universally accepted (Ball et al. 1970; Boullin et al. 1972). Even more controversial has been the question of whether or not aggregating agents decrease intracellular cyclic AMP levels below the resting level and, if so, whether this causes or promotes platelet aggregation (Salzman & Neri 1969; Haslam & Taylor 1971a; Salzman et al. 1972; Haslam 1973). The experiments described in the first part of this paper were designed to clarify these issues.

Recently, evidence from a number of biological systems has suggested that cyclic GMP may promote cellular events that are opposite to those mediated by cyclic AMP (Goldberg et al. 1973). Thus, contraction of smooth muscle induced by a variety of agonists is associated with increases in cyclic GMP (Lee et al. 1972; Goldberg et al. 1973; Schultz et al. 1973; Dunham et al. 1974). In addition, the immunological release of histamine from sensitized lung tissue (Kaliner et al. 1972) and the release of lysosomal enzymes during phagocytosis by neutrophil leucocytes (Zurier et al. 1974; Ignarro et al. 1974) are promoted by agents that increase cyclic GMP levels. Thus, it is as appropriate to look for increased platelet cyclic GMP levels as decreased cyclic AMP levels in association with platelet aggregation and the platelet release reaction. Our own studies (Haslam & McClenaghan 1974; Haslam et al. 1975a; Haslam & Say 1975) and brief reports from other laboratories (White et al. 1973; Jakobs et al. 1974) have already shown that under some conditions platelet aggregation and the release reaction are associated with increases in cyclic GMP concentration. The experiments described in the last part of this paper were designed to investigate more closely the relationships between platelet aggregation, the release reaction and platelet cyclic GMP levels.

MATERIALS AND METHODS

Human heparinized platelet-rich plasma (PRP) containing $3.5–5.0 \times 10^8$

platelets/ml was prepared as described by Haslam & Rosson (1972) and was used in all the experiments with human platelets. For experiments with dog platelets, citrated PRP, prepared from 9 vol. blood mixed with 1 vol. 3.13% trisodium citrate, or suspensions of twice-washed platelets in Tyrode's solution, pH 7.35, containing 0.35% bovine serum albumin but lacking $CaCl_2$, were used. The latter suspensions were prepared by the method of Ardlie *et al.* (1970). PRP and washed platelet suspensions were stored at 37 °C until used and all incubations were performed at this temperature.

Platelet aggregation was recorded turbidometrically using an aggregation module made by Payton Associates Ltd., Scarborough, Ontario. When quantitative studies were required the decrease in extinction from the maximum value attained to the value at the chosen time of measurement was noted. Percentage inhibition of aggregation was calculated with respect to the decrease in extinction in appropriate controls. The platelet release reaction was measured by the percentage release of ^{14}C from platelets that had been preincubated with 1 μM [^{14}C]5-hydroxytryptamine ([^{14}C]5HT), as described fully elsewhere (Haslam & Rosson 1972).

Changes in platelet cyclic AMP and cyclic GMP concentrations were measured by prelabelling methods in almost all experiments. In the prelabelling assay for cyclic AMP used, PRP was incubated for 80–90 min at 37 °C with purified 2 μM [U-^{14}C]adenine (287 mCi/mmol) before experiments. Cyclic [^{14}C]AMP was isolated either (Method 1) as described by Haslam & Taylor (1971*b*) but with the addition of further purification by t.l.c. in a second dimension on cellulose (Haslam & McClenaghan 1974) or (Method 2) by a modification (Haslam & Rosson 1975) of the method of Krishna *et al.* (1968). Both methods usually gave values for cyclic [^{14}C]AMP in unstimulated PRP equivalent to 0.025–0.035% of the ^{14}C incorporated into the platelets. In one experiment described in this paper, preincubation with 2 μM [U-^{14}C]adenosine (533 mCi/ mmol) was also used to label the platelet nucleotides. In the prelabelling assay for cyclic GMP, PRP or the washed platelet suspension was incubated for 60 min at 37 °C with 2 μM [8-^3H]guanine (3–4 Ci/mmol) before experiments and cyclic [^3H]GMP was isolated by column chromatography followed by t.l.c. (Haslam & McClenaghan 1974). With both prelabelling assays little or no labelled cyclic nucleotide was found outside the platelets and the material assayed as cyclic [^{14}C]AMP or cyclic [^3H]GMP was almost completely degraded by cyclic nucleotide phosphodiesterase. In one experiment reported in this paper unlabelled cyclic AMP was measured by the protein-binding method of Brown *et al.* (1971) as modified by Haslam & Goldstein (1974).

RESULTS AND DISCUSSION

Lack of effects of aggregating agents on basal cyclic AMP levels in platelets

In a previous report from my laboratory it was shown that aggregating agents, including ADP and adrenaline, did not significantly decrease the concentration of cyclic [^{14}C]AMP in platelets labelled with [^{14}C]adenine although the latter two agents did markedly inhibit the increase in cyclic [^{14}C]AMP caused by PGE_1 (Haslam & Taylor 1971*a*). In view of these apparently conflicting results and evidence from other laboratories using different techniques that aggregating agents may decrease cyclic AMP levels (Salzman & Neri 1969; Salzman *et al.* 1972), I have reinvestigated this problem using a method for isolating cyclic [^{14}C]AMP which involves three separate chromatographic steps. The results (Table 1) confirm that none of the aggregating agents tested have

TABLE 1

Lack of effects of aggregating agents on cyclic [^{14}C]AMP levels in human platelets

Aggregating agent	*Cyclic [^{14}C]AMP after 20 s (% of platelet ^{14}C)*	*Cyclic [^{14}C]AMP after 60 s (% of platelet ^{14}C)*
None	0.031 ± 0.001(3)	0.031 ± 0.001(4)
ADP (4 μM)	0.030 ± 0.001(4)	0.032 ± 0.001(4)
(–)-Adrenaline (4 μM)	0.031 ± 0.001(4)	0.030 ± 0.001(4)
(–)-Noradrenaline (4 μM)	0.030 ± 0.001(4)	0.029 ± 0.001(4)
5-Hydroxytryptamine (10 μM)	0.030 ± 0.002(3)	0.029 ± 0.001(4)
Arg^8-vasopressin (100 mU/ml)	0.033 ± 0.004(4)	0.032 ± 0.002(4)

Incubation mixtures contained 0.9 ml human heparinized platelet-rich plasma labelled with [^{14}C]adenine and 0.1 ml 0.154 M-NaCl containing the indicated aggregating agents. Cyclic [^{14}C]AMP was isolated by Method 1. Values expressed as percentage of platelet ^{14}C are means ± S.E.M. from the number of incubation mixtures indicated in parentheses.

any significant effect on cyclic [^{14}C]AMP levels. The accuracy of the method is such that a change of 10 % or greater would have been detected. Salzman *et al.* (1972) have reported that while they similarly were unable to detect a change in cyclic [^{14}C]AMP on addition of aggregating agents to platelets labelled with [^{14}C]adenine, decreases were observed when the platelets were labelled with [^{14}C]adenosine. They suggested that different pools of precursor ATP were labelled. However, studies in my laboratory showed no significant effect of ADP or adrenaline on cyclic [^{14}C]AMP levels in platelets labelled with [^{14}C]adenosine for 30 or 90 min. As shown in Table 2, the d.p.m. found

TABLE 2

Lack of effect of ADP or adrenaline on cyclic [^{14}C]AMP levels in human platelets labelled with [^{14}C]adenine or [^{14}C]adenosine

Aggregating agent	Cyclic [^{14}C]AMP in PRP incubated with [^{14}C]adenine (d.p.m.)		Cyclic [^{14}C]AMP in PRP incubated with [^{14}C]adenosine (d.p.m.)	
	30 min	90 min	30 min	90 min
None	135 ± 5	284 ± 17	128 ± 44	142 ± 13
ADP (4 μM)	123 ± 1	281 ± 12	139 ± 17	136 ± 8
(–)-Adrenaline (4 μM)	138 ± 1	258 ± 24	110 ± 13	139 ± 12

Incubation mixtures contained 0.9 ml human heparinized platelet-rich plasma (PRP) that had been preincubated for 30 min or 90 min with [^{14}C]adenine or [^{14}C]adenosine and 0.1 ml 0.154 M-NaCl with or without the indicated aggregating agents. Incubations were terminated after 20 s and cyclic [^{14}C]AMP was isolated by Method 1. Values for cyclic [^{14}C]AMP (d.p.m.) are means ± s.e.m. from three identical incubation mixtures.

in cyclic [^{14}C]AMP in PRP labelled with [^{14}C]adenosine did not increase after 30 min, probably because of the complete breakdown of the adenosine in plasma, with the result that prelabelling with [^{14}C]adenine for 90 min was a more effective method of labelling platelet cyclic AMP and permitted more accurate determination of changes in cyclic AMP level. A further complication to the use of labelled adenosine is the ability of this compound to increase cyclic AMP levels in platelets (Mills & Smith 1971), an effect which is inhibited by ADP (Haslam & Rosson 1975), with the result that information relevant to the basal levels of cyclic AMP cannot be obtained if unmetabolized adenosine remains in the platelet suspension.

Attempts at measuring changes in unlabelled cyclic AMP in platelets during aggregation have led to conflicting results. High levels of cyclic AMP in PRP which decreased on incubation with ADP or adrenaline were reported by one group (Salzman & Neri 1969; Salzman et al. 1972), while others found lower basal levels of platelet cyclic AMP, which were unaffected by these aggregating agents (Cole et al. 1971; McDonald & Stuart 1973). In studies in my laboratory using a protein-binding method for estimation of cyclic AMP, ADP did not affect cyclic AMP levels in PRP, while adrenaline caused a decrease of marginal significance (Table 3). As these studies are complicated by the presence of relatively large amounts of cyclic AMP in plasma (Broadus et al. 1970), which prevents detection of small changes in platelet cyclic AMP, experiments were also carried out on PRP that had been preincubated with cyclic nucleotide phosphodiesterase (Table 3). These indicated that 75% of the cyclic AMP in the PRP used was extracellular and that ADP and adrenaline had no measurable

TABLE 3

Effects of ADP and of adrenaline on cyclic AMP levels in PRP pre-incubated with or without cyclic nucleotide phosphodiesterase

Aggregating agent	Cyclic AMP in untreated PRP (pmol/ml)		Cyclic AMP in PRP treated with phosphodiesterase (pmol/ml)	
	20 s	60 s	20 s	60 s
None	17.6 ± 1.7	18.6 ± 0.3	4.5 ± 0.9	4.5 ± 0.3
ADP (4 μM)	17.9 ± 0.4	17.8 ± 2.4	4.4 ± 0.6	4.2 ± 0.2
(−)-Adrenaline (4 μM)	17.7 ± 2.3	15.4 ± 0.9	5.0 ± 0.3	4.8 ± 0.3

Heparinized human platelet-rich plasma (PRP) was incubated for over 30 min at 37 °C with Sigma cyclic nucleotide phosphodiesterase (0.05 units/ml). Samples (0.9 ml) of this material or of untreated PRP were mixed with 0.1 ml 0.154 M-NaCl with or without ADP or adrenaline and incubated for 20 s or 60 s, after which cyclic AMP was extracted and assayed by a protein-binding method (Haslam & Goldstein 1974). Values (pmol/ml) are means ± S.E.M. from three identical incubation mixtures each containing 3.4×10^8 platelets.

effect on the residual platelet cyclic AMP (13.2 ± 0.9 pmol/10^9 platelets). These results also show that release of platelet cyclic AMP phosphodiesterase activity into plasma or on to the platelet surface during aggregation (Salzman 1972) could account for any decrease in cyclic AMP levels in PRP.

This failure to detect a change in platelet cyclic AMP concentration by any method during exposure to aggregating agents, despite marked changes in adenylate cyclase activity (see later), strongly argues for structural or functional compartmentation of platelet cyclic AMP. Cyclic AMP is known to be present in the platelet granule fraction (Da Prada et al. 1972) but as cyclic [14C]AMP is not released by collagen after prelabelling platelets with [14C]adenine for 90 min (Haslam, unpublished results), there must be further compartmentation of cyclic [14C]AMP within the cytoplasm, possibly due to firm protein binding. The results suggest that the functional pool of platelet cyclic [14C]AMP is likely to be only a small fraction of that labelled by [14C]adenine under basal conditions. The question of whether this cyclic AMP exerts a tonic inhibitory effect on platelet function, which is diminished in the presence of some aggregating agents, remains unresolved.

Effects of aggregating agents on the adenylate cyclase activity of intact platelets

Previous studies have shown that the cyclic [14C]AMP level in platelets labelled with [14C]adenine increases linearly for at least 1 min in the presence of a high concentration of an inhibitor of cyclic AMP phosphodiesterase such

TABLE 4

Effects of aggregating agents on the adenylate cyclase activity of intact platelets

Additions	Cyclic [^{14}C]AMP (% of platelet ^{14}C)	Change in adenylate cyclase activity (%)
None	0.030 ± 0.001	–
Papaverine (2 mM)	0.059 ± 0.001	–
ADP (2 μM) + papaverine	0.042 ± 0.001	– 59 ± 5[a]
(–)-Adrenaline (10 μM) + papaverine	0.077 ± 0.002	+ 62 ± 8[a]
(–)-Noradrenaline (10 μM) + papaverine	0.059 ± 0.002	0 ± 8
5-Hydroxytryptamine (10 μM) + papaverine	0.061 ± 0.001	+ 7 ± 5
Arg^8-vasopressin (30 mU/ml) + papaverine	0.061 ± 0.001	+ 7 ± 5

[a] $2P < 0.005$.

Incubation mixtures contained 0.85 ml human heparinized platelet-rich plasma labelled with [^{14}C]adenine and 0.15 ml 0.154 M-NaCl containing the indicated additions. Incubations were terminated after 1 min. Cyclic [^{14}C]AMP was isolated by Method 2. The increases in cyclic [^{14}C]AMP in the presence of 2 mM-papaverine relative to the control with no additions were taken as equivalent to intracellular adenylate cyclase activities. Values are means ± S.E.M. from three identical incubation mixtures.

as 2 mM-papaverine or 20 mM-caffeine (Haslam 1973). This provides a measure of the endogenous adenylate cyclase activity of the platelets and permits analysis of the effects of aggregating agents on the unstimulated enzyme. Table 4 shows that 2 μM-ADP inhibited platelet adenylate cyclase by about 60%, while 10 μM-adrenaline stimulated the enzyme by the same amount. Noradrenaline, 5-hydroxytryptamine (5HT) and Arg^8-vasopressin had no significant net effects at the concentrations tested. Previous studies on the effects of catecholamines on adenylate cyclase in intact platelets have shown that the net effect observed depends on the balance of α- and β-adrenergic receptor stimulation, the former receptors tending to mediate an inhibition of adenylate cyclase and the latter an activation (Haslam & Taylor 1971b). With adrenaline the balance of these two effects favoured activation of platelet adenylate cyclase, while with noradrenaline little or no net effect was observed. Although the results show that 5HT and vasopressin probably have no effect on platelet adenylate cyclase, the possibility that each of these also acts on two receptor types with opposing but balanced effects on the enzyme has not been eliminated. The fact that the aggregating agents tested have diverse effects on platelet adenylate cyclase indicates that platelet aggregation cannot be a function of the activity of this enzyme alone. Aggregating agents and particularly adrenaline (Amer & Marquis 1972) may, of course, affect the hypothetical small functional pool of platelet cyclic AMP through effects on cyclic AMP phosphodiesterase, as well as on adenylate cyclase.

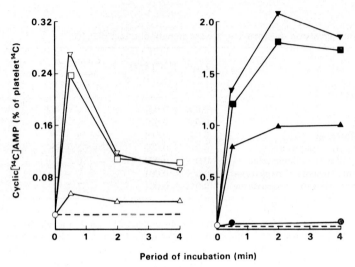

FIG. 1. Effects of ADP and of Arg[8]-vasopressin on the increases in platelet cyclic [^{14}C]AMP caused by PGE$_1$ in the presence and absence of caffeine. Incubation mixtures contained 0.85 ml human heparinized PRP labelled with [^{14}C]adenine, 0.1 ml 200mM-caffeine as indicated, and other additions in 0.154 M-NaCl, giving a final volume of 1 ml. Open symbols, caffeine absent; closed symbols, caffeine present. Other additions: ○, ●, none; □, ■, 0.2 μM-PGE$_1$; △, ▲, 0.2 μM-PGE$_1$ + 1 μM-ADP; ▽, ▼, 0.2 μM-PGE$_1$ + Arg[8]-vasopressin (30 mU/ml).

PGE$_1$ activates adenylate cyclase in platelet particulate fractions (Wolfe & Shulman 1969). This is also readily demonstrated in intact platelets (Fig. 1) in which PGE$_1$ causes an increase in cyclic AMP levels with a characteristic time course (Ball *et al.* 1970); inhibitors of cyclic AMP phosphodiesterase greatly enhance this increase. Several workers using different methods have shown that the increase in platelet cyclic AMP caused by PGE$_1$ is greatly reduced in the presence of adrenaline or noradrenaline (Robison *et al.* 1969; Marquis *et al.* 1970; Haslam & Taylor 1971a; Harwood *et al.* 1972). This α-adrenergic effect appears to be due to both an inhibition of adenylate cyclase and an activation of cyclic AMP phosphodiesterase. Thus, the weak β-adrenergic activation of platelet adenylate cyclase by these compounds is suppressed in the presence of PGE$_1$, a much more powerful activator of the enzyme, while the α-adrenergic action of the catecholamines is still fully expressed. It has been shown (Haslam & Taylor 1971a) that ADP markedly reduces the increases in cyclic [^{14}C]AMP caused by PGE$_1$ in both the presence and absence of caffeine in platelets labelled with [^{14}C]adenine, while vasopressin does not do so and may increase cyclic [^{14}C]AMP levels slightly (Fig. 1). This action of

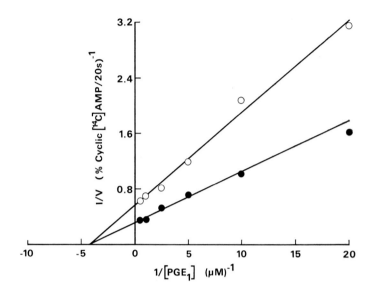

FIG. 2. Double reciprocal plots of the effects of PGE_1 concentration on the formation of cyclic $[^{14}C]AMP$ in platelets in the presence and absence of ADP. Incubation mixtures consisted of 0.85 ml human heparinized platelet-rich plasma labelled with $[^{14}C]$adenine, 0.1 ml 200 mM-caffeine and 0.05 ml 0.154 M-NaCl containing various PGE_1 concentrations with or without 0.9 μM-ADP. Incubations were terminated after 20 s by addition of $HClO_4$ and cyclic $[^{14}C]AMP$ was isolated by Method 2. The cyclic $[^{14}C]AMP$ levels found after 20 s with caffeine in the absence of PGE_1 were subtracted from those found in the presence of PGE_1 to give measures of the PGE_1-activated adenylate cyclase activities of the platelets, the reciprocals of which were calculated. ●, ADP absent; ○, ADP present. The kinetic parameters calculated from this experiment were: K_a for PGE_1, 0.23 μM; K_i for ADP, 1.1 μM.

ADP has been confirmed by measurements of total cyclic AMP levels (McDonald & Stuart 1973). As in the presence of caffeine the increases in cyclic $[^{14}C]AMP$ caused by PGE_1 with and without ADP are linear with respect to time for at least 20 s, it is possible to carry out a kinetic analysis of the effect of ADP (Fig. 2). In confirmation of previous results (Haslam 1973), it was found that ADP is a non-competitive inhibitor (K_i approximately 1 μM) of the activation of adenylate cyclase in intact platelets by PGE_1. This finding contradicts the claim of Boullin et al. (1972) that PGE_1 competes with ADP for the same receptor. The difference between the effects of ADP and vasopressin on platelet adenylate cyclase suggests that this action of ADP may be a specific effect of the ADP receptor mechanism within the platelet membrane, as events subsequent to receptor action are likely to be the same for both agonists. The non-competitive effect of ADP on the activation of adenylate cyclase could result from competition for ATP between adenylate cyclase and the ADP

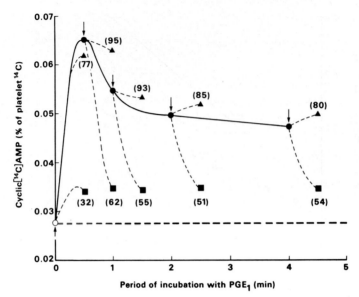

FIG. 3. Platelet cyclic [^{14}C]AMP and the inhibition of ADP and vasopressin-induced platelet aggregation after different periods of incubation with 0.1 μM-PGE$_1$. Incubation mixtures consisted of 0.9 ml human heparinized platelet-rich plasma labelled with [^{14}C]adenine and a final total of 0.1 ml additions in 0.154 M-NaCl. PGE$_1$ was added from 0 to 4 min before the aggregating agent. Mixtures were stirred in an aggregation module for 0.5 min before and 0.5 min after addition of the aggregating agent, at which time HClO$_4$ was added to extract cyclic [^{14}C]AMP. Controls without aggregating agents were stirred for 0.5 min before the addition of HClO$_4$. Cyclic [^{14}C]AMP was isolated by Method 2. The level of cyclic [^{14}C]AMP in the absence of any addition is indicated by the horizontal dashed line. Values for percentage inhibition of the extent of platelet aggregation after 0.5 min corresponding to particular values of cyclic [^{14}C]AMP are given in parentheses. ●, no aggregating agent; ■, 1 μM-ADP; ▲, 50 mU Arg^8-vasopressin/ml; ↓, times of addition of ADP or vasopressin.

receptor, if the latter is a nucleosidediphosphate kinase, as has been suggested (Guccione *et al.* 1971).

Relationships between increased cyclic AMP levels in platelets and the inhibition of aggregation

Several workers have noted a qualitative correlation between the abilities of many drugs to increase cyclic AMP levels in platelets and to inhibit platelet aggregation, though in a number of instances quantitative discrepancies have been observed (Ball *et al.* 1970; Mills & Smith 1971; McDonald & Stuart 1973). In previous reports from my laboratory it has been suggested that these discrepancies can largely be accounted for by a failure to allow for the effects of aggregating agents on cyclic AMP levels (Haslam & Taylor 1971a; Haslam 1973). For example, if ADP is added with or at any time after the addition of PGE_1, the inhibition of the extent of the aggregation is much lower than is observed with a concentration of vasopressin which causes the same extent of aggregation as the ADP in the absence of PGE_1. As shown in Fig. 3 this difference reflects the ability of ADP but not vasopressin to lower the cyclic $[^{14}C]AMP$ level. In contrast to ADP, vasopressin causes small increases in cyclic $[^{14}C]AMP$. These results show that the cyclic $[^{14}C]AMP$ level before the addition of the aggregating agent does not determine the inhibition of aggregation. Equally, Fig. 3 shows that the inhibitions of the extent of aggregation after 30 s do not correlate with the cyclic $[^{14}C]AMP$ levels measured at the same time. Thus, a substantially greater inhibition occurred when PGE_1 was added 30 s before either ADP or vasopressin instead of with the aggregating agent, despite the fact that the cyclic $[^{14}C]AMP$ levels at the times the inhibitions were measured were virtually identical (Fig. 3). These observations can readily be explained if the mean cyclic $[^{14}C]AMP$ concentration over a period intermediate between the addition of the aggregating agent and the measurement of the inhibition of aggregation 30 s later determines the extent of the inhibition. Thus, the inhibition observed was not determined by the peak cyclic AMP concentration encountered in the presence of PGE_1 alone, as claimed by McDonald & Stuart (1973). Moreover, in contrast with the results of others (Ball et al. 1970; McDonald & Stuart 1973), Fig. 3 shows that the extent of inhibition of both ADP- and vasopressin-induced aggregations declined with increasing periods of preincubation with PGE_1 after the first 30 s. This correlates with the decrease in the mean concentration of cyclic $[^{14}C]AMP$ between addition of the aggregating agent and measurement of the inhibition of aggregation.

Difficulties have been encountered in correlating the increases in cyclic $[^{14}C]AMP$ caused by PGE_1 in the presence and absence of an inhibitor of cyclic AMP phosphodiesterase with the inhibition of ADP-induced aggregation (Ball et al. 1970; Mills & Smith 1971). In these latter studies the cyclic $[^{14}C]$-AMP found in the presence of PGE_1 alone appeared to be less effective in inhibiting aggregation than that found when a phosphodiesterase inhibitor was also present. This discrepancy may also be due to measurement of cyclic $[^{14}C]AMP$ before rather than after addition of ADP, as cyclic $[^{14}C]AMP$ levels would be expected to fall more rapidly and proportionally further on addition of ADP in the absence of a phosphodiesterase inhibitor. The experiments reported here show the relationships between the increases in platelet cyclic $[^{14}C]AMP$ levels 30 s after simultaneous addition of ADP and various PGE_1 concentrations with and without papaverine and the associated inhibitions of

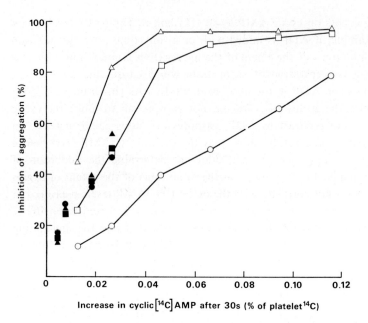

FIG. 4. Relationships between the increases in platelet cyclic [^{14}C]AMP 30 s after the simultaneous addition of 2 μM-ADP and 0.025-2.0 μM-PGE$_1$ with or without 0.2 mM-papaverine and the inhibitions of ADP-induced aggregation by the same agents. Incubation mixtures consisted of 0.85 ml human heparinized platelet-rich plasma (PRP) and 0.15 ml 0.154 M-NaCl containing the additions. One set of incubation mixtures containing PRP labelled with [^{14}C]adenine were terminated after 30 s for determination of cyclic [^{14}C]AMP (Method 2), while an identical set containing unlabelled PRP was stirred in an aggregation module for determination of the percentage inhibition of the extent of aggregation after 30 s (○, ●), 45 s (□, ■) and 60 s (△, ▲). Open symbols, increases in cyclic [^{14}C]AMP with PGE$_1$; closed symbols, increases in cyclic [^{14}C]AMP with PGE$_1$ + papaverine.

aggregation (Fig. 4). In the absence of papaverine the relationship observed was not significantly affected by the time at which the extent of inhibition of aggregation was measured, but in the presence of papaverine three entirely different relationships were obtained when the inhibition of aggregation was measured 30, 45 and 60 s after addition of ADP. Only when the inhibition was measured after 45 s were coincident relationships obtained in both the presence and absence of papaverine (Fig. 4). The reasons for these findings can be more readily understood after reference to Fig. 5, which shows that the shapes of the aggregation curves and of the time courses of cyclic [^{14}C]AMP accumulation are entirely different with a high concentration of PGE$_1$ in the absence of papaverine and a low concentration of PGE$_1$ in the presence of papaverine. The cyclic [^{14}C]AMP concentration rose much more rapidly in the former case

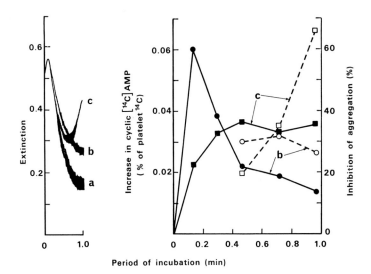

Period of incubation (min)

FIG. 5. Relationships between the increases in platelet cyclic [^{14}C]AMP caused by PGE$_1$ and by PGE$_1$ with papaverine and the associated inhibitions of ADP-induced aggregation. Incubation mixtures consisting of 0.85 ml human heparinized platelet-rich plasma labelled with [^{14}C]adenine and 0.15 ml of additions in 0.154 M-NaCl were stirred in an aggregation module for the indicated periods before addition of HClO$_4$ and determination of cyclic [^{14}C]AMP by Method 2 (closed symbols). The inhibition of the extent of aggregation immediately before addition of HClO$_4$ was also measured (open symbols); aggregation recordings from the 1 min incubations are shown on the left. Additions (final concentrations) were: a, 2 μM-ADP; b, 2 μM-ADP + 2 μM-PGE$_1$ (●, ○); c, 2 μM-ADP + 0.05 μM-PGE$_1$ + 0.2 μM-papaverine (■, □).

with the result that its inhibitory effect was initially greater. However, in the absence of papaverine the cyclic [^{14}C]AMP level soon fell again, with the result that the inhibition did not increase above the initial level. In the presence of both papaverine and PGE$_1$, the cyclic [^{14}C]AMP concentrations rose more slowly to a steady state, which was associated with increasing inhibition and reversal of aggregation. The cross-over points in Fig. 5 suggest that there is at least a 15 s (0.25 min) gap between achievement of a particular cyclic [^{14}C]AMP level and its full expression in terms of inhibition of aggregation.

A further factor influencing the inhibitory effectiveness of a particular level of cyclic [^{14}C]AMP appears to be the concentration of ADP used. Fig. 6 shows that different relationships were obtained between the increases in cyclic [^{14}C]AMP and the inhibitions of platelet aggregation, when different ADP concentrations were added simultaneously with a range of PGE$_1$ concentrations and papaverine. This was the case whether the inhibitions of aggregation were

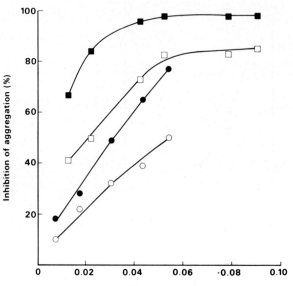

FIG. 6. Inhibitory effect of increased platelet cyclic AMP levels on aggregation induced by different ADP concentrations. Incubation mixtures consisted of 0.85 ml human heparinized platelet-rich plasma (PRP) and 0.15 ml 0.154 M-NaCl containing the indicated additions. Cyclic AMP levels were increased by addition of a range of concentrations of PGE_1 (0.025-0.8 μM) with 0.1 mM-papaverine at the same time as 0.5 μM or 2 μM-ADP. One set of incubations with labelled PRP was terminated after 30 s for determination of cyclic [14C]AMP (Method 2). Identical incubation mixtures but with unlabelled PRP were stirred in an aggregation module for determination of the percentage inhibition of the extent of aggregation observed 30 s (open symbols) and 45 s (closed symbols) after addition of ADP. □, ■, 0.5 μM-ADP; ○, ●, 2 μM-ADP.

measured at the same time as, or 15 s after, the time at which cyclic [14C]AMP was determined. This discrepancy could reflect the arbitrariness of the measure of platelet aggregation used or alternatively could imply some interaction between the mechanisms of action of cyclic AMP and ADP, as has been suggested by Booyse *et al.* (1973).

The evidence that the inhibition of platelet aggregation by PGE_1 is most closely related to the increase in cyclic [14C]AMP level about 15 s before the inhibition is measured is consistent with the view that cyclic AMP may inhibit platelet aggregation by activation of a protein kinase, which then phosphorylates a regulatory protein in a time-consuming reaction. The lack of any persistent inhibitory effects of the relatively high cyclic [14C]AMP levels achieved with PGE_1 alone after addition of ADP implies that this hypothetical phosphoprotein

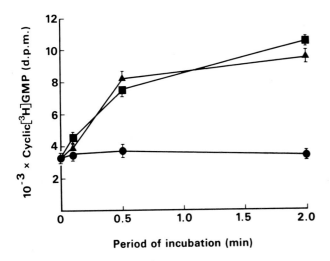

FIG. 7. Effects of ADP on cyclic [³H]GMP levels in human platelets. Incubation mixtures contained 0.85 ml heparinized platelet-rich plasma labelled with [³H]guanine and 0.15 ml 0.154 M-NaCl with or without ADP. These were stirred in an aggregation module for the indicated times before addition of HClO₄ to extract cyclic [³H]GMP. Values for cyclic [³H]GMP (d.p.m.) are means ± S.E.M. from three identical incubation mixtures. ●, no ADP; ▲, 0.4 μM-ADP; ■, 4 μM-ADP.

turns over rapidly, presumably as a result of the action of a phosphatase. The results also show that relatively small increases in platelet cyclic [¹⁴C]AMP ($<100\%$) have potent inhibitory effects on aggregation. This provides further evidence for compartmentation of platelet cyclic [¹⁴C]AMP and emphasizes the importance of using highly sensitive methods for measuring changes in platelet cyclic AMP. Increases in platelet cyclic AMP which cause a significant inhibition of aggregation can probably not be detected by measurement of total unlabelled cyclic AMP in PRP. As appreciable aggregation could still occur with significantly elevated levels of cyclic [¹⁴C]AMP, a fall in cyclic AMP level is very unlikely to be required for the initiation of platelet aggregation.

Effects of aggregating agents on cyclic GMP levels in human platelets

In marked contrast to its lack of effect on cyclic AMP levels, ADP caused a roughly three-fold increase in the concentration of cyclic [³H]GMP in heparinized human PRP labelled with [³H]guanine (Haslam *et al.* 1975a). The time course of this increase (Fig. 7) closely paralleled that of aggregation, the major part occurring between 6 and 30 s after addition of the ADP. The same maximum response was obtained with all ADP concentrations above about

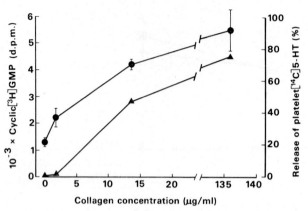

FIG. 8. Effects of the concentration of collagen on cyclic [³H]GMP levels in human platelets and on the release of [¹⁴C]5HT. Incubation mixtures contained 0.85 ml heparinized platelet-rich plasma labelled with both [³H]guanine and [¹⁴C]5HT and 0.15 ml 0.154 M-NaCl with or without collagen. These were stirred in an aggregation module for 2 min, after which either HClO₄ was added to extract cyclic [³H]GMP (●) or they were centrifuged to measure release of [¹⁴C]5HT (▲). Values for cyclic [³H]GMP (d.p.m.) are means ± S.E.M. from three identical incubation mixtures.

0.4 μM, which caused a slightly submaximal extent of aggregation. ADP caused no release of [¹⁴C]5HT from platelets in heparinized PRP at any concentration. Thus, in this system the increase in cyclic GMP could be involved in controlling the aggregation response or alternatively could be a parallel event with no functional significance. When collagen was used as the aggregating agent a significant increase in cyclic [³H]GMP was observed just before aggregation at the time at which the platelets first showed changes in shape, but after that the increase closely paralleled aggregation (Haslam & McClenaghan 1974). Maximum increases in cyclic [³H]GMP of up to four-fold were encountered with high collagen concentrations and in general these increases paralleled the extent of the release reaction (Fig. 8). The question arises of the extent to which the increase in platelet cyclic [³H]GMP with collagen is an effect of the ADP released or a direct effect of the collagen stimulus and therefore possibly involved in initiating the release reaction. In an attempt to resolve this problem, inhibitors of the release reaction (aspirin or indomethacin) were included in the incubation mixtures (Table 5). It was found that even when release of [¹⁴C]5HT was inhibited by 90% the increase in cyclic [³H]GMP caused by collagen was not reduced. This suggests that collagen itself can increase the platelet cyclic [³H]GMP concentration, but is not conclusive as only very low ADP concentrations are required to increase platelet cyclic [³H]GMP. However,

TABLE 5

Effects of inhibitors of the platelet release reaction on cyclic [³H]GMP levels in platelets incubated with and without collagen

Additions		Cyclic [³H]GMP	Release of
Inhibitor	Aggregating agent	(d.p.m.)	[¹⁴C]5HT (%)
None	None	1617 ± 140	–
Aspirin (0.02 mM)	None	1565	0
Aspirin (0.1 mM)	None	607	0
Indomethacin (0.04 mM)	None	1205	0
Indomethacin (0.2 mM)	None	1085	0
None	Collagen	3669 ± 669	44
Aspirin (0.02 mM)	Collagen	3690	21
Aspirin (0.1 mM)	Collagen	4479	5
Indomethacin (0.04 mM)	Collagen	4478	4
Indomethacin (0.2 mM)	Collagen	4058	6

Incubation mixtures consisted of 1.0 ml human heparinized platelet-rich plasma containing platelets labelled with both [³H]guanine and [¹⁴C]5HT, and a total of 0.2 ml additions in 0.154 M-NaCl. Inhibitors were added 10 min before collagen and the samples were stirred in an aggregation module from 0.5 min before addition of collagen until 2 min afterwards, when either $HClO_4$ was added to extract cyclic [³H]GMP or samples were centrifuged to determine the release of [¹⁴C]5HT. Control incubations without inhibitors were performed in triplicate; mean values ± s.e.m. for cyclic [³H]GMP (d.p.m.) are given.

as the ADP released by collagen may have an important role in potentiating the release reaction (Packham et al. 1973), cyclic [³H]GMP could still be involved in this process, even if collagen is not a direct stimulus to its formation. So far it has only been possible to resolve more clearly the question of which, if any, aspect of platelet function involves cyclic GMP using the dog platelet system (see later).

An unexpected observation was the finding that aspirin and some related drugs depress the basal unstimulated level of cyclic [³H]GMP in platelets labelled with [³H]guanine (Haslam & McClenaghan 1974; Haslam et al. 1975b). This is illustrated in Table 5, which also shows that aspirin is more effective in lowering cyclic [³H]GMP levels than indomethacin. Thus, contrary to our first impression (Haslam & McClenaghan 1974), this effect does not correlate with the inhibition of the release reaction, in which indomethacin is more potent than aspirin. It now appears that these drugs may act by displacing cyclic [³H]GMP from non-specific binding sites to be then rapidly broken down by cyclic GMP phosphodiesterase (Haslam et al. 1975b). If correct, this implies that the increases in cyclic [³H]GMP in the presence of aggregating agents, which are not decreased by aspirin, occur in a different functional compartment

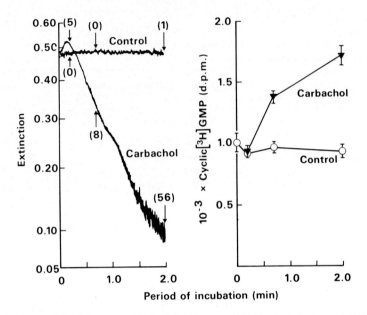

FIG. 9. Increase in cyclic [³H]GMP in citrated dog platelet-rich plasma (PRP) induced by 1 mM carbachol in relation to platelet aggregation and the release reaction. Incubation mixtures consisted of 0.85 ml PRP, containing platelets labelled with both [³H]guanine and [¹⁴C]5HT, and 0.15 ml 0.154 M-NaCl with or without carbachol. These were stirred in an aggregation module for the indicated times before addition of HClO₄ for extraction of cyclic [³H]GMP or centrifugation to determine release of [¹⁴C]5HT. Aggregation recordings and percentage release of [¹⁴C]5HT (in parentheses) are shown on the left and platelet cyclic [³H]GMP levels (d.p.m.) on the right (mean values ± S.E.M. from three identical incubation mixtures).

of the platelet in which proportionately far larger changes in cyclic GMP concentration may occur than can be measured in whole platelets.

Effects of cholinergic agonists on cyclic GMP levels in dog platelets

Two recent reports have indicated that high concentrations of cholinergic agonists induce both aggregation of dog platelets and the release of granule constituents from them (Shermer & Chuang 1973; Chuang *et al.* 1974). These effects were mediated by classical muscarinic receptors. In view of the evidence that activation of muscarinic receptors causes an increase in cyclic GMP in a variety of biological systems (Goldberg *et al.* 1973) and the specific suggestion that cyclic GMP may mediate muscarinic effects (Lee *et al.* 1972), we have investigated the changes in cyclic [³H]GMP concentration in dog platelets labelled with [³H]guanine (Haslam & Say 1975). The effects of adding 1 mM-

TABLE 6

Role of Ca^{2+} ions in the increase in platelet cyclic GMP and release of 5HT induced by addition of cholinergic agonists to dog washed platelets

Cholinergic agonist	$CaCl_2$ concentration (mM)	Cyclic $[^3H]GMP$ (d.p.m.)	Change in cyclic $[^3H]GMP$ (%)	Release of $[^{14}C]5HT$ (%)
None	0	445 ± 58	–	–
	0.1	448 ± 31	+ 1 ± 15	0
	1.0	338 ± 24	− 24 ± 14	0
Acetylcholine	0	417 ± 9	− 6 ± 13	6
(1mM)	0.1	984 ± 80	+ 121 ± 22[a]	43
	1.0	1111 ± 57	+ 150 ± 18[a]	59
Carbachol	0	600 ± 15	+ 35 ± 13	9
(1mM)	0.1	1313 ± 75	+ 195 ± 21[a]	48
	1.0	1666 ± 134	+ 274 ± 33[a]	60

[a] $2P < 0.01$.

The platelets were incubated for 1 h at 37 °C with $[^3H]$guanine and $[^{14}C]5HT$ during the second wash. Incubation mixtures consisted of 0.95 ml of the final platelet suspension in calcium-free Tyrode's solution containing albumin (2.5×10^8 platelets/ml) and 0.05 ml 0.154 M-NaCl containing a cholinergic agonist and/or $CaCl_2$ as indicated. These samples were stirred in an aggregation module for 3 min before addition of $HClO_4$ for extraction of cyclic $[^3H]GMP$ or centrifugation to determine release of $[^{14}C]5HT$. Values for cyclic $[^3H]GMP$ (d.p.m.) are means ± S.E.M. from three identical incubation mixtures.

carbachol to labelled citrated PRP are shown in Fig. 9. The compound caused a change in platelet shape followed by primary aggregation and finally secondary aggregation associated with the release of $[^{14}C]5HT$. An increase in cyclic $[^3H]GMP$ occurred during primary and secondary aggregation with a time course that was consistent with a mediating or potentiating role for the compound in either of these processes. However, when this experiment was repeated several times using 1mM-acetylcholine as the agonist, increases in cyclic $[^3H]GMP$ were only observed occasionally, although the drug always caused considerable aggregation and release. Clearly, an increase in the cyclic GMP level was not essential for either of these processes. These negative experiments represent the first instances in which muscarinic effects have been observed without an associated increase in cyclic GMP. In view of evidence that Ca^{2+} ions may be required for an increase in tissue cyclic GMP levels (Schultz et al. 1973), it seemed possible that the variable results obtained with acetylcholine in dog citrated PRP could be due to variations in Ca^{2+} ion concentration around a threshold value, which might be different for acetylcholine and carbachol. This hypothesis was confirmed by experiments with washed platelets

(Table 6), in which no significant increases in cyclic [³H]GMP concentration occurred with either acetylcholine or carbachol, unless Ca^{2+} ions were included in the incubation mixtures, although marked aggregation and some release of [¹⁴C]5HT were observed in the absence of Ca^{2+} ions. Addition of Ca^{2+} ions alone had no effect on cyclic [³H]GMP levels. In the presence of the cholinergic agonists increases in cyclic [³H]GMP were readily detected on addition of 0.1 mM-$CaCl_2$, which also caused a marked potentiation of the release reaction. In the presence of Ca^{2+} ions, carbachol was more effective in increasing cyclic [³H]GMP and in causing release of [¹⁴C]5HT than acetylcholine. The addition of ADP to these preparations of washed platelets neither caused aggregation nor increased cyclic [³H]GMP levels, which suggests that the increases in cyclic [³H]GMP observed with cholinergic agonists were not a secondary effect of the ADP liberated in the release reaction. As a whole, these results suggest that in the dog platelet an increase in cyclic GMP levels is not necessary for either aggregation or the release reaction to occur but may have some role secondary to Ca^{2+} ions in potentiating release.

CONCLUSION

As little is known about the mechanisms of action of cyclic nucleotides in platelets, it seems justified to offer some speculations as a stimulus to further work in this area. It is known that platelets possess cytoplasmic and membrane-bound protein kinases which are activated by cyclic AMP and that these enzymes can phosphorylate a specific protein in isolated platelet membranes (Booyse et al. 1973). Although aggregating agents appear to decrease the level of phosphorylation of this protein (Booyse et al. 1973), the mechanism by which they do so and the physiological significance of these observations are still obscure. Progress with other biological systems, particularly with the sarcoplasmic reticulum of the heart (Kirchberger et al. 1974), suggests that control of Ca^{2+} ion kinetics by phosphorylation of membrane protein by cyclic AMP-activated protein kinases may be a fundamental biological control mechanism. In this connection, evidence from studies with calcium ionophores (Massini & Lüscher 1974; White et al. 1974) supports the view that Ca^{2+} ions are the primary mediators in platelet function. Moreover, platelets possess a calcium-binding membrane fraction analogous to sarcoplasmic reticulum (Statland et al. 1969). It is therefore reasonable to suggest that cyclic AMP may stimulate the removal of Ca^{2+} ions from the platelet cytoplasm by activation of a calcium pump. As phosphorylation of certain membrane proteins in smooth muscle has recently been shown to be activated by cyclic GMP (Casnellie & Greengard 1974), it might also seem likely that cyclic GMP could promote release of Ca^{2+} ions by a similar mechanism. However, as Ca^{2+} ions are required for cyclic GMP formation this would result in a positive feedback loop which would rapidly increase the cytoplasmic Ca^{2+} ion concentration and cause an all-or-none reaction, which is not in fact observed. I, therefore, tentatively suggest that cyclic GMP is more likely to facilitate an *action* of Ca^{2+} ions, possibly the activation of the contractile protein system in the platelets. In this connection, Adelstein *et al.* (1975) have recently observed that phosphorylation of one of the light chains of platelet myosin promotes its actin-activated ATPase activity.

ACKNOWLEDGEMENTS

This work was supported by grants from the Medical Research Council of Canada (DG 94) and the Ontario Heart Foundation (15-6). I wish to express my gratitude for the experimental assistance of P. Crossland, M. M. L. Davidson, M. D. McClenaghan, A. Say and A. Taylor.

References

ADELSTEIN, R. S., DANIEL, J. L., CONTI, M. A. & ANDERSON, W. JR (1975) Platelet myosin phosphorylation: studies on the kinase, substrate and effect of phosphorylation. *Proc. Fed. Europ. Biochem. Socs., 9th Meeting*, vol. 31, pp. 177-186, North-Holland, Amsterdam.

AMER, M. S. & MARQUIS, N. R. (1972) The effect of prostaglandins, epinephrine and aspirin on cyclic AMP phosphodiesterase activity of human blood platelets and their aggregation In *Prostaglandins in Cellular Biology* (Ramwell, P. W. & Pharris, B. B., eds.), pp. 93-110 Plenum Press, New York

ARDLIE, N. G., PACKHAM, M. A. & MUSTARD, J. F. (1970) Adenosine diphosphate-induced platelet aggregation in suspensions of washed rabbit platelets. *Br. J. Haematol. 19*, 7-17

BALL, G., BRERETON, G. G., FULWOOD, M., IRELAND, D. M. & YATES, P. (1970) Effect of prostaglandin E_1 alone and in combination with theophylline or aspirin on collagen-induced platelet aggregation and on platelet nucleotides including adenosine $3' : 5'$-cyclic monophosphate. *Biochem. J. 120*, 709-718

BOOYSE, F. M., GUILIANI, D., MARR, J. J. & RAFELSON, M. E. (1973) Cyclic adenosine $3'$, $5'$-monophosphate dependent protein kinase of human platelets: membrane phosphorylation and regulation of platelet function. *Ser. Haematol. 6*, 351-366

BOULLIN, D. J., GREEN, A. R. & PRICE, K. S. (1972) The mechanism of adenosine diphosphate-induced platelet aggregation: binding to platelet receptors and inhibition of binding and aggregation by prostaglandin E_1. *J. Physiol. (Lond.) 221*, 415-426

BROADUS, A. E., KAMINSKY, N. I., HARDMAN, J. G., SUTHERLAND, E. W. & LIDDLE, G. W. (1970) Kinetic parameters and renal clearances of plasma adenosine $3',5'$-monophosphate and guanosine $3',5'$-monophosphate in man. *J. Clin. Invest. 49*, 2222-2236

BROWN, B. L., ALBANO, J. D. M., EKINS, R. P., SGHERZI, A. M. & TAMPION, W. (1971) A simple and sensitive saturation assay method for the measurement of adenosine $3':5'$-cyclic monophosphate. *Biochem. J. 121*, 561-562

CASNELLIE, J. E. & GREENGARD, P. (1974) Guanosine $3':5'$-cyclic monophosphate-dependent phosphorylation of endogenous substrate proteins in membranes of mammalian smooth muscle. *Proc. Natl. Acad. Sci. U.S.A. 71*, 1891-1895

CHUANG, H. Y. K., SHERMER, R. W. & MASON, R. G. (1974) Acetylcholine-induced release reaction of canine platelets. *Res. Commun. Chem. Pathol. Pharmacol. 7*, 333-346

COLE, B., ROBISON, A. & HARTMANN, R. C. (1971) Studies on the role of cyclic AMP in platelet function. *Ann. N.Y. Acad. Sci. 185*, 477-487

DA PRADA, M., BURKARD, W. P. & PLETSCHER, A. (1972) Cyclic AMP of blood platelets: accumulation in organelles storing 5-hydroxytryptamine and ATP. *Experientia 28*, 845-846

DUNHAM, E. W., HADDOX, M. K. & GOLDBERG, N. D. (1974) Alteration of vein cyclic 3′:5′-nucleotide concentrations during changes in contractility. *Proc. Natl. Acad. Sci. U.S.A. 71*, 815-819

GOLDBERG, N. D., O'DEA, R. F. & HADDOX, M. K. (1973) Cyclic GMP. In *Advances in Cyclic Nucleotide Research*, vol. 3 (Greengard, P. & Robison, G. A., eds.), pp. 155-223, Raven Press, New York

GUCCIONE, M. A., PACKHAM, M. A., KINLOUGH-RATHBONE, R. L. & MUSTARD, J. F. (1971) Reactions of ^{14}C-ADP and ^{14}C-ATP with washed platelets from rabbits. *Blood 37*, 542-555

HARWOOD, J. P., MOSKOWITZ, J. & KRISHNA, G. (1972) Dynamic interaction of prostaglandin and norepinephrine in the formation of adenosine 3′,5′-monophosphate in human and rabbit platelets. *Biochim. Biophys. Acta 261*, 444-456

HASLAM, R. J. (1973) Interactions of the pharmacological receptors of blood platelets with adenylate cyclase. *Ser. Haematol. 6*, 333-350

HASLAM, R. J. & GOLDSTEIN, S. (1974) Adenosine 3′:5′-cyclic monophosphate in young and senescent human fibroblasts during growth and stationary phase *in vitro*. Effects of prostaglandin E$_1$ and of adrenaline. *Biochem. J. 144*, 253-263

HASLAM, R. J. & McCLENAGHAN, M. D. (1974) Effects of collagen and of aspirin on the concentration of guanosine 3′:5′-cyclic monophosphate in human blood platelets: measurement by a prelabelling technique. *Biochem. J. 138*, 317-320

HASLAM, R. J. & ROSSON, G. M. (1972) Aggregation of human blood platelets by vasopressin. *Am. J. Physiol. 223*, 958-967

HASLAM, R. J. & ROSSON, G. M. (1975) Effects of adenosine on levels of adenosine 3′:5′-cyclic monophosphate in human blood platelets in relation to adenosine incorporation and platelet aggregation. *Mol. Pharmacol. 11*, 528-544

HASLAM, R. J. & SAY, A. (1975) Effects of acetylcholine and carbachol on cyclic GMP levels in dog blood platelets in relation to platelet function: role of extracellular Ca^{2+} ions. *Fed. Proc. 34*, 231 (abs.)

HASLAM, R. J. & TAYLOR, A. (1971a) Role of cyclic 3′,5′-adenosine monophosphate in platelet aggregation. In *Platelet Aggregation* (Caen, J., ed.), pp. 85-93, Masson, Paris

HASLAM, R. J. & TAYLOR, A. (1971b) Effects of catecholamines on the formation of adenosine 3′:5′-cyclic monophosphate in human blood platelets. *Biochem. J. 125*, 377-379

HASLAM, R. J., DAVIDSON, M. & McCLENAGHAN, M. D. (1975a) Cytochalasin B, the blood platelet release reaction and cyclic GMP. *Nature (Lond.) 253*, 455-457

HASLAM, R. J., McCLENAGHAN, M. D. & ADAMS, A. (1975b) Depression of cyclic GMP levels in blood platelets by acetylsalicylic acid (ASA) and related drugs. In *Advances in Cyclic Nucleotide Research*, vol. 5 (Greengard, P. & Robison, G. A., eds.), p. 821, Raven Press, New York

IGNARRO, L. J., LINT, T. F. & GEORGE, W. J. (1974) Hormonal control of lysosomal enzyme release from human neutrophils. Effects of autonomic agents on enzyme release, phagocytosis, and cyclic nucleotide levels. *J. Exp. Med. 139*, 1395-1414

JAKOBS, K. H., BÖHME, E. & MOCIKAT, S. (1974) Cyclic GMP formation in human platelets. *Naunyn-Schmiedebergs Arch. Pharmakol.* Suppl. *282*, R40

KALINER, M., ORANGE, R. P. & AUSTEN, K. F. (1972) Immunological release of histamine and slow reacting substance of anaphylaxis from human lung. IV. Enhancement by cholinergic and alpha adrenergic stimulation. *J. Exp. Med. 136*, 556-567

KIRCHBERGER, M. A., TADA, M. & KATZ, A. M. (1974) Adenosine 3′:5′-monophosphate-dependent protein kinase-catalyzed phosphorylation reaction and its relationship to calcium transport in cardiac sarcoplasmic reticulum. *J. Biol. Chem. 249*, 6166-6173

KRISHNA, G., WEISS, B. & BRODIE, B. B. (1968) A simple sensitive method for the assay of adenylate cyclase. *J. Pharmacol. Exp. Therap.* *163*, 379-385

LEE, T.-P., KUO, J. F. & GREENGARD, P. (1972) Role of muscarinic cholinergic receptors in regulation of guanosine $3':5'$-cyclic monophosphate content in mammalian brain, heart muscle, and intestinal smooth muscle. *Proc. Natl. Acad. Sci. U.S.A.* *69*, 3287-3291

MARQUIS, N. R., BECKER, J. A. & VIGDAHL, R. L. (1970) Platelet aggregation. III. An epinephrine-induced decrease in cyclic AMP synthesis. *Biochem. Biophys. Res. Commun.* *39*, 783-789

MASSINI, P. & LÜSCHER, E. F. (1974) Some effects of ionophores for divalent cations on blood platelets. Comparison with the effects of thrombin. *Biochim. Biophys. Acta 372*, 109-121

McDONALD, J. W. D. & STUART, R. K. (1973) Regulation of cyclic AMP levels and aggregation in human platelets by prostaglandin E_1. *J. Lab. Clin. Med. 81*, 838-849

MILLS, D. C. B. & SMITH, J. B. (1971) The influence on platelet aggregation of drugs that affect the accumulation of adenosine $3':5'$-cyclic monophosphate in platelets. *Biochem. J. 121*, 185-196

PACKHAM, M. A., GUCCIONE, M. A., CHANG, P.-L. & MUSTARD, J. F. (1973) Platelet aggregation and release: effects of low concentrations of thrombin or collagen. *Am. J. Physiol. 225*, 38-47

ROBISON, G. A., ARNOLD, A. & HARTMANN, R. C. (1969) Divergent effects of epinephrine and prostaglandin E_1 on the level of cyclic AMP in human blood platelets. *Pharmacol. Res. Commun. 1*, 325-332

SALZMAN, E. W. (1972) Cyclic AMP and platelet function. *N. Engl. J. Med. 286*, 358-363

SALZMAN, E. W. & NERI, L. L. (1969) Cyclic $3',5'$-adenosine monophosphate in human blood platelets. *Nature (Lond.) 224*, 609-610

SALZMAN, E. W., KENSLER, P. C. & LEVINE, L. (1972) Cyclic $3',5'$-adenosine monophosphate in human blood platelets. IV. Regulatory role of cyclic AMP in platelet function. *Ann. N.Y. Acad. Sci. 201*, 61-71

SCHULTZ, G., HARDMAN, J. G., SCHULTZ, K., BAIRD, C. E. & SUTHERLAND, E. W. (1973) The importance of calcium ions for the regulation of guanosine $3':5'$-cyclic monophosphate levels. *Proc. Natl. Acad. Sci. U.S.A. 70*, 3889-3893

SHERMER, R. W. & CHUANG, H. Y. (1973) Acetylcholine-induced aggregation of canine platelets. *Fed. Proc. 32*, 844 abs

STATLAND, B. E., HEAGAN, B. M. & WHITE, J. G. (1969) Uptake of calcium by platelet relaxing factor. *Nature (Lond.) 223*, 521-522

STORMORKEN, H. (1969) The release reaction of secretion. *Scand. J. Haematol.* Suppl. 9

WHITE, J. G. (1968) Fine structural alterations induced in platelets by adenosine diphosphate. *Blood 31*, 604-622

WHITE, J. G., GOLDBERG, N. D., ESTENSEN, R. D., HADDOX, M. K. & RAO, G. H. R. (1973) Rapid increase in platelet cyclic $3',5'$-guanosine monophosphate (cGMP) levels in association with irreversible aggregation, degranulation, and secretion. *J. Clin. Invest. 52*, 89a

WHITE, J. G., RAO, G. H. R. & GERRARD, J. M. (1974) Effects of the ionophore A23187 on blood platelets. I. Influence on aggregation and secretion. *Am. J. Pathol. 77*, 135-149

WOLFE, S. M. & SHULMAN, N. R. (1969) Adenyl cyclase activity in human platelets. *Biochem. Biophys. Res. Commun. 35*, 265-272

ZURIER, R. B., WEISSMANN, G., HOFFSTEIN, S., KAMMERMAN, S. & TAI, H. H. (1974) Mechanisms of lysosomal enzyme release from human leukocytes. II. Effects of cAMP and cGMP, autonomic agonists, and agents which affect microtubule function. *J. Clin. Invest. 53*, 297-309

Discussion

Mills: Why do you express cyclic [³H]guanosine monophosphate levels in d.p.m.? And what is the relationship between the counts and the total amount of tritium in the guanine nucleotides in your platelets?

Haslam: The cyclic [³H]GMP in control incubations usually amounted to about 0.08% of the [³H]guanine taken up by the platelets. However, as this value was more variable than the corresponding figure for cyclic [¹⁴C]AMP in platelets labelled with [¹⁴C]adenine, I have chosen to express the results as d.p.m. I have also found considerable variation in the amount of [³H]guanine taken up during preincubation with different platelet preparations for one hour (3–12%).

Mills: Have you any information on variations in the total quantity of guanine nucleotides in the platelets?

Haslam: No; we have shown that GTP and GDP are indeed labelled in platelets incubated with [³H]guanine, as you would expect, but we have not determined if there are variations in the total amounts present under different conditions.

Born: By labelling the nucleotide di- and triphosphates with ³²P we found a ratio of adenine to guanine nucleotides greater than 10 to 1 (Born & Esnouf 1958).

Nachman: You mentioned that aspirin and other non-steroidal anti-inflammatory agents shifted cyclic GMP out of a storage compartment. Is this specific to platelets?

Haslam: We have not yet looked at any other tissue. I would not go so far as to say that aspirin displaces cyclic [³H]GMP out of a *storage* compartment. It may displace cyclic [³H]GMP from binding sites on proteins. We have looked at the mechanism responsible for this effect but it has been difficult to get a clear answer. However, the reproducibility of the phenomenon is very good; we can always lower the control cyclic [³H]GMP level by 90–95% with salicylate or aspirin. This effect is clearly not related to any inhibition of the release reaction. On the other hand, the increases in cyclic [³H]GMP during aggregation or release are clearly associated with these functional changes, even if they do not cause them.

Holmsen: I have one comment and one question. I think it would be a good idea to keep in mind what older workers found. Hellem (1960) routinely adjusted the citrate concentration for variations in the haematocrit when preparing platelet-rich plasma (PRP) from citrated blood. In this way the calcium concentration in PRP was always the same. Application of this simple adjustment would probably have prevented the variations in cyclic

GMP formation. My question is: was guanine present extracellularly during your experiments?

Haslam: That depended on whether we were using platelet-rich plasma or washed platelets. In the former case, [³H]guanine was present throughout the experiment, while in the latter case the extracellular [³H]guanine was washed away in the preparation of the final platelet suspension.

Holmsen: The reason I ask is the following. When platelet functions such as shape change, aggregation and release are induced in the presence of extra-cellular radioactive adenine, there is a burst in the uptake of this nucleotide precursor. When the release reaction, for example, is induced *after* all radio-active adenine has been taken up by the platelets, the level of radioactive ATP decreases, whereas when release takes place with radioactive adenine present no change, or even an increase in radioactive ATP, is often seen, because of the burst in adenine uptake (Holmsen *et al.* 1972). Do you think there may be a similar burst in guanine uptake which could cause the observed increase in cyclic GMP?

Haslam: I think that is unlikely. We have obtained similar results with platelet-rich plasma which contained [³H]guanine and washed platelet suspensions which did not, provided the extracellular Ca²⁺ ion concentrations were the same.

Holmsen: You showed an experiment (Fig. 7, p. 135) with ADP-induced aggregation in heparinized PRP, a condition in which release (secondary aggregation) should not take place, according to what we have heard from Dr Mustard. If I am not wrong, there was an accumulation of cyclic GMP. Then you showed another experiment with collagen (Fig. 8, p. 136) which only aggregates platelets through release of ADP, where cyclic GMP accumulated. You conclude that cyclic GMP formation is related to the release rather than aggregation, but how does this conclusion follow from these experiments?

Haslam: On the evidence we have at present, the increase in cyclic GMP with collagen is the product of direct effects of both the collagen and the ADP released. So far, the only way we have attempted to eliminate the effect on human platelets of ADP released by collagen is by using aspirin-like drugs (Table 5, p. 137). In these experiments we observed the same increase in cyclic [³H]GMP whether the drug was present or not, so that we can say that this increase is probably related to the collagen stimulus. However, there is no doubt that ADP can produce a similar effect and in some circumstances can be responsible for part of the effect of collagen on cyclic [³H]GMP levels. For example, when we use a very low dose of collagen, cytochalasin B greatly potentiates the release reaction. This is associated with a potentiation of the cyclic [³H]GMP response. We believe that this is an effect of the released ADP and not a cause of the potentiation of the release by cytochalasin B (Haslam *et al.* 1975). Only with dog platelets have we been able to observe aggregation without an increase in cyclic [^{3}H]GMP. However, this does suggest that cyclic GMP may not be required for aggregation to occur.

Born: If you added a phosphatase that broke down ADP in the plasma, would that be a useful experiment?

Haslam: Yes. However, we haven't done that yet.

Packham: I am interested in your graph of cyclic [^{3}H]GMP formation after the addition of ADP (Fig. 7, p. 135). In the time interval that you studied the reaction, the cyclic [^{3}H]GMP level continued to rise and you did not reach a point where it levelled off or began to fall. Have you followed the reaction in terms of the platelets becoming refractory to ADP? Is there any correlation between cyclic GMP levels and refractoriness or de-aggregation?

Haslam: So far, we have only followed the changes in cyclic [^{3}H]GMP with ADP for two minutes, at which time neither de-aggregation nor a decrease in cyclic [^{3}H]GMP had occurred.

Mills: Have you looked at the effect of ascorbic acid?

Haslam: No.

Mustard: Didn't Jim White report that vitamin C causes platelet cyclic GMP levels to rise?

Mills: Yes (D. Glass, J. G. White & N. Goldberg, personal communication, 1974), but it does not have any detectable effect on platelet function.

Adelstein: You mentioned the effect of cyclic GMP on smooth muscle. Can you elaborate?

Haslam: The observations most pertinent to ours are those of Schultz *et al.* (1973), who showed that in rat ductus deferens, stimulation by acetylcholine produced an increase in cyclic GMP only when extracellular calcium was present. This relates closely to our observations with washed dog platelets. There are many other close parallels that can be drawn between the molecular pharmacology of the blood platelet and smooth muscle (Haslam & Rosson 1972).

Crawford: Regarding the phosphodiesterase, is there any evidence for the presence of a low K_m enzyme and, if so, do the inhibitors you used (papaverine and caffeine) operate equally effectively against the two forms?

Haslam: We have not done any work with the platelet cyclic AMP phosphodiesterases ourselves but I do not question the evidence (Amer & Mayol 1973) that both low and high K_m forms of the enzyme are present. From the effects of papaverine and of caffeine on the increases in cyclic [^{14}C]AMP observed in the presence of weak and strong activation of platelet adenylate cyclase, I would guess that, at the concentrations we used, caffeine may be a less effective inhibitor of the low K_m phosphodiesterase than papaverine, though it may be a more effective inhibitor of the high K_m enzyme.

Smith: You said that adrenaline increases cyclic AMP in the presence of the phosphodiesterase inhibitor and lowers it in the presence of PGE_1; you postulated that this is because adrenaline activates phosphodiesterase. Surely another explanation could be that PGE_1 is a powerful β-adrenergic agonist and that adrenaline acts at the same site.

Haslam: I agree that in the presence of PGE_1 it is possible that the β-adrenergic effect of catecholamines cannot be expressed. PGE_1 and β-adrenergic agonists may well activate the same adenylate cyclase in platelets. However, I do not think this invalidates my argument that one of the α-adrenergic effects of adrenaline may be to increase cyclic AMP phosphodiesterase activity.

Holmsen: You presented data (Table 4, p. 127) on the effect of various aggregating agents on the increase or reduction in the steady-state levels of platelet cyclic AMP in the presence of papaverine. These changes were referred to as reflecting changes in the activity of adenylate cyclase. I don't think this is correct, since the levels of cyclic AMP are regulated by the enzyme's activity *and* the level of substrate ATP as well as by other factors (i.e. Mg^{2+}). For example, Dr Mills (1973) has shown that ADP causes an immediate fall in the total level of metabolic ATP, and this might involve the same ATP pool that is used for cyclic AMP synthesis. In this case a reduction in the level of cyclic AMP one minute after the addition of aggregating agent is probably caused by ATP storage, rather than reduction in the cyclase activity.

Haslam: When I referred to inhibition of platelet adenylate cyclase by ADP, I did not mean to imply that the mechanism was necessarily direct. In fact, as several workers including ourselves have previously noted, competition for ATP between adenylate cyclase and some aspect of the aggregation mechanism would provide a plausible explanation for the inhibition by ADP of adenylate cyclase in intact platelets that I have described. However, as vasopressin causes a platelet aggregation very similar to that induced by ADP but does not inhibit the adenylate cyclase, it is likely that the ADP receptor is specifically and intimately linked in some way with adenylate cyclase. For example, if the ADP receptor is a nucleosidediphosphate kinase, as Dr Mustard's results suggest, then competition between the cyclase and the kinase for ATP in a local membrane compartment would be feasible.

Caen: To return to the question of the effect of adenosine on rat and human platelets (adenosine is an inhibitor of ADP-induced aggregation in human and not in rat platelets), we were interested in using [^{3}H]- or [^{14}C]adenosine or cold adenosine and seeing whether adenosine is able to change cyclic AMP levels in rat platelets, as in human platelets. Using the same amounts of the nucleoside we have found the same increase in the two species. Adenosine increases cyclic AMP in rat platelets as much as in the human, without any inhibition of aggregation. How can this be explained?

Haslam: We haven't done that experiment but we have very substantial evidence that the inhibitory effect of adenosine on the aggregation of human platelets *is* mediated by cyclic AMP (Haslam & Rosson 1975).

Born: One would like to know, then, why in species such as the rat, in which aggregation is not inhibited by adenosine, it increases the concentration of cyclic AMP very much like the increase in human platelets which *are* inhibited by adenosine.

Haslam: There are a number of possible explanations. With human platelets the inhibition of ADP-induced aggregation by adenosine relates not to the cyclic AMP level observed with adenosine by itself, but to the level observed with adenosine in the presence of ADP. Thus, the effectiveness of ADP in blocking the increase in cyclic AMP with adenosine could be greater in rat than in human platelets.

Pletscher: The time of incubation may be critical in your incubation experiments, Dr Haslam. This is an important point, because the interchange between the metabolic and the storage nucleotide pools might be relatively slow.

Haslam: I agree. In the experiments in which we found no release of labelled cyclic AMP, we preincubated with [^{14}C]adenine for 90 minutes.

Pletscher: Perhaps that is not long enough. For instance, with the ATP storage pool we showed in rabbit platelets that there is an exchange, and I think Dr Mustard has similar evidence.

Mustard: Yes, that is so (Reimers *et al.* 1975).

Haslam: I agree. In fact we were glad to be able to prevent labelling of the storage pool of adenine nucleotides because we wished to look at the cyclic AMP in the metabolic pool alone, if at all possible. I assume that if we preincubated with [^{14}C]adenine for much longer we would, as you suggest, label the granule pool of adenine nucleotides, including cyclic AMP, as well.

Mustard: You have clearly demonstrated that ADP does not cause a measurable fall in the cyclic AMP level in resting platelets. However, papaverine increases the cyclic AMP levels, presumably by inhibiting the phosphodiesterase, without increasing the rate of formation of cyclic AMP. When you add ADP to platelets in the presence of papaverine, cyclic AMP falls. I am left with the interpretation that ADP causes some change in cyclic AMP levels; therefore your failure to demonstrate it without papaverine leaves us with the problem that ADP *has* some effect, perhaps on the turnover of cyclic AMP, which may be a crucial control.

Haslam: I don't think the turnover of cyclic AMP is likely to be important, except in so far as it determines the cyclic AMP concentration, because in the systems studied so far cyclic AMP expresses itself through activation of protein kinases in a manner that depends on its concentration. I agree that there are likely to be changes in a small pool of platelet cyclic AMP during aggregation which we can't measure. However, I think it would be wrong to generalize on the direction in which these changes might occur. When we measure adenylate cyclase in intact platelets, we get very diverse effects depending on the aggregating agent used.

Cohen: I would like to stress the relationship between calcium and cyclic AMP. On the one hand, calcium decreases the activity of adenylate cyclase (Vigdahl *et al.* 1969); on the other hand, cyclic AMP increases the uptake of calcium by the smooth muscle sarcoplasmic reticulum (Andersson & Nilsson 1972). Thus, increased cyclic AMP is related to relaxation.

Haslam: That is exactly my present working hypothesis on the mechanism of action of cyclic AMP, namely that it enhances the activity of a calcium pump. What is more puzzling is what cyclic GMP could do, because if it opposes the action of cyclic AMP on this same system, we would have both an activation of guanylate cyclase by calcium and a potentiation of the release of calcium by cyclic GMP. This would constitute a positive feedback loop and lead to an all-or-none effect, which apparently does not occur. So, if cyclic GMP has a function in platelets, I do not see how it can act to control the movement of calcium.

Born: I agree with Dr Haslam that the absolute levels of cyclic AMP at the time of measurement and the inhibition of aggregation bear very little relation to each other. The inhibition of aggregation produced by adenosine at first increases rapidly with time (Born 1964) and so does inhibition produced by PGE$_1$ (Macfarlane 1975). Furthermore, adenosine added to platelet-rich plasma disappears much more rapidly than the inhibition of aggregation that it causes. Therefore, whatever cyclic AMP does as an intermediate in the inhibitory mechanism, the time constants of one or more subsequent reactions leading to inhibition as well as to its disappearance seem to be considerably longer than the time constants for the rise or fall of cyclic AMP itself.

Haslam: Actually, my experiments suggest that the lag before a change in cyclic AMP concentration in platelets fully expresses itself as a change in platelet function is only about 15 seconds, so that it is the cyclic AMP level during the course of aggregation that determines what happens only slightly later. How else can one explain the differences between the inhibitions of vasopressin- and ADP-induced aggregations by PGE$_1$ and the relationships between the extent of inhibition and the period of pre-incubation with PGE$_1$ (Fig. 3, p. 130)?

Born: The results with adenosine and 2-chloroadenosine are rather different. The increase in inhibition is fast with adenosine but not quite so fast as with 2-chloroadenosine. But there is no reason why the time courses of inhibition and cyclic AMP rise should necessarily be the same. There are presumably one or more steps in the sequence activated by cyclic AMP and resulting ultimately in inhibition of aggregation which may have different time constants of activation.

Haslam: Our results with adenosine (Haslam & Rosson 1975) are very similar to those with PGE$_1$. Again, I think it is the cyclic AMP level about 15 seconds before measurement of the inhibition of aggregation that matters. Presumably, with both inhibitors the time required for activation of the protein kinase and phosphorylation of the hypothetical regulatory protein is about 15 seconds. There is another important point. This phosphoprotein must be turning over rapidly, because otherwise we would not see less inhibition with ADP than with vasopressin after preincubation with PGE$_1$. It must be possible for this protein to be dephosphorylated during the fall in cyclic AMP level caused by ADP. In other words, the platelet has only a short memory for cyclic AMP, perhaps about 15 seconds.

References

AMER, M. S. & MAYOL, R. F. (1973) Studies with phosphodiesterase. III. Two forms of the enzyme from human blood platelets. *Biochim. Biophys. Acta 309*, 149-156

ANDERSSON, R. & NILSSON, K. (1972) Cyclic AMP and calcium in relaxation in intestinal smooth muscle. *Nature (Lond.) 238*, 119-120

BORN, G. V. R. (1964) Strong inhibition by 2-chloroadenosine of the aggregation of blood platelets by adenosine diphosphate. *Nature (Lond.) 202*, 95-96

BORN, G. V. R. & ESNOUF, M. P. (1958) Biochemical changes in platelet-rich plasma during clotting. In *Proceedings of the 4th International Congress of Biochemistry*, vol. 10, pp. 97-104, Pergamon, Oxford

HASLAM, R. J. & ROSSON, G. M. (1972) Aggregation of human blood platelets by vasopressin. *Am. J. Physiol. 223*, 958-967

HASLAM, R. J. & ROSSON, G. M. (1975) Effects of adenosine on levels of adenosine 3':5'-cyclic monophosphate in human blood platelets in relation to adenosine incorporation and platelet aggregation. *Mol. Pharmacol. 11*, 528-544

HASLAM, R. J., DAVIDSON, M. M. L. & MCCLENAGHAN, M. D. (1975) Cytochalasin B, the blood platelet release reaction and cyclic GMP. *Nature (Lond.) 253*, 455-457

HELLEM, A. J. (1960) The adhesiveness of human blood platelets *in vitro*. *Scand. J. Clin. Lab. Invest. 12*, Suppl. 51

HOLMSEN, H., DAY, H. J. & SETKOWSKY, C. A. (1972) Secretory mechanisms. Behaviour of adenine nucleotides during the platelet release reaction induced by adenosine diphosphate and adrenaline. *Biochem. J. 129*, 67-82

MACFARLANE, D. E. (1975) Personal communication

MICHEL, H., CAEN, J. P., ANGLES D'AURIAC, G., MEYER, P. & BORN, G. V. R. (1975) Cyclic AMP in platelet aggregation. *Br. J. Haematol.* in press

MILLS, D. C. B. (1973) Changes in the adenylate energy charge in human blood platelets induced by adenosine diphosphate. *Nature New Biol. 243*, 220-222

SCHULTZ, G., HARDMAN, J. G., SCHULTZ, K., BAIRD, C. E. & SUTHERLAND, E. W. (1973) The importance of calcium ions for the regulation of guanosine 3':5'-cyclic monophosphate levels. *Proc. Natl. Acad. Sci. U.S.A. 70*, 3889-3893

REIMERS, H. J., MUSTARD, J. F. & PACKHAM, M. A. (1975) Transfer of adenine nucleotides between the releasable and non-releasable compartments of rabbit blood platelets. *J. Cell Biol.* in press

VIGDAHL, R. L., MARQUIS, N. R. & TAVORMINA, P. A. (1969) Platelet aggregation II. Adenyl cyclase, prostaglandin E_1 and calcium. *Biochem. Biophys. Res. Commun. 37*, 409-415

Initial biochemical responses of platelets to stimulation

D. C. B. MILLS

Specialized Center for Thrombosis Research, Temple University Hospital, Philadelphia, Pennsylvania

Abstract Cyclic AMP formation and adenine nucleotide metabolism have been studied in human platelet-rich plasma using adenine as a radioactive nucleotide precursor. ADP and adrenaline rapidly reduce the formation of cyclic AMP in platelets stimulated by prostaglandin E_1. Other aggregating agents, including collagen, 5-hydroxytryptamine and vasopressin, do not inhibit this effect of prostaglandin E_1. The inhibitory effect of ADP is blocked by the thiol reagent N-ethyl maleimide which also enhances the stimulation of cyclic AMP formation by prostaglandin E_1. ADP also affects intracellular adenine nucleotides in platelets, lowering the adenylate energy charge. This effect is associated with the induction of platelet shape change rather than with aggregation, and occurs with other aggregating agents, including 5-hydroxytryptamine, vasopressin and thrombin, which also induce the shape change. Reduction of the adenylate energy charge also occurs on treatment with metabolic inhibitors (antimycin plus deoxy-D-glucose) which do not cause shape change, and so is not a mediator of this effect. Prostaglandin E_1, which stimulates ATP use by activating adenylate cyclase, does not lower the energy charge in untreated platelets but does so in the presence of metabolic inhibitors. Metabolic inhibitors enhance the lowering of the energy charge by ADP, indicating that this effect is due to increased ATP consumption. N-Ethyl maleimide at concentrations which block the effect of ADP on the adenylate cyclase does not prevent the reduction of energy charge, showing that these two effects have independent mechanisms.

The initial response of platelets to exposure to ADP is a morphological change from their normal disk shape to a more isotropic but irregular form which is basically spherical with pseudopods (Zucker & Borrelli 1954; MacMillan & Oliver 1965; Born 1970) and this change is associated with a detectable alteration in the turbidity of platelet-rich plasma (PRP). The baseline oscillations seen in the aggregometer with stirred PRP at 37 °C disappear and the average optical density increases (O'Brien 1965). This change is associated with various ultrastructural modifications, suggesting that the process is a contractile one

(White 1968); the marginal band of microtubules appears to contract, pseudo-pods are formed and the various types of granule are gathered together in the central part of the cell. This shape change is independent of subsequent aggregation; it occurs in the presence of EDTA, and when the pH is lowered to 6.4, both of which treatments inhibit aggregation. Also, platelets from patients with thrombasthenia (Glanzmann's disease), which do not aggregate, change shape normally (Mills 1973).

The first biochemical evidence that this reaction involves the utilization of energy was the observation of D. M. Ireland (personal communication) that ADP causes a reduction of the ratio of ATP to ADP in the intracellular nucleotides of platelets labelled with radioactive adenine. We have confirmed Ireland's observation and found evidence directly associating increased ATP utilization with the shape change.

It is generally accepted that agents that act on platelets to cause an increase in the intracellular concentration of cyclic AMP, inhibit aggregation (Mills & Smith 1971; Haslam 1973). Considerable interest and controversy has been raised by observations that aggregating agents can inhibit adenylate cyclase (Zieve & Greenough 1969; Marquis et al. 1970; Brodie et al. 1972) and reduce the basal concentration of cyclic AMP in platelets (Salzman & Neri 1969; Salzman 1972). While it is no longer thought that the reduction of cellular cyclic AMP levels is a plausible mechanism for the action of aggregating agents (Haslam 1973 and this symposium, pp. 121–143; Mills 1974) the ability of ADP and adrenaline to inhibit the stimulation of platelet adenylate cyclase (Mills & Smith 1972) still represents one of the earliest detectable biochemical actions of these aggregating agents.

We have examined the possible relationships between the effects of ADP on metabolic ATP utilization and on shape change and its effects on the adenylate cyclase, both of which systems require ATP.

METHODS

Platelet aggregation and the shape change were studied using the apparatus and methods previously described (Mills & Roberts 1967). The adenylate cyclase system in intact platelets in PRP has been examined by the technique of following the incorporation of radioactivity into cyclic AMP in platelets previously labelled by incubation with [U-^{14}C]adenine (Mills & Smith 1971) or [2-^{3}H]adenine (Macfarlane & Mills 1975). Blood from volunteers is collected in citrate (1 volume of 3.8% Na_3 citrate to 9 volumes blood), and PRP is prepared by low speed centrifugation, and incubated with labelled adenine (0.51-μM) for 30 min–1 hour at 37°C. By this time between 85 and 95% of the added radioactivity is found in the form of intracellular nucleotides. Samples of this labelled PRP (usually 0.5 ml) are then exposed to various additions and then the reaction is stopped with perchloric acid containing cyclic AMP and an appropriate standard (either tritium- or carbon-labelled cyclic AMP) to allow correction for the variation in recovery in the subsequent procedures. Cyclic AMP is purified from the perchloric acid extracts by column chromatography on Dowex AG 50 W × 4 and elution with water followed by precipitation of remaining non-cyclic nucleotides with barium hydroxide and zinc sulphate (Krishna et al. 1968). Results obtained by this method are generally in close agreement with measurements of total cyclic AMP concentrations made by the protein-binding assay (Harwood et al. 1972; McDonald & Stuart 1973). Measurements of the basal cyclic AMP level in platelets are probably overestimated by this method (Haslam 1973) and have not been attempted in this investigation.

The effects of aggregating agents on platelet energy metabolism have been investigated by measuring the distribution of radioactivity among the adenine nucleotides of platelets prelabelled by incubation with $[U^{-14}C]$ adenine as described above. After various treatments, the labelled PRP is mixed with a small volume (usually 20 µl per 200 µl of PRP) of $5N-HClO_4$ containing 5–10 mM of non-radioactive carriers (ATP, ADP, AMP, IMP, inosine, hypoxanthine, adenine and adenosine). The extract is neutralized with potassium carbonate and the individual nucleotides are separated by paper chromatography (Mills 1973) or by high voltage paper electrophoresis in citrate buffer, pH 4.05 (Macfarlane & Mills 1975). Results are usually expressed as the Adenylate Energy Charge (AEC), where AEC = $1/2$ (2ATP + ADP)/(ATP + ADP + AMP). This function is directly related to the phosphate bond energy in ATP that is available to the cell for metabolic processes (Atkinson 1968).

RESULTS

Platelets exposed to prostaglandin E_1 (PGE_1) show a dramatic increase in the rate of incorporation of radioactivity from labelled nucleotides into cyclic AMP (Mills & Smith 1971, 1972). This is illustrated in Fig. 1 which shows that the peak of radioactive cyclic AMP was reached less than a minute after 1.65 µM-PGE_1, and that the radioactivity declined subsequently to a relatively stable state. In the presence of RA 233, an inhibitor of cyclic nucleotide phosphodiesterase, a smaller dose of PGE_1 caused a greater increase in cyclic AMP which was sustained. The addition of a low concentration of either ADP or adrenaline at times when the cyclic AMP concentration was fairly stable, caused a rapid and profound reduction of cyclic AMP radioactivity, even in

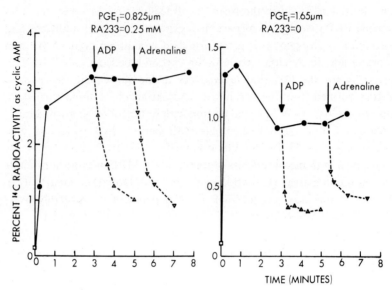

FIG. 1. Effect of ADP and adrenaline (final concentration 5 μM) on cyclic AMP radioactivity in platelets incubated with either PGE₁ (*right*) or PGE₁ plus RA 233 (*left*). (Reprinted from Mills & Smith 1972, with permission of the New York Academy of Sciences.)

the presence of a powerful phosphodiesterase inhibitor. This effect is interesting because it appears to be confined to the two aggregating agents ADP and adrenaline, and to occur at concentrations similar to those necessary for aggregation. Also, it occurs extremely quickly, and is in fact one of the earliest biochemical changes in stimulated platelets that can be detected. ADP or adrenaline can antagonize the action of PGE₁ even when added simultaneously with the cyclase stimulator. However, other aggregating agents such as thrombin, 5-hydroxytryptamine (5HT), vasopressin and collagen, though they have in some cases been shown to inhibit adenylate cyclase in platelet membrane fragments (for review see Salzman & Weisenberger 1972), do not have much effect on the adenylate cyclase system of intact cells (Mills 1974; Macfarlane & Mills 1975). Taken together with other available evidence (Haslam 1973 and this symposium, pp. 121–143) this strongly argues agains the proposal that reduction of cyclic AMP concentrations is a common mechanism of the action of aggregating agents.

The second of the early metabolic effects of aggregating agents that we have studied is their effect on adenine nucleotide metabolism. When ADP is added to ¹⁴C-labelled platelets, there is a rapid fall in the adenylate energy charge (AEC) which normally has a value of 0.92–0.94 in resting platelets. This is shown in

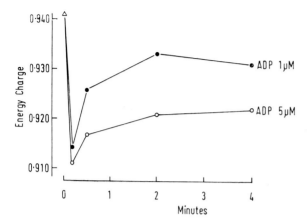

FIG. 2. Adenylate energy charge in platelets exposed for various times to ADP.

Fig. 2, where the AEC is seen to fall by nearly 0.03 in the first ten seconds after addition of ADP. During the next few minutes there is a partial recovery of AEC towards the resting level, which occurs more rapidly at lower concentrations of added ADP. We have previously shown (Mills 1973) that this effect can be demonstrated as early as 0.5 second after ADP and that it reaches its maximum within 2 seconds. This effect is in many ways associated with the induction of platelet shape change. It occurs in the presence of EDTA, and with thromb-asthenic platelets. 5HT, thrombin and vasopressin, all of which agents cause a shape change before aggregation, all induce a similar fall in the AEC (Macfarlane & Mills 1975). Adrenaline, which causes aggregation without a shape change (O'Brien 1965), has no effect on the AEC (Mills 1973). The concentration of ADP that causes one half of the maximal change in AEC is about 1 μM (Fig. 3), which is close to the value found by Born (1970) for induction of shape change in rabbit platelets (0.6 μM).

The effect of ADP on the energy charge is specific for this nucleotide, and although small reductions in AEC are sometimes observed with ATP, other nucleoside diphosphates did not cause a comparable lowering at concentrations 100-fold in excess of the ADP concentration required (Table 1). AMP was also inactive.

A reduction of the AEC might occur either through stimulation of ATP consumption, or by inhibition of ATP regeneration. As expected, a variety of metabolic poisons are able to cause progressive lowering of the AEC, along with the degradation of adenine nucleotides, first to inosine monophosphate (IMP) and finally to inosine and hypoxanthine which, being able to penetrate

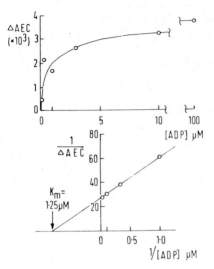

FIG. 3. Effect of ADP at different concentrations on the adenylate energy charge (AEC) measured after 5 seconds. *Top curve*: linear plot of the change in AEC against ATP concentration. *Lower curve:* double reciprocal plot of the same data.

TABLE 1

Effect of nucleoside diphosphates on adenylate energy charge

	Compound						
	Control ADP	ADP	CDP	UDP	IDP	GDP	XDP
Nucleotide concentration (μM)		1	10	100	100	100	100	100
Adenylate energy charge	0.912	0.890	0.891	0.901	0.913	0.904	0.914	0.915
Difference from control		−0.022	−0.021	−0.011	+0.001	−0.008	+0.002	+0.003

Samples of labelled PRP (0.20 ml) were added to 10 μl of Tris-saline containing the various nucleotides, and incubated for 5 seconds at 37 °C before the reaction was stopped with 20 μl cold perchloric acid. The nucleotides were: CDP, cytosine 5′-diphosphate; UDP, uridine 5′-diphosphate; IDP, inosine 5′-diphosphate; GDP, guanosine 5′-diphosphate and XDP, xanthosine 5′-diphosphate. Radioactive nucleotides were separated by paper chromatography.

the cell membrane, leak into the plasma. The combination of antimycin A (ANT) and deoxy-D-glucose (DOG) is an effective way of inhibiting ATP resynthesis (Holmsen *et al.* 1974), and its effect on platelet nucleotides is shown in Fig. 4. ANT is an inhibitor of mitochondrial oxidative phosphorylation at the 'site 2' level (Slater 1973), and DOG inhibits glycolysis by competing with glucose for hexokinase, and by the accumulation of its metabolite (deoxy-

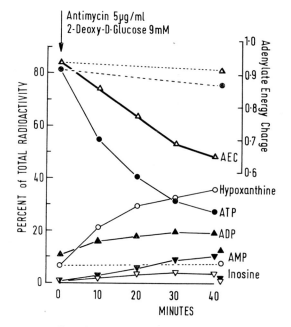

FIG. 4. Effect of a combination of antimycin A and deoxy-D-glucose added at zero time on the concentrations of ATP ($\bullet$—$\bullet$), ADP ($\blacktriangle$—$\blacktriangle$), AMP ($\blacktriangledown$—$\blacktriangledown$), inosine ($\triangledown$—$\triangledown$) and hypoxanthine ($\bigcirc$—$\bigcirc$) plotted as a percentage of the total radioactivity in platelets labelled with [^{14}C]adenine as a nucleotide precursor (left-hand axis). The adenylate energy charge (AEC, $\triangle$—$\triangle$) is plotted on the right-hand axis. The points beyond the end of the time axis indicate measurements made on a control sample incubated at 37 °C without additions.

D-glucose 6-phosphate) which inhibits phosphohexoseisomerase (Detwiler1971). The resting platelet appears to be well able to maintain its internal energy economy if either glycolysis or oxidative phosphorylation are inhibited singly (Fig. 6) but when both systems are inhibited together, as in Fig. 4, there follows a slow and almost linear fall in AEC accompanied by the formation of hypoxanthine and a small increase of ADP, AMP and inosine. High concentrations of the thiol reagent N-ethylmaleimide (NEM) can also block ATP resynthesis and cause loss of ATP and a fall in the AEC (Fig. 5). In this case the AEC falls precipitously, and there is a rapid, transient increase in ADP with a slower, larger increase in AMP and IMP. The very rapid degradation of ATP that occurs with NEM may be due to more than just the inhibition of ATP resynthesis, as several thiol reagents are able to activate ATPases (Jocelyn 1972), and it is possible that cellular disorganization by NEM might lead to the unmasking of ATPases normally sequestered in various intracellular compartments.

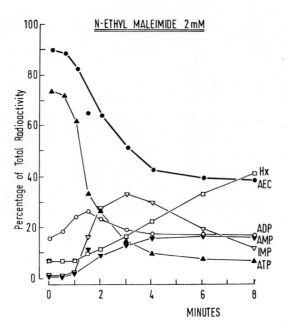

F<small>IG</small>. 5. Effect of *N*-ethylmaleimide added at zero time on the concentrations of radioactive ATP (▲—▲), ADP (○—○), AMP (▼—▼), IMP (▽—▽) and hypoxanthine (Hx, □—□) plotted as a percentage of total radioactivity. The adenylate energy charge (AEC, ●—●) is shown multiplied by 100 and plotted on the same scale.

Neither the combination of ANT and DOG nor 2 m<small>M</small>-NEM causes platelet aggregation (though the latter does induce a shape change) so it is clear that ADP does not induce the shape change and aggregation solely as a result of its effect on the AEC and it is likely that the lowering of AEC is a consequence of the shape change. It is necessary then to decide whether ADP acts by reducing ATP resynthesis or by accelerating ATP breakdown. In the first case, we would expect the effects of ADP to be reduced by other inhibitors of resynthesis, and in the second case we would expect them to be increased. We therefore measured the lowering of the energy charge by ADP in the presence of ANT and DOG. But first of all we tested the effects of ANT and DOG on another system in which ATP use is known to be increased.

PGE$_1$, by stimulating adenylate cyclase, causes an increase in ATP use equivalent to approximately 5–6% of the ATP pool per minute during the first 30 or 50 seconds (Fig. 1). This is roughly 0.25 μmoles ATP per minute for 10^{11} platelets. When PGE$_1$ was added to labelled platelets either untreated or incubated with antimycin, no fall in the energy charge could be detected (Fig. 6). During incubation with deoxy-D-glucose in this experiment a slow steady

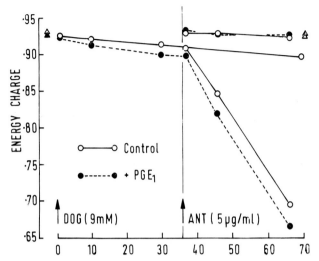

FIG. 6. Effect of PGE$_1$ (2 μM) on the adenylate energy charge of platelets incubated at 37 °C with antimycin A (ANT) or deoxy-D-glucose (DOG) or both together. The closed points represent the energy charge measured in subsamples from the bulk incubation which were added to 1/20 volume of Tris-saline containing PGE$_1$ and incubated for a further 45 seconds. Open points refer to control subsamples added to Tris-saline alone. Triangles represent subsamples from a control incubation without ANT or DOG, taken at the beginning and end of the experiment. In the right-hand half of the figure the top two curves had ANT added at the arrow. The middle and lower two curves all had DOG added at 0 minutes and the lower two curves had ANT added at 36 minutes.

reduction of the energy charge occurred, and when PGE$_1$ was added during this incubation, a further small reduction of AEC occurred within 30 seconds. When antimycin was added after 36 minutes incubation with DOG, the energy charge immediately started to fall quite rapidly, and addition of PGE$_1$ at this stage caused a further fall in AEC which was greater than the change caused by PGE$_1$ in the presence of DOG alone. This experiment confirmed the supposition that the initiation of a process of accelerated ATP breakdown would lead to a more pronounced fall in energy charge when performed in the presence of inhibitors of ATP resynthesis.

A similar experiment was then conducted with ADP (Fig. 7). In this experiment, ADP added at intervals during a control incubation of labelled PRP caused the usual fall in AEC of only about 0.02 units. When added to PRP during incubation with ANT and DOG, ADP caused a greater reduction in AEC at a time when the metabolic inhibitors had not yet caused any lowering, and the effect of ADP became more marked as the incubation continued. It is true that during incubation with ANT and DOG, as the energy charge falls

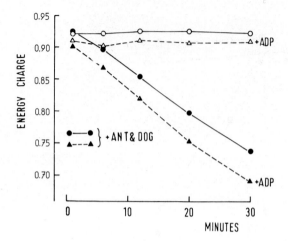

FIG. 7. Effect of ADP on the adenylate energy charge (AEC) of platelets incubated with antimycin A (ANT, 5 μg/ml) and deoxy-D-glucose (DOG, 9 mM) at 37 °C. As in Fig. 6, subsamples were added to Tris-saline containing ADP (10 μM, triangles) or to Tris-saline (circles) and incubated for a further 30 seconds. ANT and DOG were added at 0 minutes to the incubation shown by filled points, and the open points represent a control incubation.

the total pool size of the metabolic nucleotides is reduced, because of the formation of degradation products. However, at an AEC of 0.75 (after 30 min with ANT and DOG in the experiment of Fig. 7) the pool size has been decreased by only about 30% while the effect of ADP on the energy charge was increased to roughly three times its effect on control platelets. This experiment therefore supports the conclusion that ADP causes a lowering of the energy charge by stimulating ATP breakdown, as would be expected if ADP triggers an active contractile process related to the initial shape change rather than by reducing the rate of ATP resynthesis.

In addition, it can be reasoned that the rate of stimulated ATP breakdown in platelets exposed to ADP is considerably greater than that which occurs during the action of PGE_1, as ADP causes a detectable fall in the AEC of platelets in the absence of metabolic poisons, while PGE_1 does not. An alternative explanation, namely that PGE_1 causes an acceleration of ATP resynthesis as well as an increase in ATP consumption, should be considered. Cyclic AMP formed by the action of PGE_1 may well stimulate glycolytic metabolism, as it stimulates glycogenolysis (Deisseroth et al. 1970), and thus compensate for the excess ATP use. However, ADP also stimulates glycolysis in platelets (Karpatkin 1967), though the exact quantitative comparison of these two effects is not possible. Calculations from the initial rate of fall of AEC observed with ADP

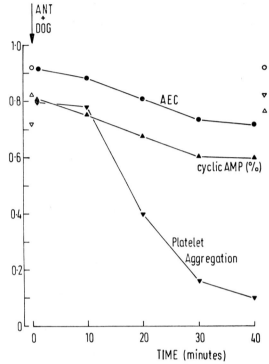

FIG. 8. Effect of PGE$_1$ on cyclic AMP formation during incubation of platelets with anti-mycin A (ANT; 5μg/ml) and deoxy-D-glucose (DOG 9 mM). At various times after the addition of ANT and DOG to a bulk sample of platelet-rich plasma at 37 °C, subsamples were removed and used for the following determinations: (1) Rate of platelet aggregation with 10 μM-ADP, expressed as the steepest slope of the aggregation curve in arbitrary units (▼—▼); (2) AEC in the bulk incubation (●—●); and (3) increase in radioactivity of cyclic AMP during 30 seconds incubation of subsamples with 2 μM-PGE$_1$ (▲—▲).

(Mills 1973) lead to a minimum rate of increased ATP breakdown of 6 μmoles per minute for 10^{11} platelets during the first two seconds after ADP, a rate far higher than the observed maximum rate of cyclic AMP formation after PGE$_1$ (0.25 μmol/min). Whether or not this high rate is sustained while the AEC remains depressed is uncertain.

We must now consider the possibility that the two actions of ADP discussed above are causally linked. Against this view is the fact that adrenaline can inhibit the effect of PGE$_1$ on the platelet adenylate cyclase system to a similar extent as ADP but without causing shape change or reduction of AEC. Conversely, thrombin, vasopressin and 5HT, which all induce the shape change and a fall in the energy charge, have a much smaller effect than ADP on the adenylate cyclase. However, these facts do not preclude the possibility that ADP has a unique action in which the fall in AEC is directly related to the inhibition of adenylate cyclase.

Two further experiments appear to make this unlikely. In the first of these, formation of cyclic AMP was measured after brief exposure to PGE$_1$ during an incubation with ANT and DOG (Fig. 8). ANT and DOG caused a much larger fall in the AEC than was seen with ADP, but had considerably less effect on the ability of the platelets to synthesize cyclic AMP when stimulated with PGE$_1$. Thus if depletion of ATP by the shape change/aggregation mechanism triggered by ADP is to explain the inhibition of cyclic AMP synthesis, the concept of a small pool of ATP associated with the platelet membrane has to be invoked. If this pool, rather than the bulk of intracellular ATP, acted as the source of substrate for both the adenylate cyclase and the shape change mechanism, only a small change in the energy charge measured in the whole cell might represent a severe depletion of the postulated membrane pool. We attempted to test this theory by using N-ethylmaleimide, a thiol reagent that is known as a powerful inhibitor of contractile protein ATPase.

Using low concentrations of NEM, below those that cause a fall in the energy charge, we examined its effect on the response of the adenylate cyclase of platelets to PGE$_1$ and ADP (Mills & Smith 1972). NEM inhibits platelet aggregation, and we anticipated that it might, by preventing the ADP-induced stimulation of ATP breakdown, also inhibit the antagonism between ADP and PGE$_1$ on the adenylate cyclase if this was mediated by substrate deprivation. The results of a typical experiment are shown in Fig. 9. NEM at concentrations between 0.1 and 0.4 mM not only inhibited the effect of ADP on the adenylate cyclase as expected, but also caused a marked stimulation of the amount of cyclic AMP formed in response to PGE$_1$. At higher concentrations NEM was inhibitory. This result does not justify our substrate competition theory, however. A companion experiment showed (Fig. 10) that NEM at these concentrations did not block the ability of ADP to lower the energy charge. We have also found that NEM does not inhibit the shape change caused by ADP, though higher concentrations of NEM (0.5–2 mM) themselves induce a shape change.

Although they do not completely rule out the possibility of substrate competition as an explanation of the action of ADP on the cyclase, our experiments with NEM have led to a novel approach to the investigation of control mechanisms acting on the platelet adenylate cyclase. To summarize briefly our recent work, we have found that the ability of various thiol reagents to block the inhibitory effect of ADP on the adenylate cyclase, and to stimulate the response to PGE$_1$, varies according to the specific structures of the reagents and their ability to penetrate the platelet membrane.

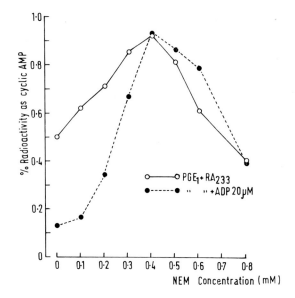

FIG. 9. Effect of *N*-ethylmaleimide (NEM) on the stimulation of cyclic AMP formation by 2μM-PGE₁ in the presence and absence of 20 μM-ADP. Samples of labelled platelet-rich plasma were incubated with the indicated concentration of NEM for 3 minutes at 37 °C and then we added either 2 μM-PGE₁ and 0.2 mM-RA 233 (○—○) or PGE₁ and RA 233 and 20 μM-ADP (●----●). The samples were incubated for a further 1 minute. Results are expressed as the percentage of the total radioactivity in the platelets recovered as cyclic AMP.

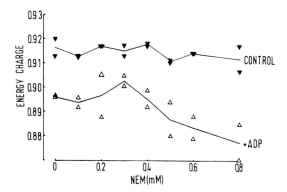

FIG. 10. Effect of *N*-ethylmaleimide (NEM) on the lowering of platelet energy charge by ADP. Samples of labelled platelet-rich plasma containing 4 mM-EDTA were incubated at 37 °C for 10 seconds with NEM and then for a further 10 seconds with either Tris-saline (▼) or Tris-saline containing ADP (final concentration = 10 μM) (△).

CONCLUSIONS

We have investigated four changes in platelets that occur rapidly after their exposure to aggregating agents. These are (1) aggregation, (2) shape change, (3) lowering of adenylate energy charge, and (4) inhibition of PGE_1-stimulated accumulation of cyclic AMP. We have shown that there is a close association between the ability of an agent to cause shape change and its effect on the energy charge, but little relation to its ability to inhibit adenylate cyclase. The observed reduction of energy charge by ADP is probably due to the stimulation of ATP consumption. This may be related to the mechanism of the shape change. Thiol reagents that block the effect of ADP on adenylate cyclase do not necessarily also prevent shape change and lowering of energy charge. A causal relationship between the energy charge effect of ADP and its adenylate cyclase effect, through substrate competition for ATP, is, though not excluded, considered to be improbable.

ACKNOWLEDGEMENTS

I thank Mrs Carol Lipson and Miss Sheila Gardner for technical assistance, and Dr D. E. Macfarlane for help in preparing the manuscript. Prostaglandins were given by Dr J. E. Pike, Upjohn Co., Kalamazoo, Michigan, and RA 233 (2,6-bis-(diethanolamino)-4-piperidino-pyrimido [5,4d] pyrimidine) was a gift from Dr J. W. Bell, Boehringer Ingelheim Ltd., Isleworth, Middlesex.

This work was supported by grant no. HL 14217 from the National Heart and Lung Institute.

References

ATKINSON, D. E. (1968) The energy charge of the adenylate pool as a regulatory parameter. *Biochemistry 7*, 4030-4034

BORN, G. V. R. (1970) Observations on the change in shape of blood platelets brought about by adenosine diphosphate. *J. Physiol. (Lond.) 209*, 487-511

BRODIE, G. N., BAENZIGER, N. L., CHASE, L. R. & MAJERUS, P. W. (1972) The effect of thrombin on adenyl cyclase activity and a membrane protein from human platelets. *J. Clin. Invest. 51*, 81-88

DETWILER, T. C. (1971) Effects of deoxyglucose on platelet metabolism. *Biochim. Biophys. Acta 244*, 303-310

DEISSEROTH, A., WOLFE, S. M. & SHULMAN, N. R. (1970) Platelet phosphorylase activity in the presence of activators and inhibitors of aggregation. *Biochem. Biophys. Res. Commun. 39*, 551-557

HARWOOD, J. P., MOSKOWITZ, J. & KRISHNA, G. (1972) Dynamic interactions of prostaglandin and norepinephrine in the formation of adenosine 3':5'-monophosphate in human and rabbit platelets. *Biochim. Biophys. Acta 261*, 444

HASLAM, R. J. (1973) Interactions of the pharmacological receptors of blood platelets with adenylate cyclase. *Ser. Haematol. 6*, 121-143

HASLAM, R. J. (1975) This volume, pp. 121-143

HOLMSEN, H., SETKOWSKY, C. A. & DAY, H. J. (1974) Effects of antimycin and 2-deoxyglucose on adenine nucleotides in human platelets. Role of metabolic ATP in primary aggregation, secondary aggregation and shape change of platelets. *Biochem. J. 144*, 385-396

JOCELYN, P. C. (1972) *Biochemistry of the SH Group*, Academic Press, London

KARPATKIN, S. (1967) Studies on human platelet glycolysis. Effect of glucose, cyanide, insulin, citrate, and agglutination and contraction on platelet glycolysis. *J. Clin. Invest. 46*, 409-417

KRISHNA, G., WEISS, B. & BRODIE, B. B. (1968) A simple, sensitive method for the assay of adenyl cyclase. *J. Pharmacol. Exp. Therap. 163*, 379-385

MACFARLANE, D. E. & MILLS, D. C. B. (1975) The effects of ATP on platelets: evidence against the role of released ADP in primary aggregation. *Blood*, in press

MACMILLAN, D. C. & OLIVER, R. T. (1965) The initial changes in platelet morphology following the addition of adenosine diphosphate. *J. Atheroscler. Res. 5*, 440-444

MARQUIS, N. R., BECKER, J. R. & VIGDAHL, R. L. (1970) Platelet aggregation III. An epinephrine induced decrease in cyclic AMP synthesis. *Biochem. Biophys. Res. Commun. 39*, 783-789

MCDONALD, J. W. D. & STUART, R. K. (1973) Regulation of cyclic AMP levels and aggregation in human platelets by prostaglandin E_1. *J. Lab. Clin. Med. 81*, 838-849

MILLS, D. C. B. (1973) Changes in the adenylate energy charge in human blood platelets induced by adenosine diphosphate. *Nature (Lond.) 243*, 220-222

MILLS, D. C. B. (1974) Factors influencing the adenylate cyclase system in human blood platelets. In *Platelets and Thrombosis* (Sherry, S. & Scriabine, A., eds.), pp. 45-67, University Park Press, Baltimore

MILLS, D. C. B. & ROBERTS, G. C. K. (1967) Effects of adrenaline on human blood platelets. *J. Physiol. (Lond.) 193*, 443-453

MILLS, D. C. B. & SMITH, J. B. (1971) The influence on platelet aggregation of drugs that affect the accumulation of adenosine 3′:5′-cyclic monophosphate in platelets. *Biochem. J. 121*, 185-196

MILLS, D. C. B. & SMITH, J. B. (1972) The control of platelet responsiveness by agents that influence cyclic AMP metabolism. *Ann. N.Y. Acad. Sci. 201*, 391

O'BRIEN, J. R. (1965) Effect of adenosine diphosphate and adrenaline on mean platelet shape. *Nature (Lond.) 207*, 306-307

SALZMAN, E. W. (1972) Cyclic AMP and platelet function. *N. Engl. J. Med. 286*, 358-363

SALZMAN, E. W. & NERI, L. L. (1969) Cyclic 3′,5′-adenosine monophosphate in human blood platelets. *Nature (Lond.) 224*, 609-610

SALZMAN, E. W. & WEISENBERGER, H. (1972) Role of cyclic AMP in platelet function. *Adv. Cyclic Nucleotide Res. 1*, 231

SLATER, E. C. (1973) The mechanism of action of the respiratory inhibitor antimycin. *Biochim. Biophys. Acta 301*, 129-154

WHITE, J. G. (1968) Fine structural alterations induced in blood platelets by adenosine diphosphate. *Blood 31*, 604-622

ZIEVE, P. D. & GREENOUGH, W. B. III (1969) Adenyl cyclase in human platelets: activity and responsiveness. *Biochem. Biophys. Res. Commun. 35*, 462-466

ZUCKER, M. B. & BORRELLI, J. (1954) Reversible alterations in platelet morphology produced by anticoagulants and by cold. *Blood 9*, 602-608

Discussion

Crawford: Do you do your experiments in a controlled oxygen environment? In your Fig. 6 (p. 161) the evidence suggests that the substrate for the adenylate cyclase was substantially of mitochondrial origin. Also you didn't show the effect of adding the inhibitors in the reverse order; I presume you did this. What was the effect then?

Mills: I have tried adding the inhibitors simultaneously: the effect here is the same as when deoxyglucose is added first, except that there is a lag of about five minutes before the energy charge starts to fall. The effect of the glycolytic inhibitor, deoxyglucose, was greater than the effect of antimycin (Fig. 6). Antimycin by itself does not cause any reduction of the energy charge in platelet-rich plasma; presumably, therefore, the balance of nucleotides in the platelet can be sustained entirely by glycolytic metabolism. Deoxyglucose, by itself, causes a slow reduction in the adenylate energy charge (AEC), which suggests that oxidative metabolism cannot entirely compensate for inhibition of glycolysis. That may be due to the non-specificity of the action of deoxyglucose.

Detwiler: One must keep in mind the fact that deoxyglucose uses a tremendous amount of ATP for its own phosphorylation (Detwiler 1971) and you have to consider whether you are lowering the energy charge simply by phosphorylating deoxyglucose.

Mills: Why should the energy charge be lowered so much more rapidly in the presence of antimycin and deoxyglucose, if the effect of the accumulation of deoxyglucose-6-phosphate is a major consideration?

Detwiler: In the absence of antimycin, you can phosphorylate deoxyglucose *and* maintain the energy charge with oxidative metabolism, but if you inhibit oxidative phosphorylation during phosphorylation of some dead-end product, you might expect a lowering of the energy charge. I am not saying that this is the explanation, but it has to be considered.

Holmsen: In ascites tumour cells Yushok (1971) has shown that deoxyglucose causes a rapid depletion of both ATP and inorganic phosphate, the latter trapped as 2-deoxyglucose-6-phosphate. As in platelets, the ATP lost from the tumour cells could be accounted for by the hypoxanthine formed, which indicates that the ATP–hypoxanthine conversion in the tumour cells also occurred via AMP deaminase. Yushok suggested that the removal of inorganic phosphate relieved the phosphate inhibition of AMP deaminase, and this enzyme now became active and drained the adenine nucleotide pool. We have shown (Holmsen *et al.* 1974) that in platelets there is an increase of almost 100% in inorganic phosphate during ATP depletion caused by incubation with antimycin *plus* deoxyglucose. So, for platelets this trapping of phosphate as 2-deoxyglucose-6-phosphate does not seem to be so important.

Detwiler: Have you measured the amount of deoxyglucose-6-phosphate? There is a lot of it!

Holmsen: No, we did not measure it. However, with an increase in the level of inorganic phosphate during incubation the ATP depletion can hardly be caused by removal of the phosphate inhibition of AMP deaminase.

Born: If the deoxyglucose phosphate is not metabolized further would you expect the process to come to an equilibrium after a short time?

Mills: It depends on what is the limiting factor, which could be the availability of phosphate. It is certainly clear that deoxyglucose phosphate inhibits the phosphohexose isomerase reaction (Detwiler 1971) and consequently inhibits glycolysis. Deoxyglucose also competes with the hexose transport system.

Holmsen: Dr Mills, I still do not understand why you assume that ADP induces ATP consumption, and not inhibition of production. You showed that PGE_1, which induces ATP consumption, gave the same changes in AEC as ADP, and by analogy you suggest that ADP causes consumption. Have you done any experiments to see what happens with a sudden stop in ATP production?

Mills: I don't know how rapidly antimycin and deoxyglucose work. In the experiments with antimycin and deoxyglucose, ATP resynthesis is severely reduced, if not completely prevented.

Feinberg: Although PGE_1 may induce the conversion of ATP to cyclic AMP the activation of phosphorylase by cyclic AMP can bring about the rapid synthesis of ATP from glycogen and glucose utilization; thus PGE_1 might not, on balance, be a net consumer of ATP.

Mills: That might well explain why deoxyglucose is more effective in revealing an action of PGE_1 on the energy charge than is antimycin.

Mustard: McElroy *et al.* (1971), using washed rabbit platelets and [6-^{14}C]glucose, found that prostaglandin E_1 depressed the production of $^{14}CO_2$. When ADP was added, the ADP-induced increase in $^{14}CO_2$ production was inhibited by prostaglandin E_1. The net effect of PGE_1 as measured by the production of $^{14}CO_2$ from labelled glucose is to depress ATP consumption rather than increase it.

Mills: Our evidence suggests that PGE_1 provokes a net consumption of ATP, but the argument is somewhat circular, I admit.

Feinberg: I wonder whether phosphodiesterase activity is an important consideration, since the use of an inhibitor of phosphodiesterase lessens the availability of AMP as a substrate for adenylate kinase activity.

Secondly, contractile processes usually have a low K_M for ATP, and therefore contractile phenomena ought not to be measurably affected by the small drop in energy charge you found.

Mills: Dr Holmsen has information on that. How far does the energy charge have to fall before the shape change mechanism fails?

Holmsen: Shape change becomes completely inhibited when the ATP level drops below 25% of normal. This critical level corresponds, when we use deoxyglucose and antimycin, to an AEC of 0.65.

Mills: So that is in agreement with Dr Feinberg's comment.

Detwiler: Dr Mazhar Malik (Malik *et al.* 1974) has shown that the K_m for ATP or platelet actomyosin is two orders of magnitude higher than that of muscle actomyosin, but it is impossible to say what the physiological significance of this is.

Mills: We have some interesting observations on the effect of cytochalasin A (D. C. B. Mills & D. E. Macfarlane, unpublished). It is a thiol reagent, and it has very similar effects to those of *N*-ethylmaleimide (NEM) on the platelet adenylate cyclase. Cytochalasin A causes less, if any, stimulation of the response to PGE_1 and the effect of ADP is completely blocked.

Haslam: Thrombosthenin extracted from human platelets which have been incubated with cytochalasin A at a concentration just sufficient to prevent aggregation completely (20 µg/ml, 42 µM) will neither clear nor superprecipitate with ATP (Haslam 1972). This is at least consistent with a role for thrombosthenin in aggregation, though, of course, cytochalasin A is probably not a very specific thiol reagent.

Nachman: Has anyone been able to label cytochalasin A?

Haslam: Not yet, so far as I know.

Adelstein: Have you extracted thrombosthenin first and then tried to see the effect of cytochalasin A?

Haslam: Yes. It also inhibits clearing and superprecipitation under these conditions, just as most thiol reagents do. However, there is very little evidence that this effect of cytochalasin A on thrombosthenin is connected with its 'cytochalasin-like' activities, particularly as cytochalasin B is not a thiol reagent and does not affect the superprecipitation of thrombosthenin (Haslam 1972).

Holmsen: In order to label actomyosin one could perhaps utilize the property of this platelet protein of binding metabolic ADP. As I will discuss in my paper (pp. 175–196), when platelets are labelled with radioactive adenine, 20–50% of the total radioactive ADP formed is associated with an ethanol-insoluble fraction. French & Wachowicz (1974) have recently shown that the major part of this ADP is associated with actomyosin.

Crawford: We may be in danger of overlooking another equally important platelet polymeric protein system which could also be involved in phosphate exchange. We have recently been working with a protein purified from pig platelets which resembles, in many of its properties, the microtubule subunit 'tubulin' of brain, cilia and flagella (Castle & Crawford 1975a, b). This platelet protein has a monomer molecular weight of around 55 000, binds colchicine as the 6S dimer, and will undergo a temperature-dependent polymerization to give long fibres resembling the microtubule subfilaments seen by Behnke & Zelander (1967) in their electron micrographs of mammalian platelets. If the analogies between this platelet protein and brain tubulin can be shown to extend further, then the platelet tubulin will have GTP and GDP binding sites, a proportion of which have exchangeable phosphate groups. Moreover, associated with the tubulin from platelets are a small number of higher molecular weight polypeptides which could be dynein-like components. These dynein proteins in other systems have ATPase activity and are believed to be involved in the energetics of polymer assembly or dissociation.

Now, the way in which you have implicated the actomyosin-like contractile proteins in your concepts of platelet phosphate dynamics is most interesting and certainly important, but I feel we may well have to include this other important polymeric protein system in our hypotheses since it too may play a part in controlling or modulating the exchangeable phosphate pool of the cell.

Mills: Holmsen and I have looked for changes in the guanylate energy charge and found much smaller changes which follow those in the adenylate energy charge after exposure of phosphate-labelled platelets to ADP.

Nachman: I am interested in your results with adrenaline. I think you showed evidence that adrenaline affected the cyclase system differently from vasopressin?

Mills: There are two kinds of effect, and they are complicated. We find that all agents which themselves cause a shape change, including 5HT, thrombin, vasopressin and ADP, cause a similar lowering of the energy charge and that this is not inhibited by EDTA. Adrenaline, which does not cause the shape change, has no effect on the energy charge. But when we look at the adenylate cyclase system, ADP and adrenaline are very powerful inhibitors; vasopressin, 5HT, thrombin and collagen are not. So there are two groupings.

Nachman: Is there any system which suggests that vasopressin and ADP should be grouped together, separate from the other activators?

Mills: No.

Haslam: I think it may be wrong to suggest that the α-adrenergic depression of cyclic AMP levels by adrenaline is entirely due to inhibition of adenylate cyclase. This may occur but there is good evidence that adrenaline also activates phosphodiesterase (Harwood *et al.* 1972).

Packham: In this experiment you used collagen or thrombin at concentrations that appeared to give the same extent of aggregation as ADP. There are synergistic effects between collagen and ADP, or thrombin and ADP (Niewiarowski & Thomas 1966; Packham *et al.* 1973). With a very low concentration of ADP combined with a very small amount of thrombin or collagen, one can cause extensive aggregation although, by itself, neither agent at these low concentrations has much effect. Could your observations that thrombin or collagen has little inhibitory effect on the adenylate cyclase system be explained on the basis that there was actually very little ADP released from the platelets, but the extent of aggregation was similar to that caused by a much higher concentration of ADP (added by itself) because of a synergistic effect on aggregation between collagen and ADP or thrombin and ADP?

Mills: This could explain the results of the aggregation experiments, but is not relevant, I think, to the effects on the cyclase system.

Packham: Did you measure the concentration of ADP outside the platelets after adding collagen or thrombin?

Mills: We did not measure the ADP outside, because we are talking about very small amounts of ADP.

Mustard: I am sure you are aware that comparing the effects of collagen or thrombin with ADP is like comparing oranges and thumbtacks! If you measure the effect of thrombin or collagen on the energy charge over a longer period of time, do you see a greater effect than with ADP by itself?

Mills: Much bigger, but this effect is related to the induction of the release reaction.

Mustard: So you feel you are looking at the changes in the energy charge which occur at the beginning of the thrombin and collagen effect?

Mills: Certainly; but there is a large difference in the time courses of the two effects. The fall in energy charge induced by ADP takes about two seconds, and the later effects of thrombin and collagen occur over several minutes.

Cohen: I am a bit confused: you said that the fall in adenylate energy charge is related to ATP consumption. But although ATP is needed for all the steps of platelet activation, I think you showed that ATP is utilized only during the shape change. Is that so?

Mills: No. With large amounts of ADP the energy charge falls by about 0.02–0.04 units and the lower level persists, but I cannot say whether the rate of ATP turnover is the same after the fall or higher than in the resting platelet. You can argue both ways. A homeostatic mechanism might restore the energy charge to the resting level as soon as the induced ATP consumption ceased; alternatively, the homeostatic mechanism might be more flexible, so that the energy charge would return to the resting level only slowly.

Born: There are experiments that could distinguish between those possibilities.
Mills: They are rather hard experiments to do.

References

BEHNKE, O. & ZELANDER, T. (1967) Filamentous substructure of microtubules of the marginal bundle of mammalian blood platelets. *J. Ultrastruct. Res. 19*, 147-165

CASTLE, A. G. & CRAWFORD, N. (1975*a*) Preparation of a tubulin-rich protein fraction from pig platelets. *Biochem. Soc. Trans. 3*, 164-167

CASTLE, A. G. & CRAWFORD, N. (1975*b*) Isolation of tubulin from pig platelets. *FEBS Lett. 51*, 195-198

DETWILER, T. C. (1971) Effects of deoxyglucose on platelet metabolism. *Biochim. Biophys. Acta 244*, 303-310

FRENCH, P. C. & WACHOWICZ, B. (1974) Investigations of the binding component of the ethanol insoluble metabolic ADP of human platelets and its relation to the release reaction. *Haemostasis 3*, 271-281

HASLAM, R. J. (1972) Inhibition of blood platelet function by cytochalasins: effects on thrombosthenin and on glucose metabolism. *Biochem. J. 127*, 34P

HARWOOD, J. P., MOSKOWITZ, J. & KRISHNA, G. (1972) Dynamic interaction of prostaglandin and norepinephrine in the formation of adenosine 3′:5′-monophosphate in human and rabbit platelets. *Biochim. Biophys. Acta 261*, 444-456

HOLMSEN, H., SETKOWSKY, C. A. & DAY, H. J. (1974) Effects of antimycin and 2-deoxyglucose on adenine nucleotides in human platelets. Role of metabolic adenosine triphosphate in primary aggregation, secondary aggregation and shape change of platelets. *Biochem. J. 144*, 385-396

McELROY, F. A., KINLOUGH-RATHBONE, R. L. ARDLIE, N. G., PACKHAM, M. A. & MUSTARD, J. F. (1971) The effect of aggregating agents on oxidative metabolism of rabbit platelets. *Biochim. Biophys. Acta 253*, 64-77

MALIK, M. N., ROSENBERG, S., DETWILER, T. C. & STRACHER, A. (1974) Role of Ca^{2+} in the allosteric regulation of platelet actomyosin. *Biochem. Biophys. Res. Commun. 61*, 1071-1075

NIEWIAROWSKI, S. & THOMAS, D. P. (1966) Platelet aggregation by ADP and thrombin. *Nature (Lond.) 212*, 1544-1547

PACKHAM, M. A., GUCCIONE, M. A., CHANG, P.-L. & MUSTARD, J. F. (1973) Platelet aggregation and release: effects of low concentrations of thrombin or collagen. *Am. J. Physiol. 225*, 38-47

YUSHOK, W. D. (1971) Control mechanisms of adenine nucleotide metabolism of ascites tumor cells. *J. Biol. Chem. 246*, 1607-1617

Biochemistry of the platelet release reaction

HOLM HOLMSEN

Specialized Center for Thrombosis Research, Temple University, Philadelphia and Institute for Thrombosis Research, University of Oslo, Norway

Abstract   The term 'platelet release reaction' describes the specific extrusion to the platelets' environment of the content of platelet storage granules. The process is analogous to several stages of secretion in typical secretory cells. The mechanism may involve a rise in the concentration of cytoplasmic calcium which triggers the ATP-consuming contractile process that brings the granule membrane and invaginations of the plasma membrane into such close contact that they fuse, and the granule contents become extracellular. In the platelets two different storage granules, dense granules and α-granules, are present, and evidence indicates that the mechanisms underlying dense granule release (Release I) differ in part from those underlying α-granule release (Release II). Some release inducers induce release I only, whereas others induce both release I and II. During the release reaction metabolic ATP is converted to IMP and hypoxanthine, and to the same extent during release I and release I + II. Antimycin inhibits the conversion of AMP to IMP during release, showing that deamination of AMP is not necessary for release. In the absence of antimycin, increased lactate formation starts 10 seconds after exposure of platelets to thrombin, and the entire pool of metabolic ATP can be shown to turn over 2–3 times during the release process. The ATP converted to IMP and hypoxanthine may represent that amount of ATP utilized during release which is *not* rephosphorylated to ATP during release. In the presence of antimycin no stimulation of lactate production takes place during release, whereas the decrease in the steady-state level of ATP and degree of release are normal. At 28 °C no stimulation of lactate production occurs and little reduction in steady-state ATP levels is seen, whereas release I is the same as at 37 °C. After release, platelets have lost their control of the maintenance of the levels of adenine nucleotides, since ATP is slowly exhausted, and less ATP is synthesized from adenine than in control platelets. It is possible, thus, that other reactions than those directly connected with the release process are responsible for the decrease in steady-state levels of ATP and increase in lactate production. When platelets are incubated with radioactive adenine, the specific radioactivity in ethanol-insoluble ADP, which contains actomyosin-bound ADP, increases in parallel to that of bulk adenine nucleotides. This indicates that actomyosin-bound ADP is turning over in the *resting* platelet, and this might have a connection with the ATP-requiring part of the release reaction. The calcium ionophore A 23187 induces release I and II, but without a decrease in steady-state ATP levels. In the presence of antimycin, A 23187 causes normal release I concomitant with a decrease in steady-state ATP levels. The use of calcium ionophores in the elucidation of the release mechanism is discussed.

Interaction between platelets and certain substances causes the release of intracellular constituents to the medium. The released constituents are localized in subcellular platelet granules, whereas the retained constituents are found in membranes, mitochondria and cytosol. The specific release of granular material from platelets has been termed the *platelet release reaction* (Grette 1962; Holmsen *et al.* 1969). The granules (storage granules) can be subdivided in two types, dense granules and α-granules. Table 1 shows their content, and indicates release inducers which can evoke release from each of the two types of granules. These data show that all inducers that release material from the α-granules always induce release from the dense granules. On the other hand, there are substances (ADP, adrenaline) that appear to induce release of constituents only from the dense granules.

Are release from the dense granules and release from the α-granules governed by different mechanisms? Thrombin, the most studied release inducer (for ref. see Holmsen *et al.* 1969), causes release from both dense and α-granules, but higher thrombin concentrations are needed for α-granule release than for dense granule release (Holmsen *et al.* 1975). Futhermore, material from dense granules is released more rapidly than that from the α-granules (Holmsen & Day 1970). Aspirin, a known inhibitor of dense granule release (Mustard & Packham 1970), appears not to inhibit release of α-granule material. Finally, in some patients with storage pool disease (Holmsen *et al.* 1975), release from α-granules is severely impaired, whereas release of ATP is normal. It seems therefore that the release from the dense granules and from the α-granules are governed by different mechanisms, which will be referred to as *release I* and *release II*, respectively.

The platelet release reaction resembles the first two steps in 'the secretory cycle' of the generalized secretory cell (Kirshner & Viveros 1972), the induction and extrusion steps. The circulating platelet differs, however, from prototype secretory cells by *not synthesizing* the material stored in granules. This makes the platelet an ideal model for study of the first two steps in secretion without interference from the synthesis or recovery (Kirshner & Viveros 1972) step.

Production of energy in the form of ATP is absolutely required for the platelet release reaction (for ref. see Day & Holmsen 1971). Energy is necessary if the release reaction depends on cellular contraction, as suggested in the

TABLE I

Substances released during the platelet release reaction: subcellular localization and specific release inducers

Subcellular localization	Constituent	Release inducer[a]								
		Ref.	T	C	L	AG	F	Z	ADP	Adr
Dense granules	5-Hydroxytryptamine		+	+	+	+	+	+	+	+
	ADP and ATP		+	+	+	+	+	+	+	+
	Calcium	1	+	+	+	?	+	?	+	+
	Pyrophosphate	2	+	?	?	?	?	?	?	?
	Antiplasmin	3	+	+	?	?	?	?	?	?
α-Granules	Acid hydrolases	4	+	+	+	?	?	−	−	−
	Potassium	5	+	+	?	?	?	?	−	−
	Fibrinogen		+	+	?	?	?	?	−	−
	Permeability factor	6	+	?	?	?	?	?	?	?
	Chemotactic factor	7	+	+	?	?	?	?	−	+
Unknown	Growth factor	8	+	+						
	Bactericidal factor	9	+	?	?	?	?	?	?	?
	Platelet factor 4	10	+	+	?	+	?	+	+	+

Actual release is designed +, demonstrated absence of release is designed —, whereas ? designates that release has not been investigated. Reference is made to Holmsen et al. (1969) or to the specific comments listed below.

[a] The release inducers are: T, thrombin; C, collagen; L, polystyrene latex particles; AG, aggregated gamma globulin; F, fluoride; Z, zymosan (Zucker & Grant 1974); ADP, adenosine diphosphate; Adr, adrenaline.

1. X-ray analysis has demonstrated Ca in the dense bodies (Martin et al. 1974), and several characteristics of Ca release in gel-filtered platelets have recently been demonstrated by Dr B. Lages (unpublished) in our laboratories.
2. Silcox et al. (1973) have demonstrated release of 50% of platelet pyrophosphate with thrombin and shown that platelets from patients with storage pool disease have greatly reduced levels of pyrophosphate. These patients have few, if any, dense granules in their platelets (Weiss & Ames 1973), indicating that pyrophosphate is located in these granules.
3. Antiplasmin has recently (Joist et al. 1975) been shown to be located together with 5-hydroxytryptamine in the dense granules.
4. The main acid hydrolases that are released are: β-N-acetylglucosaminidase, β-galactosidase, β-glucuronidase and α-arabinosidase. Acid phosphatase is present in the α-granules, but not released.
5. The exact subcellular localization of potassium is not clearly established, but since platelets from patients with storage pool disease have normal levels of K, and lack dense granules, the localization of K in the α-granules has been suggested (Lages et al. 1975). The characteristics of release of K from gel-filtered platelets are now under study (B. Lages, unpublished).
6. A factor that increases vascular permeability in skin is present in the α-granules (Nachman et al. 1970) and released during formation of the haemostatic plug, presumably through the action of thrombin.
7. Weksler & Coupal (1973).
8. Ross et al. (1974).

continued bottom page 178

secretion-coupling hypothesis for general secretion (Poisner & Trifaro 1967). In contrast to other secretory cells, the platelet release reaction takes place in the presence of extracellular EDTA, and transport of calcium into platelets during release does not occur (Mürer & Holme 1970), showing that the process is not dependent on the influx of calcium. Thus, if the release reaction depends on contractile mechanisms and hence on an increase of the cytosolic calcium concentration, the platelets must provide their own calcium for this purpose. The platelet release reaction can be considered to occur in three stages (Day & Holmsen 1971):

1. *Induction* (*or initiation*). Interaction between extracellular inducer and membrane which leads to liberation of transmitter substance from the membrane.

2. *Transmission*. Transfer of transmitter substances from membrane to contractile system.

3. *Extrusion*. Relative movement of membrane and granule (supported by contraction) until they meet and fuse; this results in the emptying of the granular contents to the extracellular space.

Evidence that shows that contraction is directly involved in the extrusion step of the platelet release reaction is scarce but there seems to be no doubt that actomyosin-containing filaments become apparent when platelets are 'activated' (White 1971). During release, the storage granules move and congregate in the centre of the platelet, where their contours become more and more diffuse as the release reaction proceeds (fusion?). A number of vacuoles appear in this central mass of granules, and specific staining has shown that some of them are transversely sectioned channels with openings to the extracellular space (White 1971). These channels lead the platelet fibrinogen out of the platelet during thrombin-induced release (Holme *et al.* 1973).

Thus, storage granules and channels (open canalicular system) move towards each other, and after contact is achieved, fusion takes place. Do the granules move towards a channel in a fixed position, or does a channel move towards granules in fixed positions? There are no adequate electron microscopic techniques available for observation of the first alternative, and we proposed (Holmsen 1973) a mechanism in which the granules were anchored by con-

---

9. Weksler & Nachman (1971).
10. Platelet factor 4 (antiheparin activity) has been reported to be present in both the dense granules and the α-granules. Platelets from patients with storage pool disease have normal amounts of platelet factor 4 (Weiss & Rogers 1973), and since these platelets lack dense granules, these organelles can hardly be the storage site for platelet factor 4. The time course of release of platelet factor 4 is different from that of 5-hydroxytryptamine (Walsh & Gagnatelli 1974), and different from that of β-N-acetylglucosaminidase, indicating a localization different from both dense granules and α-granules (S. Niewiarowski, unpublished).

tractile elements to stationary channels. When calcium becomes available in the cytoplasm, the elements contract, and the granule is rapidly pulled into the channel, fusion occurs and the granule's content is emptied into the channel. (Such a mechanism has recently been favoured for exocytosis in general [Durham 1974].) The other mechanism, movement of channels towards stationary granules, has more experimental support, since there are more pseudopods and channels (vacuoles) in the activated than in the resting platelet (White 1971). The pseudopods contain contractile elements (Zucker-Franklin *et al.* 1967) and, as suggested by Dr G. Stewart from our Research Center, a channel could be regarded as an inverted pseudopod; that is, a membrane invagination moving into cytoplasm centripetally, filled with extracellular medium, in contrast to the 'usual' pseudopod that moves centrifugally, into the extracellular medium, and filled with cytoplasm. This is illustrated schematically in Fig. 1. On activation, the resting cell, formed as an ellipsoid-like disk, is transformed into a sphere, with pseudopods directed both outwards and inwards. The inward-seeking pseudopods (channels) are fixed in three stages: one is on its way in, towards a granule; another has just reached a granule and fusion of channel and granule membrane has started; a third channel already contains the releasable material after fusion has been completed. Such a mechanism requires contractile elements in the membrane that are able to change the shape and size of the membrane. This hypothetical element is shown in Fig. 2, and will be used below as representing the ATP-consuming part of the extrusion step of the platelet release reaction.

Platelets easily incorporate radioactive adenine, adenosine or inorganic phosphate into their adenine nucleotides *in vitro*. During the release reaction such labelled platelets will, however, release *non*-labelled adenine nucleotides and retain the labelled pool. This has made it possible to distinguish between two pools of adenine nucleotides in platelets, the *metabolic* (labelled, retained) and the *non-metabolic* or *storage* (non-labelled, releasable) pool. The non-metabolic pool is localized in the dense granules, whereas the metabolic pool is present in the cytosol, mitochondria and membranes. During release, metabolic ATP is rapidly degraded in the platelets via ADP, AMP, IMP and inosine to hypoxanthine. This conversion has been suggested (Holmsen & Day 1971) to involve an initial hydrolysis of ATP to ADP by the ATPase activated by the transmitter substance. Two molecules of ADP are converted to one molecule of ATP and one molecule of AMP by adenylate kinase. ATP re-enters the reaction, whereas an increase of AMP is prevented by AMP deaminase which converts AMP to IMP. IMP is then slowly dephosphorylated to inosine which is finally phosphorolysed to hypoxanthine.

The steady-state levels of the metabolic adenine nucleotides during the

RESTING STATE

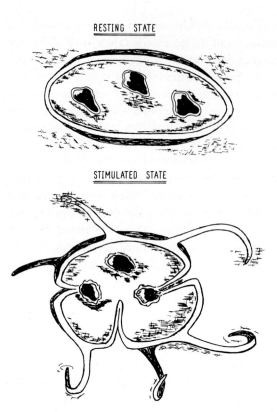

STIMULATED STATE

FIG. 1. Schematic illustration of a platelet in the resting and in the stimulated state. The resting platelet is in an ellipsoidal shape, and is shown in cross-section so that three dense granules (for simplicity) are visible. When stimulated by a release inducer the platelet changes its shape to a sphere and peudopods grow out from the cell and into the cell (invagination of the membrane, channels). Three such invaginations are seen, and represent three stages in the process: the invagination coming from below is on its way to the uppermost granule. The invagination coming from the left has reached a granule and fusion of the granule's and the invagination's membrane has started. The invagination coming from the right has already fused completely with the granule, and the contents of the granule are on the way out of the cell, through the channel.

release reaction induced by ADP and adrenaline have been measured. The ATP–hypoxanthine conversion was found to be intimately connected with the release step and not with the shape change or aggregation which also takes place. The magnitude of the ATP–hypoxanthine conversion obtained with ADP and adrenaline was the same as that obtained during release induced with thrombin and collagen (Holmsen *et al.* 1972). Detailed time-course studies of the interaction between washed platelets and thrombin reveal that the accumulation of non-metabolic ATP, ADP and β-*N*-acetylglucosaminidase

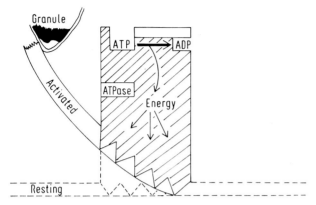

FIG. 2. Schematic representation of a contractile element in the membrane. In the resting state the membrane (broken line) is seen flattened out with the contractile element attached. By stimulation, the contractile element (actomyosin) hydrolyses ATP and some of the energy liberated transforms the element as shown in the figure so that the membrane changes its form, and might eventually reach a granule.

extracellularly is temporally closely correlated with the decrease in the steady-state level of metabolic ATP (M. H. Fukami & H. Holmsen, unpublished).

ATP–HYPOXANTHINE CONVERSION AS THE ENERGIZING STEP, WITH ENZYMES STRUCTURALLY BOUND

It was first thought that the ATP converted to hypoxanthine represented a specific 'release energy' pool of ATP, and that the conversion was specific for energizing the release reaction (Holmsen et al. 1969). In Fig. 3, the first three enzymes of such a pathway, ATPase, adenylate kinase and AMP deaminase, are linked together in such a way that the product is 'delivered' from the active site of one enzyme directly to the active site of the next enzyme in the chain. Such structurally coupled enzyme chains, for example the electron transfer and fatty acid oxidation in mitochondria, and certain glycolytic enzymes in the erythrocyte membrane (Green et al. 1965), are extremely efficient, and would explain how ATP energy can be so rapidly utilized in the platelet release reaction. Also, the efficiency obtained by combining ATPase, adenylate kinase and AMP deaminase is noteworthy, because AMP is removed from the adenylate kinase system, making the ATP–IMP conversion unidirectional, with utilization of both the energy-rich phosphoryl groups in ATP.

The ATP–hypoxanthine conversion in platelets is, however, not specific for the release reaction. It occurs slowly in the resting platelet (Holmsen & Rozenberg 1968) and rapidly during metabolic stress, such as that caused by

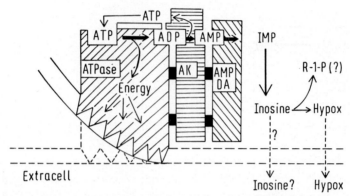

FIG. 3. Schematic illustration showing the contractile element (ATPase, see Fig. 2) bound to adenylate kinase (AK) which in turn is bound to AMP deaminase (AMP DA). When activated the contractile element hydrolyses ATP to ADP and changes the form of the membrane. The ADP produced is not set free, but captured by AK, of which the active site is located in close vicinity to the locus on the ATPase where ADP is released. AK delivers one product, ATP, close to the ATP-binding site on the ATPase, and the other product, AMP, is not set free in solution but delivered directly to the active site of AMP DA. The product of the AMP DA reaction, IMP, is set free in the cytoplasm and degraded via inosine to hypoxanthine. It is unclear whether inosine can leave the cell, or has to be broken down to hypoxanthine + ribose-1-phosphate (R-1-P) before the hypoxanthine nucleus diffuses through the membrane.

incubating platelets with 2-deoxyglucose plus antimycin A (Holmsen *et al.* 1974) or by treating washed platelets with Ca^{2+} (Holmsen, unpublished). Release does not occur under either of these circumstances. Furthermore, incubation of washed platelets with antimycin does not affect the release ability, but inhibits the conversion of AMP to IMP for unexplained reasons (Fukami & Holmsen, unpublished). This strongly indicates that deamination of AMP is not necessary for release and raises doubt about whether the coupled enzyme system in Fig. 3 energizes release.

ATP-HYPOXANTHINE CONVERSION AS A 'NON-COMPENSATION' PHENOMENON

Ball *et al.* (1969) have shown that more metabolic ATP is converted to IMP and hypoxanthine during the release reaction when glycolysis and respiration are inhibited than when ATP regeneration is undisturbed. This suggests that ATP resynthesis *during* release is of importance for the degree of conversion of ATP to hypoxanthine. Thus, as illustrated in Fig. 4, if more ATP is consumed in the release-supporting contraction process than is immediately compensated for through ATP resynthesis via glycolysis and oxidative phosphorylation, this ATP would be converted to AMP and further degraded via IMP to hypoxan-

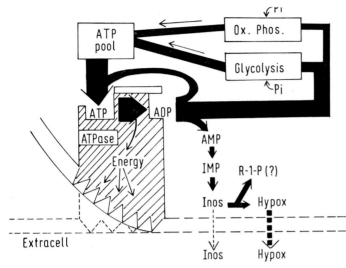

FIG. 4. Schematic illustration showing the contractile element (see Fig. 2) in the activated state, hydrolysing ATP to ADP which is set free and available for rephosphorylation in glycolysis and oxidative phosphorylation. The ADP that is not immediately rephosphorylated is seen to be converted into ATP and AMP (adenylate kinase). Accumulation of AMP is prevented by AMP deaminase which deaminates AMP to IMP, and further degradation to hypoxanthine, which diffuses out of the cell, is shown.

thine. Therefore, the ATP–hypoxanthine conversion represents the ATP used but *not compensated for* through ATP resynthesis during the release process itself. It is well known that platelet glycolysis and respiration are stimulated after treatment of platelets with agents causing the release reaction (Warshaw *et al.* 1966; Karpatkin 1967; Detwiler 1972). Detwiler (1972) has shown that the rates of glycogenolysis and glycolysis increased 2.5 and 10 seconds, respectively, after addition of thrombin to rat platelets; he suggested that this burst in metabolism was a result of an increase in intracellular Ca^{2+} (phosphorylase activation) and a decrease in the adenylate energy charge (phosphofructokinase activation).

We have correlated the time course of release I and II with that of the ATP–hypoxanthine conversion and lactate production in washed platelets treated with thrombin (Fukami & Holmsen, unpublished). In these experiments the exact size of the metabolic adenine nucleotide pool was determined as total platelet adenine nucleotides minus that released by thrombin under optimal conditions, and shown to be 12.5 nmol/mg protein. With no metabolic inhibitors present, about 2 nmol metabolic ATP was consumed within the first 10 seconds of the platelet–thrombin interaction, without significant increase in the lactate production. However, after 30 seconds the steady-state ATP level had decreased by 4 nmol/mg protein and the lactate produced was 10 nmol/mg protein above the control. After 60 seconds, when release I and II were terminated, these values were 5 and 15 nmol/mg protein, respectively. After release was terminated, the ATP level decreased slowly by 1 nmol/mg protein in the next four minutes, and the rate of lactate production was only slightly greater than the control. This indicates that the onset of the increased lactate production occurs early during the release period and that it might be initiated by the change in the adenylate energy charge occurring within the first 10 seconds of the reaction, as was suggested by Holmsen *et al.* (1969) and Detwiler (1972). Our studies show that the greatest burst in anaerobic ATP resynthesis occurs between the 10th and 60th second of the interaction, and little difference from controls was found *after* release had been terminated.

The amounts of ATP resynthesized per mole lactate are 2 and 3 moles for glucose and glycogen as substrates respectively. The variations with time in the ATP equivalents (above control) synthesized and in the steady-state level of metabolic ATP during the platelet–thrombin interaction are shown in Fig. 5. Clearly, the amounts of ATP consumed through the ATP–hypoxanthine conversion are minute compared with those produced through glycolysis. Actually, within the first 30 seconds, during which 90% release is achieved, the entire ATP pool has turned over two or three times, depending on whether glucose or glycogen is the substrate, respectively. These results favour the non-compensation phenomenon illustrated in Fig. 4. It is possible that *all* ATP synthesized during release is used for the release process, at the expense of other processes in the cell that continuously use ATP in the resting state. From our experiments this would mean 30% more ATP is produced than that given in Fig. 5. In addition, ATP is also produced through oxidative phosphorylation, although a major part of the burst in O_2 uptake occurring during the thrombin–platelet interaction appears not to be linked to mitochondrial respiration (Mürer 1968). Nevertheless, it is reasonable to assume that more ATP is resynthesized during release than is apparent from Fig. 5, and that the ATP–hypoxanthine conversion represents a very small fraction of the ATP consumed.

IS ATP ACTUALLY CONSUMED IN REACTIONS DIRECTLY CONNECTED WITH RELEASE DURING THE RELEASE PROCESS?

The platelet functions of shape change, aggregation and release I are all completely inhibited by lowering the steady-state level of metabolic ATP by incubation of platelets with metabolic inhibitors (Holmsen *et al.* 1974). However, the ability to perform individual functions disappears at different degrees

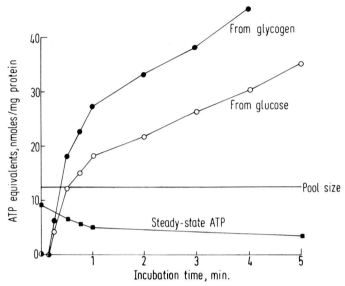

FIG. 5. Production of ATP, based on lactate measurements and assuming glucose or glycogen as substrates, during incubation of washed platelets (Holmsen & Day 1970) with thrombin at 37 °C. The platelets had been incubated with [³H]adenine before washing, and the variation of the radioactivity of ATP during the thrombin–platelet interaction was assumed to be due to variation in the steady-state level of intracellular, metabolic ATP. The size of the metabolic pool was determined as the difference between the total platelet ATP content and that release-able by excess thrombin. Amounts and radioactivity of ATP were measured as described elsewhere (Holmsen et al. 1972). Lactate was determined with lactate hydrogenase in the presence of hydrazine. Platelet protein was 8 mg/ml. The data are from recent experiments in our laboratory (M. H. Fukami & H. Holmsen, to be published).

of reduction in the ATP level. Further experiments (Holmsen, unpublished) have shown that release I and release II also differ in their requirement for metabolic ATP, with release II requiring higher ATP concentrations than release I. As shown in Table 2, thrombin, collagen and adrenaline give the same degree of ATP–hypoxanthine conversion. Thrombin and collagen induce release I and II, whereas adrenaline induces only release I. Thus, even if release II requires the *presence* of more ATP than release I, the same degree of ATP–hypoxanthine conversion takes place in the two processes. However, without knowing exactly the turnover of ATP specifically during release I and II, one does not know whether the same amount of ATP is consumed in the two instances. The apparent requirement of ATP above different levels for the various platelet functions might reflect the differences in K_m for the ATPase involved in the particular function. But it might also reflect a priority of ATP usage within the platelet; that is, when the ATP supply decreases, as during

TABLE 2

Thrombin-, collagen- and adrenaline-induced release I, release II and reduction in steady-state level of metabolic ATP in gel-filtered platelets

	Thrombin	Collagen	Adrenaline
	%	%	%
Release I (ATP + ADP)	35	33	32
Release II (β-N-acetylglucosaminidase)	31	31	4
ATP* decrease	46	45	39

Human platelet-rich plasma (6.16×10^8 cells/ml) was labelled with [^{3}H]adenine (Holmsen et al. 1972) and gel-filtered (Lages et al. 1975). Portions of the gel-filtered platelets obtained (2.36×10^8 cells/ml) were stirred in a Payton aggregometer with 1 unit/ml of thrombin, 91 μg/ml of collagen, 5 μM of adrenaline, and 0.9 % NaCl (control). Samples for determination of radioactive metabolites, i.e. metabolic ATP (Holmsen et al. 1972), were prepared immediately before addition of the release inducer and after release was terminated (3 min). After this last sample was prepared the incubation mixtures were centrifuged at 20000 g and ATP and ADP (Holmsen et al. 1972) and β-N-acetylglucosaminidase (4-Me-umbelliferone-β-N-acetylglucosaminide as substrate) were determined in the supernatants. The numbers give the % release (of total) and the decrease in radioactive ATP (ATP*) in % of initial values.

inhibition of ATP regeneration, some processes are regarded as 'less important' than others by the platelet, and their ATP supply is the first to be shut off. Thus, the meaning of different ATP level requirements for the various functions is uncertain.

When the release reaction was induced at different temperatures, 37 °C and 28°C (Fig. 6), approximately the same degree of release I was obtained, but the degree of ATP–hypoxanthine conversion at the lower temperature was four times smaller than at the higher temperature. No stimulation of lactate production *during* release was seen at the lower temperature. The total production of ATP from lactate during release was nine times less at 28 °C than at 37 °C. Under these circumstances there is a poor correlation among ATP–hypoxanthine conversion, anaerobic ATP production and release capacity.

Similarly, when release was measured at 37 °C in the presence of antimycin, the usual decrease in the steady-state level of ATP took place, but without any stimulation of lactate production (Fukami & Holmsen, unpublished). As noted above, antimycin has little, if any, effect on the release capacity and under this condition there is no contribution to ATP resynthesis from oxidative phosphorylation.

These experiments, and the finding of great variability in lactate production and ATP–hypoxanthine conversion from experiment to experiment, raise some doubt as to whether ATP actually is utilized *during* release. The requirement for a continuous production of ATP does not necessarily mean that ATP is needed

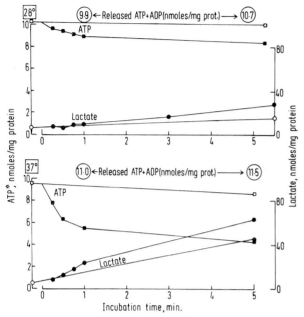

FIG. 6. Lactate production and variation in steady-state levels of metabolic ATP (ATP*) were measured during platelet–thrombin interaction at 37 °C and 28 °C. The experiment was performed as outlined in Fig. 5. Platelet protein was 9.1 mg/ml. Thrombin (5 μ/ml), ●, ■; control, ○, □.

for utilization *during* a particular function. The need could result just as well from ATP usage in processes taking place continuously in the *resting* platelet— that is, before the release reaction. These processes could be called 'maintenance of responsiveness' and should, according to the above, require different levels of metabolic ATP, and depend on the specific platelet function for which the responsiveness is maintained.

How can contraction, which requires ATP, be involved in the release reaction, if ATP is not utilized during the process? Is energy stored in the resting state and released upon stimulus? It has been shown (Yamada *et al.* 1973; Schliselfeld & Kaldor 1973; Marston & Tregar 1974) that the myosin-catalysed hydrolysis of ATP involves a myosin–ADP complex, and that the splitting of this complex is the rate-limiting step in the contraction cycle. Actually, the actomyosin–ADP complex can be regarded as an energy-storing complex of actomyosin. In platelets this complex is present in the insoluble material after ethanol ex- traction of the cells (French & Wachowicz 1974) and ADP can be extracted from the insoluble material by perchloric acid (Holmsen & Day 1971). This ethanol-insoluble ADP fraction does not change during the release reaction

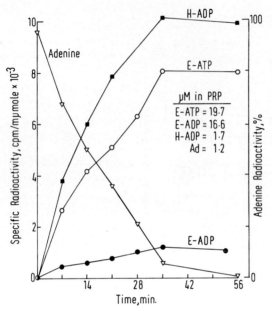

FIG. 7. [³H]Adenine was incubated with citrated human platelet-rich plasma (PRP) (6.2 × 10⁸ platelets/ml) at 37 °C for the times shown, and the specific radioactivity of ethanol-soluble (E) and -insoluble (H) ATP and ADP was determined as described elsewhere (Holmsen *et al.* 1974).

induced by thrombin (French & Wachowicz 1974), which is to be expected if all sites for ADP in the actomyosin molecule are fully saturated with ADP, as seems to be the case for skeletal muscle actomyosin (Marston & Tregar 1974). However, as shown in Fig. 7, when [³H]adenine is taken up by resting platelets, the specific radioactivity of ethanol-insoluble ADP increases in parallel with that of ATP and ADP in the ethanol-soluble fraction. The specific radioactivity of the ethanol-insoluble ADP is about 10 times higher than that of the ethanol-soluble ADP (mixture of metabolic and non-metabolic ADP), strongly indicating that after disruption of the cells with ethanol there are no further exchanges between the soluble fraction of the metabolic pool and the actomyosin-bound ADP. Therefore, exchange of radioactivity between these nucleotide fractions must have taken place *before extraction, in the intact, resting cell.* This could mean that the actomyosin-bound ADP is turning over in the resting state; that is, that ATP energy is constantly consumed in contraction or energy-storing processes. It is therefore possible that the energy-consuming part of the release reaction takes place in the resting cell, and that the energy is stored as a sort of mechanical energy that is not liberated until the cell is activated. Such a mechanism could be likened to a spring that is held in a stretched or

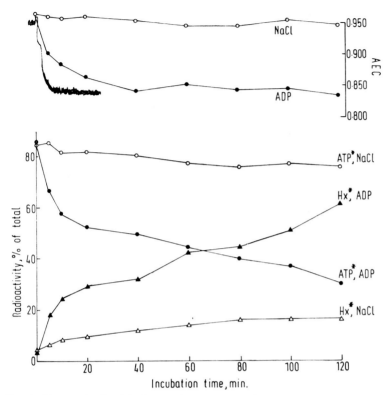

FIG. 8. Human platelet-rich plasma (citrate, 4.1×10^8 cells/ml) was labelled with [³H]adenine and one portion (ADP) was stirred with 4 μM-ADP and another (NaCl) with 0.9% NaCl in a Payton two-channel aggregometer at 37 °C. Samples were taken out of the stirred mixtures at the times indicated for measurement of adenine metabolite radioactivity. The tracing in the upper left corner is the aggregometer tracing obtained in the portion stirred with ADP, and has been omitted after secondary aggregation, after which there was no further change in optical density. The figure shows the total radioactivity of ATP (ATP*) and hypoxanthine (Hx*) in the lower panel, and the adenylate energy charge (AEC) in the upper panel. Methods described elsewhere (Holmsen *et al.* 1972, 1974) were used.

compressed position by energy-requiring processes that go on constantly, and the energy stored is liberated by 'unhooking' the spring. In light of the 'inverted pseudopod' hypothesis (Fig. 1, p. 180) it is therefore of interest that Durham (1974) in a recent review on the function of actomyosin in non-muscle cells regards the resting cell as being in the contracted state, whereas pseudopod formation results from relaxation.

THE DISTURBANCE PHENOMENON

If the ATP-consuming part of the release reaction does not take place during release, what causes the ATP–hypoxanthine conversion and increase in lactate

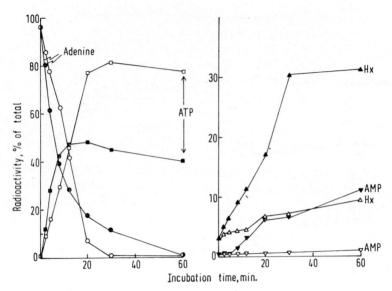

FIG. 9. Two portions of human platelet-rich plasma (citrate, 4.8×10^8 cells/ml) were stirred with 5 μM-adrenaline (filled symbols) or 0.9% NaCl (open symbols) in a Payton two-channel aggregometer at 37 °C. After secondary aggregation was completed in the adrenaline-containing portion, 0.8 μM [³H]adenine was added to both portions and samples were taken from both portions of platelet-rich plasma at the times indicated and analysed for radioactive metabolites. The variation with time in the total radioactivity of ATP, AMP, hypoxanthine (Hx) and adenine is shown. Methods are described by Holmsen *et al.* (1972).

production during the release reaction? Fig. 8 shows the variation in the levels of metabolic ATP and hypoxanthine during and after the release reaction induced by ADP in platelet-rich plasma. During the biphasic aggregation the level of metabolic ATP decreases and that of hypoxanthine increases rapidly, but after secondary aggregation (= release reaction) is terminated, the ATP and hypoxanthine levels continue to decrease and increase respectively, although more slowly than during release. The changes in ATP and hypoxanthine after release are distinctly greater than in control platelets (Fig. 8). It is noteworthy that the adenylate energy charge (Atkinson & Walton 1967) decreases during release, and does not return to that of control platelets after release, but decreases slowly and in parallel to that in the control platelets. This indicates that after release, processes in the cell are activated that keep the adenylate energy charge constant, despite the fall in ATP. The inability of platelets to maintain constant levels of ATP after release is further substantiated by the increased uptake of adenine in platelets that have undergone secondary aggregation and release; far less ATP and more IMP, AMP and hypoxanthine are formed from adenine than in non-aggregated platelets (Fig. 9).

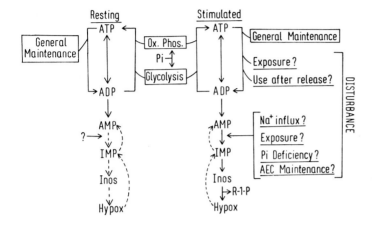

FIG. 10. Possible reactions causing conversion of ATP to IMP and hypoxanthine without utilization of ATP energy in the release process (see text). AEC, adenylate energy charge.

Thus, during the release reaction, alterations in the activity of the enzymes that maintain constant ATP levels must have occurred, which might be referred to as a 'disturbance phenomenon'. This is illustrated in Fig. 10, which indicates specific alterations that may account for the ATP–hypoxanthine conversion. These include exposure of ATPases, both those connected with the utilization of ATP energy as well as 'non-specific' ATPases. The control step in the conversion of ATP to hypoxanthine is AMP deaminase. The platelet enzyme is poorly activated by K^+, but powerfully stimulated by Na^+; it is inhibited by P_i and shows a great dependence on pH with a sharp pH optimum around pH 6.5 (Holmsen, unpublished). Although it has not been established for the platelet enzyme, the AMP deaminase from liver increases rapidly in activity as the adenylate energy charge decreases below 0.93 (Chapman & Atkinson 1973). Several factors, such as a rapid influx of Na^+ (Feinberg et al. 1974), a decrease in intracellular pH, the removal of P_i and exposure of the enzyme from a latent form in the resting cell, might therefore regulate the activity of AMP deaminase during the release reaction (Fig. 10). The exposure of both ATPases and AMP deaminase from latent forms is feasible, because with the great morphological changes taking place during release, enzymes normally shielded from their substrates by binding to subcellular sites might suddenly become exposed to the intracellular milieu.

Fig. 9 also indicates a hitherto unexplored metabolic route by which hypoxanthine is reincorporated into adenine nucleotides. It has recently been shown

(Rivard *et al.* 1975) that hypoxanthine can be taken up slowly by platelets and converted by hypoxanthine phosphoryl transferase into IMP (Jerushalmy *et al.* 1972/73), which is further converted to AMP. In resting platelets this conversion occurs extremely slowly, but it is possible that the reaction is enhanced after release, as is the adenine–ATP conversion (Fig. 9).

The ATP–hypoxanthine conversion connected with the release reaction could, therefore, be a *result* of (morphological?) changes in the platelet during release, rather than a representation of a reaction that energizes either the secretory process or the 'non-compensation phenomenon' discussed above.

RELEASE REACTION INDUCED BY CALCIUM IONOPHORE

If contraction is involved in the release process, and its activation depends on an increase in the concentration of cytosolic Ca^{2+}, release should be initiated by increasing the cytosolic Ca^{2+} concentration artificially. This could be accomplished either by transporting Ca^{2+} from the extracellular medium into platelets by specific calcium ionophores, or by allowing the ionophore to enter the cell and liberate calcium from intracellular stores. Feinman & Detwiler (1974) have demonstrated that A23187 (from Lilly) as well as X-537A (La Roche) in micromolar concentrations release ATP and calcium from washed platelets in the presence of EDTA with a time course closely resembling that obtained with thrombin as release inducer. Table 3 shows that, in addition to

TABLE 3

Release of adenine nucleotides and acid hydrolases from gel-filtered platelets by thrombin and A 23187 and the effect of antimycin A

| Constituents released | Percentage release | | | |
| | Thrombin | | A 23187 | |
	−AA	+AA	−AA	+AA
ATP + ADP	53.5	40.0	50.0	38.6
β-N-Acetylglucosaminidase	31.2	29.6	18.4	12.6
β-Galactosidase	21.6	16.9	6.1	0.7
β-Glucuronidase	24.6	15.3	12.1	8.9
ATP* decrease (%)	30	47	8	20

Human platelet-rich plasma (5.12×10^8 cells/ml) was labelled with [^{3}H]adenine and gel-filtered. Portions of the gel-filtered platelets (2.2×10^8 cells/ml) were incubated at 37 °C for 2 min with thrombin (1 unit/ml), the calcium ionophore, 23187 (1 μM) or 0.9% NaCl in the absence or presence of antimycin A (AA) (3 μg/mg protein). Samples for determination of metabolic radioactivity and released substances were prepared as outlined in Table 2. The *p*-nitrophenylglycosides were used as substrates for the acid hydrolases. The values represent % release (of total) and decrease in metabolic ATP (ATP*) in % of initial value.

inducing release I, the ionophore also induces release II, although to a smaller degree than thrombin. This table also shows that although thrombin and A23187 give the same degree of release I in the absence of antimycin, the decrease in the steady-state level of metabolic ATP during release is considerably smaller with the ionophore than with thrombin. The ionophore could thus have *by-passed* an ATP-requiring step in the release reaction, which suggests that it is the induction step that requires ATP, and not the extrusion step, as proposed above. This is not in accordance with the findings of Mürer (1972) which showed that the induction step can take place at 0 °C, whereas the extrusion step does not occur at this low temperature, but only at elevated temperatures. In agreement with the non-compensation phenomenon discussed above, little change in the steady-state level of ATP would take place if the ATP regeneration were stimulated to such an extent that it completely balanced the usage of ATP. If the ionophore-induced increase in the cytosolic Ca^{2+} concentration both induced contraction and stimulated ATP regeneration (for example, by stimulating glycogenolysis), little reduction in the steady-state ATP levels during release would be expected. It follows from Table 3 that a greater reduction in ATP takes place during release induced with ionophore when ATP regeneration from oxidative phosphorylation is inhibited by antimycin A, than occurs in the absence of antimycin. The reduction in ATP was balanced by an accumulation of IMP and hypoxanthine (values not shown). Mürer (unpublished) has clearly shown that ionophore-induced release can occur with a simultaneous conversion of ATP to IMP and hypoxanthine and that the occurrence of the conversion depends greatly on the conditions used. In the experiment shown in Table 3 gel-filtered platelets were used, with albumin in the extracellular medium. Omission of albumin and the presence of small amounts of extracellular calcium greatly enhance the degree of reduction in steady-state ATP levels (Mürer, unpublished). Mürer has also shown that in the presence of greater concentrations of extracellular Ca^{2+} (0.63 mM-$CaCl_2$ in 10 mM-citrate), 2 μM-A23187 causes cell lysis, an indication of the hazards of using ionophores. He has further shown that IMP is the main metabolite accumulated during ATP degradation when low concentrations of ionophore (0.1 μM) are used, and that part of the IMP is reconverted to ATP.

Thus, in addition to inducing release, the calcium ionophore induces many other effects in the platelet, such as an apparent stimulation of metabolism, lysis under certain circumstances, and stimulation of the IMP–ATP conversion—effects that complicate the study of the involvement of ATP in release. There is no doubt that the ionophore can induce the specific release I and II processes, since the ATP and ADP released from [³H]adenine-labelled platelets in platelet-rich plasma and in suspensions of gel-filtered or conventionally washed platelets have negligible specific radioactivity compared with the retained adenine nucleotides, and thus belong to the non-metabolic pool (Holmsen & Mürer, unpublished). It is also possible that by careful assessment of stimulation of ATP regeneration, calcium ionophores as inducers of the release reaction can be useful tools for further exploration of the involvement of ATP in the secretory process of platelets. So far, the results obtained seem to support the hypothesis (Holmsen *et al.* 1969) that mobilization of calcium intracellularly is part of the release mechanism.

CONCLUSIONS

It seems to be uncertain whether ATP is utilized in processes that are directly involved in the release mechanism *during* the release reaction. If ATP is utilized during release, the amounts required appear to vary widely, and undoubtedly depend on the experimental conditions used. Further research should therefore aim to delineate what and how intrinsic (metabolic status, etc.) or extrinsic (method of preparing platelets, extracellular substances, etc.) factors influence ATP turnover and conversion to IMP and hypoxanthine during release. The possibility that a reduction in the steady-state levels of ATP represents a 'non-compensation' phenomenon is likely and should be pursued further. Another alternative suggested here, that ATP energy is stored in the resting state to be utilized later, during release, is also attractive and could be approached by determining the turnover of ADP in actomyosin-bound ADP under various conditions.

ACKNOWLEDGEMENT

This work was supported by grant no. HL 14217 from the National Heart and Lung Institute.

References

ATKINSON, D. E. & WALTON, G. M. (1967) Adenosine triphosphate conservation in metabolic regulation. Rat liver citrate cleavage enzyme. *J. Biol. Chem. 242*, 3239-3241
BALL, G., FULWOOD, M., IRELAND, D. M. & YATES, P. (1969) Effect of some inhibitors of platelet aggregation on adenine nucleotides. *Biochem. J. 114*, 669-671
CHAPMAN, A. G. & ATKINSON, D. E. (1973) Stabilization of adenylate energy charge by the adenylate deaminase reaction. *J. Biol. Chem. 248*, 8309-8312
DAY, H. J. & HOLMSEN, H. (1971) Concepts of the platelet release reaction. *Ser. Haematol. 4*, 3-27
DETWILER, T. C. (1972) Control of energy metabolism in platelets. The effects of thrombin and cyanide on glycolysis. *Biochim. Biophys. Acta 256*, 163-174
DURHAM, A. C. H. (1974) A unified theory of the control of actin and myosin in nonmuscle movements. *Cell 2*, 123-136

FEINBERG, H., SCORER, M., LEBRETON, G., GROSSMAN, B. & BORN, G. V. R. (1974) ADP-induced ^{22}Na uptake by human platelets. *Circulation 50*, Suppl. III, 277 (abstr.)

FEINMAN, R. D. & DETWILER, T. C. (1974) Platelet secretion induced by divalent cation ionophores. *Nature (Lond.) 249*, 172

FRENCH, P. C. & WACHOWICZ, B. (1974) Investigation of the binding component of the ethanol insoluble metabolic ADP of human platelets and its relation to the release reaction. *Haemostasis 3*, 271-281

GREEN, D. E., MÜRER, E. H., HULTIN, H. O., RICHARDSON, S. H., SALMON, B., BRIERLEY, G. P. & BAUM, H. (1965) Association of integrated metabolic pathways with membranes. I. Glycolytic enzymes of the red blood corpuscle and yeast. *Arch. Biochem. Biophys. 112*, 635-647

GRETTE, K. (1962) Studies on the mechanism of thrombin-catalyzed haemostatic mechanisms in blood platelets. *Acta. Physiol. Scand. 56*, Suppl. 165

HOLME, R., SIXMA, J. J., MÜRER, E. H. & HOVIG, T. (1973) Demonstration of platelet fibrinogen secretion via the surface connecting system. *Thromb. Res. 3*, 347-356

HOLMSEN, H. (1973) Compartmentation of adenine nucleotides in platelets. In *Erythrocytes, Thrombocytes, Leukocytes: Recent Advances in Membrane and Metabolic Research* (Gerlach, E., Moser, K., Deutsch, E. & Wilmans, W., eds.), pp. 228-230, Georg Thieme, Stuttgart

HOLMSEN, H. & DAY, H. J. (1970) The selectivity of the thrombin-induced platelet release reaction: subcellular localization of released and retained substances. *J. Lab. Clin. Med. 75*, 840-855

HOLMSEN, H. & DAY, H. J. (1971) Adenine nucleotides and platelet function. *Ser. Haematol. 4*, 28-58

HOLMSEN, H., DAY, H. J. & STORMORKEN, H. (1969) The blood platelet release reaction. *Scand. J. Haematol.* Suppl. 8, 1-26

HOLMSEN, H., DAY, H. J. & SETKOWSKY, C. A. (1972) Secretory mechanisms: behaviour of adenine nucleotides during the platelet release reaction induced by adenosine diphosphate and adrenaline. *Biochem. J. 129*, 67-82

HOLMSEN, H. & ROZENBERG, M. C. (1968) Adenine nucleotide metabolism of blood platelets. III. Adenine phosphoribosyl transferase and nucleotide formation from exogenous adenine. *Biochim. Biophys. Acta 157*, 266-279

HOLMSEN, H., SETKOWSKY, C. A. & DAY, H. J. (1974) Effects of antimycin and 2-deoxyglucose on adenine nucleotides in human platelets. Role of metabolic ATP in primary aggregation, secondary aggregation and shape change of platelets. *Biochem. J. 144*, 385-396

HOLMSEN, H., SETKOWSKY, C. A., LAGES, B., DAY, H. J., WEISS, H. J. & SCRUTTON, M. C. (1975) Content and thrombin-induced release of acid hydrolases in gel-filtered platelets from patients with storage pool disease. *Blood 46*, 131-142

JERUSHALMY, Z., SPERLING, O., PINKHAS, J., KRYNSKA, M. & DEVRIES, A. (1972/73) Phosphoribosyl pyrophosphate transferase and purine phosphoribosyl transferases in human and rabbit blood platelets. *Haemostasis 1*, 279-284

JOIST, J. H., NIEWIAROWSKI, S., NATH, N. & MUSTARD, J. F. (1975) Platelet antiplasmin: its extrusion during the release reactions, subcellular localization, and relation to platelet antiheparin. *Thromb. Res.*, in press

KARPATKIN, S. (1967) Studies on human platelet glycolysis. Effect of glucose, cyanide, insulin, citrate, and agglutination and contraction on platelet glycolysis. *J. Clin. Invest. 46*, 409-17

KIRSHNER, N. & VIVEROS, O. H. (1972) The secretory cycle in the adrenal medulla. *Pharmacol. Rev. 84*, 385-398

LAGES, B., SCRUTTON, M. C., HOLMSEN, H., DAY, H. J. & WEISS, H. J. (1975) Metal ion contents of gel-filtered platelets from patients with storage pool disease. *Blood 46*, 119-130

MARSTON, S. B. & TREGAR, R. T. (1974) Nucleotide binding to myosin in calcium activated muscle. *Biochim. Biophys. Acta 333*, 581-584

MARTIN, J. H., CARSON, F. L. & RACE, G. J. (1974) Calcium-containing platelet granules. *J. Cell Biol. 60*, 775-777

MÜRER, E. H. (1972) Factors influencing the initiation and the extrusion phase of the platelet release reaction. *Biochim. Biophys. Acta 261*, 435-443

MÜRER, E. H. (1968) Release reaction and energy metabolism in blood platelets with special reference to the burst in oxygen uptake. *Biochim. Biophys. Acta 162*, 320-326

MÜRER, E. H. & HOLME, R. (1970) A study of the release of calcium from human blood platelets and its inhibition by metabolic inhibitors, N-ethylmaleimide and aspirin. *Biochim. Biophys. Acta 222*, 197-205

MUSTARD, J. F. & PACKHAM, M. A. (1970) Factors influencing platelet function: adhesion, release and aggregation. *Pharmacol. Rev. 22*, 97-187

NACHMAN, R. L., WEKSLER, B. & FERRIS, B. (1970) Increased vascular permeability produced by human platelet granule cationic extract. *J. Clin. Invest. 49*, 274-281

NACHMAN, R. L., WEKSLER, B. & FERRIS, B. (1972) Characterization of human platelet vascular permeability-enhancing activity. *J. Clin. Invest. 51*, 549-556

POISNER, A. M. & TRIFARO, J. M. (1967) The role of ATP and ATPase in the release of cate-cholamines from the adrenal medulla. I. ATP evoked release of catecholamines, ATP and protein from isolated chromaffin granules. *Mol. Pharmacol. 3*, 561-571

RIVARD, G. E., BRUNST, R. F., MC LAREN, J. D. & BERGGREN, W. R. (1975) Incorporation of hypoxanthine into adenine and guanine nucleotides by human platelets. *Biochim. Biophys. Acta 381*, 144-156

ROSS, R., GLOMSET, J., KARIYA, B. & HARKER, L. (1974) A platelet-dependent serum factor stimulates the proliferation of arterial smooth muscle cells *in vitro*. *Proc. Natl. Acad. Sci. U.S.A. 71*, 1207-1210

SCHLISELFELD, L. H. & KALDOR, G. J. (1973) Kinetic study of the pre-steady state formation and the decay of the heavy meromyosin adenosine triphosphate complex. *Biochim. Biophys. Acta 328*, 481-490

SILCOX, D. C., JACOBELLI, S. & MCCARTY, D. J. (1973) Identification of inorganic pyro-phosphate in human platelets and its release on stimulation with thrombin. *J. Clin. Invest. 52*, 1595-1604

WALSH, P. N. & GAGNATELLI, G. (1974) Platelet antiheparin activity: storage site and release mechanism. *Blood 44*, 157-168

WARSHAW, A. L., LASTER, L. & SCHULMAN, N. R. (1966) The stimulation by thrombin of glucose oxidation in human platelets. *J. Clin. Invest. 45*, 1923-1934

WEISS, H. J. & AMES, R. P. (1973) Ultrastructural findings in storage pool disease and aspirin-like defects of platelets. *Am. J. Pathol. 71*, 447-460

WEISS, H. J. & ROGERS, J. (1973) Platelet factor 4 in platelet disorders—storage location and the requirement of endogenous ADP for its release. *Proc. Soc. Exp. Biol. Med. 142*, 30-35

WEKSLER, B. B. & COUPAL, C. E. (1973) Platelet-dependent generation of chemotactic activity in serum. *J. Exp. Med. 137*, 1419-1430

WEKSLER, B. B. & NACHMAN, R. L. (1971) Rabbit platelet bactericidal protein. *J. Exp. Med. 134*, 1114-1130

WHITE, J. G. (1971) Platelet morphology. In *The Circulating Platelet* (Johnson, S. A., ed.), pp. 45-121, Academic Press, New York & London

YAMADA, T., SCHIMIZU, H. & SUGA, H. (1973) A kinetic study of the energy storing enzyme product complex in the hydrolysis of ATP by heavy meromyosin. *Biochim. Biophys. Acta 305*, 642-653

ZUCKER, M. B. & GRANT, R. A. (1974) Aggregation and release reaction induced in human blood platelets by zymosan. *J. Immunol. 112*, 1219-1230

ZUCKER-FRANKLIN, D., NACHMAN, R. L. & MARCUS, A. J. (1967) Ultrastructure of throm-bosthenin, the contractile protein of human blood platelets. *Science (Wash. D.C.) 157*, 945-946

Discussion

Feinberg: Is there any evidence of 5'-nucleotidase activity in platelets? 5'-Nucleotidase action on IMP to form inosine would be a possible pathway leading to hypoxanthine, in addition to the pathway you showed.

Holmsen: It is obvious that 5'-nucleotidase is present in platelets, since IMP is converted via inosine to hypoxanthine. However, when the cells are broken up, either by freezing and thawing or by pestle homogenization, the enzyme can be demonstrated, but the activity is *very* small (0.012 nmol/min per mg protein at pH 6.5 in the presence of Mg^{2+} and tartate) and with a 1:4 distribution between membranes and cytosol (Day *et al.* 1969). This small activity is several orders of magnitude lower than that calculated from the IMP–hypoxanthine conversion in the *intact* platelet, which indicates that the activity of this enzyme is particularly dependent on structural integrity.

But I don't think we have to look for other pathways for hypoxanthine formation. The conversion of ATP to hypoxanthine in broken platelets is qualitatively similar to that in the intact cell, but the rate constants for the individual steps are different. You might have the alternative AMP–adenosine–inosine pathway in mind. But although there are large amounts of adenosine deaminase in platelets, we have not been able to demonstrate dephosphorylation of AMP, only deamination or phosphorylation if ATP is present.

Born: I have often wondered what AMP deaminase is for, functionally, unless one supposes that the reaction product is concerned in regulating some other enzyme. Otherwise the reaction seems curiously wasteful.

Feinberg: AMP has been shown to have an excitatory or de-inhibitory effect on glycolysis. Lowenstein (1972) has proposed that the deamination of AMP to IMP in the presence of high ATP levels is a regulatory mechanism to control glycolytic flux.

Holmsen: I think one major purpose of AMP deaminase could be to keep the adenylate energy charge (AEC) constant. According to Chapman & Atkinson (1973) a decrease in AEC activates the deaminase, so that AMP is removed from the system, which results in an *increase* in AEC. However, the effect of the AEC on AMP deaminase has only been demonstrated for the liver enzyme; the effect might be different in other tissues.

Cohen: May I go back to your beautiful scheme for the turnover of ATP in the resting state of the platelet? Your 'hook' concept could be compared to an isometric contractile state maintaining the original discoid shape. But I am not sure whether there is enough evidence for associating release with the contractile process. I know that some people object to the use of cytochalasin B. But here we have a substance which prevents contractile processes and cell motility, probably, as Wessells proposed, by disorganizing microfilaments (Wessells *et al.* 1971). I agree that it does not affect the ATPase activity or superprecipitation of actomyosin from muscle or non-muscle cells, but it might act at the level of microfilament assembly. Cytochalasin B has been shown to prevent clot retraction (Shepro *et al.* 1970; Wessells *et al.* 1971). On the other hand, White (1971) has shown that thrombin-induced release is normal in platelets treated with cytochalasin B; the cells also retain their disk shape. Taking these facts into consideration, it is difficult to associate the release reaction with a contractile process. Moreover, one would expect that in the presence of cytochalasin B, release would occur without consumption of ATP. Have you studied the energetic metabolism of thrombin-induced release in the presence of cytochalasin B?

Holmsen: We have not studied the effect of cytochalasin B on changes in nucleotides during the thrombin–platelet interaction. However, Dr Mills tells me that the drug does not interfere with the adenylate energy charge in concentrations up to 112 μM.

Haslam: If you tried to do what Dr Cohen suggests, you would probably find that cytochalasin B had marked effects even in the absence of thrombin, because of the inhibition of glucose uptake. In my experiments with washed rabbit platelets, cytochalasin B at 8 μM reduced the production of metabolic $^{14}CO_2$ from [6-^{14}C]glucose by about 90% (Haslam 1972). I expect this would affect the adenine nucleotide changes seen on addition of thrombin in much the same way as a metabolic inhibitor and would make any other effects of cytochalasin B on adenine nucleotide metabolism, due for instance to effects on contractile protein function, difficult to detect.

Holmsen: There are of course other hypotheses about secretion than the excitation–secretion theory, which includes contraction. Smith (1971) has proposed the 'hit and stick' hypothesis which does *not* involve contraction. In the resting state the storage granules are in Brownian motion and hit the plasma membrane constantly. But they do not stick. When the cell is stimulated to release, the properties of the membrane change in such a way that when a granule hits, it will stick. Fusion of the plasma and granule membranes now follows automatically and the stored material diffuses out to the extracellular space. This theory has recently been questioned by Poste & Allison (1973), since the distance between membranes brought together by Brownian movement is too far to allow membrane fusion.

Haslam: This hypothesis is not inconsistent with the view that cytochalasin B promotes secretion by disrupting submembrane microfilaments, which in the unstimulated cell may prevent access of granules to the plasma membrane (Orci *et al.* 1972).

You discussed the ADP which is bound to thrombosthenin. I would not have expected this complex to survive treatment with ethanol.

Holmsen: It does, though. French & Wachowicz (1974) have purified actomyosin from platelets and this is precipitated by 43% ethanol with ADP attached.

Haslam: Are you sure this ADP is on the myosin and is not the ADP that is bound to F-actin?

Holmsen: We prepared acetone powders from platelets and extracted G-actin from this material by solutions with low ionic strength. No ADP was attached to the actin solubilized. Furthermore, when platelets are lysed in water, little ethanol-insoluble ADP is present compared to that in lysate in 0.3 or 0.6 M-KCl. Finally, after precipitation of the protein–ADP complex with 43% ethanol, most of the ADP is solubilized when the precipitate is treated with water (Holmsen 1972). This indicates that the metabolic ADP is not bound to actin.

I would like to add that when platelet actomyosin dissolved in 0.6 M-KCl is incubated with labelled ATP or ADP the ADP–actomyosin complex that can be precipitated with ethanol does not become labelled. It is *only* when the *intact* platelets contain nucleotides that the complex contains labelled ADP.

Nachman: Do you know what the relative affinity of the binding is, even if you don't know what is in the ethanol-insoluble fraction?

Holmsen: No, not yet.

Adelstein: A recent paper by Puszkin & Kochwa (1974) suggests, but by no means establishes, than an actin–relaxing factor complex, isolated from rat brain, interacts with synaptic vesicles of rat brain to release [14C]glutamate.

Crawford: Is it conceivable that Dr Holmsen's proposed sequence of events could be just as readily sustained by the Ca^{2+}-ATPase activity of unassociated myosin, not necessarily involved in a contractile complex with thin filament structures? Our current view is that the soluble phase of the platelet is a valid compartment for a significant quantity of the cell's myosin and this is present as both monomer and dimer. The equilibrium between those two forms can be directionally influenced by various factors, but in particular by the proximity of F-actin and ATP (Harris & Crawford 1975; Cove & Crawford 1975). We believe that this aggregation may be the nucleating mechanism for thick filament synthesis.

Holmsen: Yes. The ATPase action of unassociated myosin could as well have been responsible for the changes seen. However, I am not sure about the characteristics of the myosin–ADP (product) complex of free myosin—whether it is ethanol-insoluble and so on.

Shepro: Tubulin was mentioned earlier (p. 171) by Dr Crawford, and in a model system which ties adenine nucleotides to platelet structural proteins, it would be unwise to restrict the protein to actomyosin. Dr Holmsen said that early in the release reaction the granules come together in the centre of the platelets, and some change also takes place to the microtubules in that they appear to move from the periphery to the centre of the platelet. We and others have evidence that thrombin produces significant increases in colchicine uptake and binding and that colchicine binding is also increased during clot retraction; activities which directly implicate microtubules (Shepro *et al.* 1969; Chao *et al.* 1970; F. C. Chao, J. L. Tullis, D. Shepro & F. A. Belamarich, unpublished; D. M. Kenny, F. C. Chao, J. L. Tullis & G. S. Conneely, personal communication).

Lüscher: It is perhaps not quite justified to assign to the contractile system the entire responsibility for the observed alterations in nucleotide metabolism. In fact, many things happen at the same time: the resting potential breaks down; ions cross the originally almost impermeable membrane; microtubules are depolymerized, and, partly as a consequence of the altered ionic environment in the cytoplasm, an unknown number of enzyme systems will become activated or inhibited. To single out just one of these many systems is probably not quite correct.

Adelstein: I agree with Dr Lüscher's point, and I suspect that someone taking into account both microtubular proteins and contractile proteins in a process so overwhelming as the 'release reaction' may come closer to the truth than someone looking at one of these protein complexes alone.

Born: Dr Holmsen, might there be an analogy with erythrocytes? Their normal, biconcave shape is maintained as long as they contain enough ATP. It is a very static, curious shape to maintain. When the ATP is lowered, by whatever means, red cells become more spherical and crenated and this change is reversed by increasing the amount of ATP in the cells. Does this change necessarily imply that ATP is used up in the cells' contractile protein mechanism? Or could it be due to the disappearance of a structural function of ATP? That is, the shape of the normal cell may depend, among other things, on ATP bound in the membrane which becomes deformed when that ATP disappears.

Holmsen: In the red cell it has been shown that contractile proteins are present in the membrane (Marchesi *et al.* 1969) that might be responsible for maintaining the shape of this cell. Durham (1974) has recently suggested that contractile processes are continuously going on in all cells to maintain their proper shape and that the pressure inside the cell is higher than outside. The formation of pseudopods, in his opinion, is the result of relaxation, caused by a cut-off in energy (ATP) supply. He also has used the model I showed for exocytosis where the granules are anchored with contractile threads.

Sneddon: There is indirect evidence for this in the blood platelet. If you fix blood platelets for electron microscopy at 36 °C they are discoid with no pseudopodia. If you cool platelets and fix them at 0 °C, or if you poison them with dinitrophenol and sodium fluoride and then fix them at 0 °C, the cells are round and thick protuberances are seen on the surface. This would imply that the normal discoid shape requires energy for its maintenance.

If you poison platelets with metabolic inhibitors, or cool them to 4 °C, the bands of microtubules can no longer be observed.

Cohen: However, after stimulating platelets with aggregating agents you still see microtubules. You can see them in the pseudopodia.

Sneddon: In the resting state platelet microtubules form a circumferential band, and when the cell is stimulated they move towards the centre of the cell (White 1968; Sneddon 1971). This is easy to visualize. But what of the microtubules in the pseudopodia? Are they separate from the circular band of microtubules or do they represent some realignment of the circular band?

Cohen: When you take into consideration the centripetal movement of the microtubules during shape change, there appears to be a loss of structural matter. In fact it is found in the pseudopodia, following a possible rearrangement. So there is indeed conservation of structural matter!

Feinberg: The well-known action of Mg^{2+}-ATP in keeping actin and myosin dissociated may be pertinent. Thus, as long as ATP levels are kept high actin and myosin do not interact and the disk shape is maintained. Utilization of ATP leading to a depletion to a critical level may then permit the formation of actomyosin and the ensuing contractile events.

Shepro: Dr Holmsen, you mentioned that platelets don't have a recovery phase yet you showed in the model the extrusion of a granule which then refills. Isn't that recovery?

Holmsen: This must be a misunderstanding. I didn't intend to show a granule that was refilled after extrusion. We thought until six months ago that granules which had emptied their contents through the release reaction were not able to refill again. However, recently H. F. Reimers, J. F. Mustard & M. A. Packham (personal communication) have demonstrated that the adenine nucleotides in the granules and cytosol do exchange, although slowly. Whether this also indicates that an emptied granule can be refilled, I doubt; it has to be established. So I believe that circulating platelets hardly refill with calcium and adenine nucleotides.

Shepro: Perhaps only certain granules cannot be reutilized? Since the platelet carries many secretory substances, and if preferential release is a physiological phenomenon, it would be reasonable to assume that platelets have a recovery stage—even for calcium and nucleotides. Perhaps, as suggested by several investigators, platelet granules are at different stages of development, and the ability of a granule to store is a function of its development.

Holmsen: Professor Pletscher showed that ATP enters the granules in the megakaryocyte but not in the circulating platelets (see Pletscher & Da Prada, this volume, pp. 261–279).

Pletscher: In relation to that, do we have any idea of what happens to the granular membranes? According to your scheme, the contents are expelled. Are the granular membranes incorporated into the cytoplasmic membrane, or are they reutilized to form new granules, or what happens? Are there specific membrane markers—perhaps the Mg^{2+}-dependent ATPase?

Holmsen: White (1971) has already clearly demonstrated that the number of apparent 'vacuoles' is greater after release than before. However, many of the new 'vacuoles' are not vacuoles but transected channels—that is, invaginations of the plasma membrane. Whether the number of 'true' vacuoles has increased is uncertain, but some of the 'new' true vacuoles might be the emptied granules. Since the granules moved inwards, they do not become a part of the membrane at the circumference of the platelet, but might be parts of the channels in the interior of the cell, as I showed (Fig. 1, p. 180).

Mustard: Did I understand you to say that these platelet changes indicate that the platelet is on its way to destruction?

Holmsen: No, I didn't imply that.

Mustard: The experimental conditions have to be taken into account here. As I indicated earlier (p. 96), if one treats platelets with thrombin in order to release most of their 5HT and storage pool nucleotides, and recovers them, they go back to the disk shape; they respond normally to ADP; they circulate on reinfusion into an animal. There must be some restoration of their metabolism to normal. The study of platelet metabolism *in vitro* can be influenced by a number of factors; platelets in suspending media other than tissue culture medium with protein show alterations in metabolism that are due to the suspending medium (Doery *et al.* 1973). Furthermore, you are also faced with the effects of the released materials on the platelet if you do not suspend them in fresh medium. I wonder if you could try another experiment, which may also answer the question about granule resynthesis or rebuilding. Infuse thrombin-treated rabbit platelets into a thrombocytopenic rabbit and remove samples for metabolic studies after various times. This might give more specific answers about metabolism without the complexity of long incubations *in vitro*.

Holmsen: I agree that the intact animal is the best medium for the platelet. The fact that platelets that have been emptied of their granular contents have a normal survival when reinfused into animals shows, as you say, that they must have regained a normal metabolism. This is to be expected from the compartmentation of the adenine nucleotides, but not from the two experiments I showed (Figs. 8 and 9, pp. 189 and 190), where the metabolic pool continued to disappear long after the release reaction had been terminated. These experiments were done in citrated plasma and not with washed platelets, as you inferred. However, it is a very good idea to try to study the metabolic adenine nucleotides in platelets that have been through a release reaction and then reinfused into an animal.

Mills: Does aspirin have any effect on the metabolic changes that you observe during the release reaction? Is there any change in the pattern of metabolite accumulation?

Holmsen: I take it you are asking what changes may occur in aspirin-treated platelets when high thrombin or collagen concentrations are used. I am afraid we never did that experiment, but it will be done! With aspirin you have to distinguish between two extreme situations. One is when aspirin completely inhibits the release reaction, such as when one uses ADP, adrenaline and low concentrations of collagen. The other situation is when the aspirin inhibition is completely overcome by the use of high concentrations of inducer, which can be achieved with high concentrations of thrombin or collagen. Aspirin *per se* does *not* alter the levels of metabolic adenine nucleotides. With complete inhibition of release there is *no* conversion of ATP to hypoxanthine, as shown by Ireland's group (Ball *et al.* 1969) and by us (Holmsen *et al.* 1972). This indicates that aspirin inhibits a step before that involved in the ATP–hypoxanthine conversion.

Feinberg: With respect to the early events in platelet activation, we measured the uptake of ^{22}Na by platelets after adding ADP (Feinberg *et al.* 1974*b*). Platelets in plasma were incubated at 37 °C with ^{125}I-labelled human serum albumin as a marker of trapped plasma and with ^{22}NaCl. The platelets were separated by sedimentation through silicone oil (Feinberg *et al.* 1974*a*) and both ^{125}I and ^{22}Na activity were determined on the platelet pellet and on the platelet-free plasma. Using this technique we were able to measure the total ^{22}Na space (the volume occupied by the ^{22}Na in the platelet pellet calculated on the basis of the ^{22}Na concentration in the plasma) and the ^{22}Na space in the platelet (the total ^{22}Na space minus the ^{22}Na in the trapped plasma). ADP-induced aggregation led to a dose-related increase in the ^{22}Na space followed by a decrease toward the pre-ADP level; GDP had no effect. On the other hand, ^{36}Cl as NaCl did not increase after ADP—an indication that only the ^{22}Na entered the platelet. Earlier experiments (Feinberg *et al.* 1974*a*) showed that ADP-induced aggregation is not associated with an increase in platelet volume; hence it is likely that ^{22}Na entered the platelet in relation to a membrane destabilization process rather than as part of a swelling process involving the uptake of NaCl and water. If the platelets were pre-treated with ouabain (10^{-6}M) the ADP-induced increase in ^{22}Na space did not decline but continued to rise.

Nachman: What is the time sequence with respect to the magnitude of the shape change?

Feinberg: Centrifugation over silicone oil takes at least 10–15 seconds; therefore we are not able to resolve the initial rates at 37 °C. We are attempting to make measurements at reduced temperatures and in circumstances where aggregation does not occur, in order to determine whether the ^{22}Na uptake is associated with shape change.

Mills: Is ^{22}Na taken up in the presence of EDTA?

Feinberg: So far we have only tried EGTA and have found uptake of ^{22}Na in a few of these experiments. More experiments will be needed for a definite answer to be possible.

Mills: I once by mistake resuspended platelets in isotonic Tris-hydrochloride and then aggregated them with ADP. I couldn't see whether there was a shape change, but they certainly aggregated.

Feinberg: Your point is that the platelets aggregated despite the absence of Na^+. Professor Born and his co-workers (1972) showed earlier that the velocity of aggregation was the same in platelet-rich plasma dialysed against a choline-Tyrode mixture as in normal platelet-rich plasma. I don't think this procedure gets rid of all of the sodium. (We have recently shown [W. Sandler, G. LeBreton & H. Feinberg, unpublished 1975] that resuspension of human platelets in choline-containing Tyrode's solution leads to complete inhibition of ADP-induced aggregation.)

References

BALL, G., FULWOOD, M., IRELAND, D. M. & YATES, P. (1969) Effect of some inhibitors of platelet aggregation on adenine nucleotides. *Biochem. J. 114*, 669-671

BORN, G. V. R., JUENGJAROEN, K. & MICHAL, F. (1972) Relative activities on and uptake by human blood platelets of 5-hydroxytryptamine and several analogues. *Br. J. Pharmacol. 44*, 117-139

CHAO, F. C., SHEPRO, D. & YAO, F. (1970) Clot retraction. II. Theoretical model of platelet filamentogenesis. *Microvasc. Res. 2*, 61-66

CHAPMAN, A. G. & ATKINSON, D. E. (1973) Stabilization of adenylate energy charge by the adenylate deaminase reaction. *J. Biol. Chem. 248*, 8306-8308

COVE, D. H. & CRAWFORD, N. (1975) Platelet contractile proteins: separation and characterisation of the actin and myosin-like components. *J. Mechanochem. Cell Motility 3*, 123-134

DAY, H. J., HOLMSEN, H. & HOVIG, T. (1969) Subcellular particles of human platelets. *Scand. J. Haematol.* Suppl. 7

DOERY, J. C. G., HIRSH, J. & MUSTARD, J. F. (1973) Energy metabolism in washed human platelets responsive to ADP: comparison with platelets in plasma. *Br. J. Haematol. 25*, 657-673

Durham, A. C. H. (1974) A unified theory of the control of actin and myosin in nonmuscle movements. *Cell 2*, 123-136

Feinberg, H., Michel, H. & Born, G. V. R. (1974a) Determination of the fluid volume of platelets by their separation through silicone oil. *J. Lab. Clin. Med. 84*, 926-934

Feinberg, H., Scorer, M., LeBreton, G. & Born, G. V. R. (1974b) ADP-induction of ^{22}Na uptake by platelets. *Circulation 50*, 1059

French, P. C. & Wachowicz, B. (1974) Investigations of the binding component of the ethanol insoluble metabolic ADP of human platelets and its relation to the release reaction. *Haemostasis 3*, 271-281

Harris, G. L. A. & Crawford, N. (1975) The identification and subcellular localization of thrombosthenin 'M'; the myosin-like component of pig platelet. *J. Mechanochem. Cell Motility 3*, 135-145

Haslam, R. J. (1972) Inhibition of blood platelet function by cytochalasins: effects on thrombosthenin and on glucose metabolism. *Biochem. J. 127*, 34P

Holmsen, H. (1972) Ethanol-insoluble adenine nucleotides in platelets and their possible role in platelet function. *Ann. N.Y. Acad. Sci. 201*, 109-121

Holmsen, H., Day, H. J. & Setkowsky, C. A. (1972) Secretory mechanisms. Behaviour of adenine nucleotides during the platelet release reaction induced by adenosine diphosphate and adrenaline. *Biochem. J. 129*, 67-82

Lowenstein, J. M. (1972) Ammonia production in muscle and other tissues: the purine nucleotide cycle. *Physiol. Rev. 52*, 382-414

Marchesi, V. T., Sheers, E., Tillack, T. W. & Marchesi, S. L. (1969) in *Red Cell Membrane, Structure and Function* (Jamieson, G. A. & Greenwalt, T. J., eds.), pp. 117-130, Lippincott, Philadelphia-Toronto

Orci, L., Gabbay, K. H. & Malaisse, W. J. (1972) Pancreatic beta-cell web: its possible role in insulin secretion. *Science (Wash. D.C.) 175*, 1128-1130

Pletscher, A. & Da Prada, M. (1975) This volume, pp. 261-279

Poste, G. & Allison, A. C. (1973) Membrane fusion. *Biochim. Biophys. Acta 300*, 421-503

Puszkin, S. & Kochwa, S. (1974) Regulation of neurotransmitter release by a complex of actin with relaxing protein isolated from rat brain synaptosomes. *J. Biol. Chem. 249*, 7711-7714

Shepro, D., Belamarich, F. A. & Chao, F. C. (1969) Clot retraction following platelet incubation with colchicine and heavy water. *Nature (Lond.) 221*, 453-454

Shepro, D., Belamarich, F. A., Robblee, L. & Chao, F. C. (1970) Antimotility effect of cytochalasin B observed in mammalian clot retraction. *J. Cell Biol. 47*, 544-547

Smith, A. D. (1971) Summing up: some implications of the neuron as a secreting cell. *Philos. Trans. R. Soc. Lond. B. Biol. Sci. 261*, 423

Sneddon, J. M. (1971) Effect of mitosis inhibitors on blood platelet microtubules and aggregation. *J. Physiol. (Lond.) 214*, 145-158

Wessells, N. K., Spooner, B. S., Ash, J. F., Bradley, M. O., Luduena, M. A., Taylor, E. L., Wrenn, J. T. & Yamada, K. M. (1971) Microfilaments in cellular and developmental processes. *Science (Wash. D.C.) 171*, 135-143

White, J. G. (1968) Fine structural alterations induced in platelets by adenosine diphosphate. *Blood 31*, 604-622

White, J. G. (1971) Platelet microtubules and microfilaments: effects of cytochalasin B on structure and function. In *Platelet Aggregation* (Caen, J., ed.), pp. 15-52, Masson, Paris

Prostaglandins and precursors in platelet function

J. BRYAN SMITH, CAROL M. INGERMAN and MELVIN J. SILVER

Cardeza Foundation, Thomas Jefferson University, Philadelphia

Abstract The exciting developments that have taken place in platelet prostaglandin research in the past two years are presented, dealing in particular with arachidonic acid. The mechanism of bioconversion of arachidonic acid into prostaglandins is discussed, and the possible significance of prostaglandin D_2, a potent inhibitor of platelet aggregation, is considered. The transformations of added arachidonic acid by human platelets are presented and related to transformations of endogenous arachidonic acid that occur when platelets are stimulated with thrombin. Of particular importance is the indication that microgram amounts of arachidonic acid are converted into prostaglandin endoperoxides in this way. These endoperoxides are potent aggregating agents and are produced during irreversible platelet aggregation. Finally, the implications of prostaglandin formation in platelet function are considered, and it is suggested that a combination of prostaglandin formation and extracellular ADP is necessary for irreversible aggregation.

In 1970, it was shown that the stimulation of human platelets with thrombin produces small amounts of prostaglandins (PG) E_2 and $PGF_2\alpha$ (Smith & Willis 1970). This finding seemed to have little relevance to platelet function because it had been shown earlier that, while PGE_1 is a very potent inhibitor of human platelet aggregation, PGE_2 and $PGF_2\alpha$ are comparatively inactive (Kloeze 1967; Sekhar 1970). The subsequent finding that aspirin and indomethacin are strong inhibitors of platelet prostaglandin formation (Smith & Willis 1971) was, however, a clue that prostaglandin synthesis is truly involved in platelet function. This inhibition of prostaglandin formation was independently demonstrated in a cell-free system, and it was proposed that the aspirin-like drugs might act by inhibiting prostaglandin biosynthesis (Vane 1971). These initial findings and the hypothesis provide a background for the material presented in this paper, which is concerned with the abundant developments in platelet prostaglandin research that have occurred in the past two years. Most

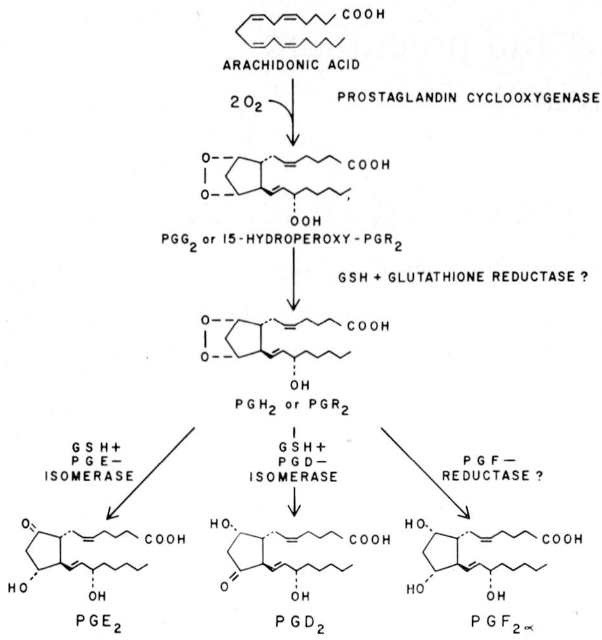

FIG. 1. Mechanism of formation of stable prostaglandins from arachidonic acid by preparations of sheep seminal vesicles.

of this work is oriented around the prostaglandin precursor arachidonic acid and, as will become apparent, this essential fatty acid is the essence of this presentation.

ARACHIDONIC ACID—A PROSTAGLANDIN PRECURSOR

In 1963, the chemical structure of several naturally occurring prostaglandins was announced (Bergström *et al.* 1963), and shortly afterwards it was shown that PGE_2 could be biosynthetically produced by incubating arachidonic acid with enzyme preparations from sheep seminal vesicles (van Dorp *et al.* 1964; Bergström *et al.* 1964). Later work has shown that $PGF_2\alpha$ and PGD_2 also are produced enzymically from arachidonic acid. Our present knowledge of this process is illustrated in Fig. 1. Two molecules of oxygen are consumed for each molecule of prostaglandin that is formed, and at least three enzymes are known to be involved in their formation. The first enzyme, a cyclooxygenase, is believed to catalyse both the incorporation of molecular oxygen into arachidonic acid and a concerted cyclization reaction to yield an intermediate

TABLE 1

Inhibition of ADP-induced platelet aggregation in different species by PGE_1 and PGD_2

Species	PGE_1	PGD_2
Human	Strong	Strong
Monkey	Strong	None
Cat	Strong	None
Rat	Strong	None
Guinea pig	Strong	None
Rabbit	Strong	Weak

Strong signifies an ID50 of about 25 nM, Weak an ID50 of about 250 nM and None an ID50 of greater than 2.5 μM. The results in monkey and cat are unpublished observations of D. C. B. Mills and D. E. Macfarlane.

endoperoxide prostaglandin that has been designated PGG_2 (Hamberg *et al.* 1974*a*) and 15-hydroperoxy-PGR_2 (Nugteren & Hazelhof 1973). The other known enzymes are a PGE-isomerase that catalyses the formation of PGE_2 from the endoperoxide, and a PGD-isomerase that catalyses the formation of PGD_2. Both of these enzymes are glutathione dependent. It is very possible that other enzymes are also involved in prostaglandin formation, such as in the reduction of PGG_2 to produce PGH_2, and the reduction of PGH_2 to produce $PGF_2\alpha$ (Nugteren & Hazelhof 1973).

As stated previously, PGE_2 and $PGF_2\alpha$ are poor inhibitors of platelet aggregation. We have recently found, however, that PGD_2 is more potent than PGE_1 as an inhibitor of human platelet aggregation (Smith *et al.* 1974*b*). The most remarkable thing about this prostaglandin is its species specificity. Table 1 shows that whereas PGE_1 strongly inhibits ADP-induced aggregation of the platelets of man, monkey, cat, rat, guinea pig and rabbit, PGD_2 only has strong activity when tested on human platelets. Both PGE_1 and PGD_2 are potent stimulators of the adenylate cyclase in human platelets, and probably act by increasing cyclic AMP (Mills & Macfarlane 1974). In the discussion of this paper, Dr Mills will present some new evidence which indicates that human platelets contain separate receptors for PGE and PGD (p. 222).

It is unlikely that PGD_2 is ever produced by human platelets in amounts sufficient to influence aggregation. The reason for this will become apparent shortly. On the other hand, it seems possible that PGD_2 is produced elsewhere in the body, because PGD-isomerase has been found to be present in several tissues of the rat, such as the lung and stomach (Nugteren & Hazelhof 1973). These tissues may release PGD_2 and thereby inhibit platelet aggregation locally.

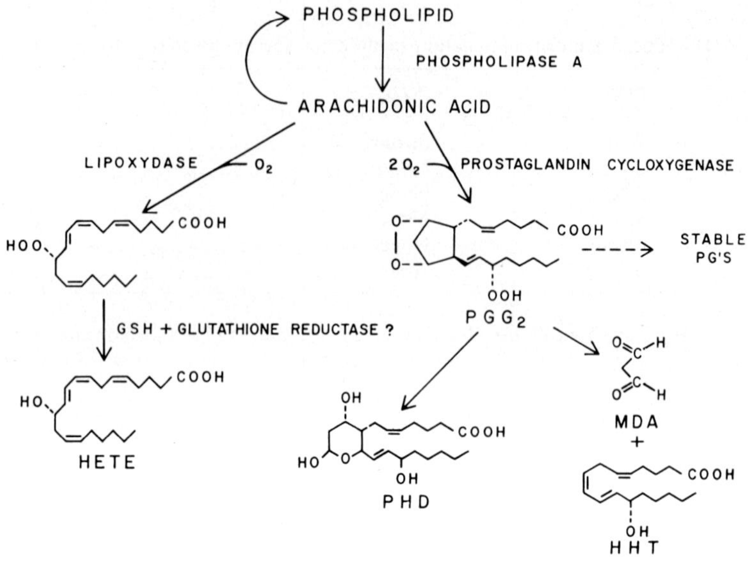

Fig. 2. Some transformations of arachidonic acid by human platelets. Abbreviations (as set forth by Hamberg & Samuelsson 1974) are HETE: 12L-hydroxy-5,8,10,14-eicosatetraenoic acid, HHT: 12L-hydroxy-5,8,10-heptadecatrienoic acid, PHD: 8-(1-hydroxy-3-oxopropyl)-9,12L-dihydroxy-5,10-heptadecadienoic acid and MDA: malondialdehyde.

EXOGENOUS ARACHIDONIC ACID—TRANSFORMATIONS IN PLATELETS

A scheme showing some of the transformation of added arachidonic acid by human platelets is presented in Fig. 2, and the chemical names of the products and their abbreviations are given in the legend. Hamberg & Samuelsson (1974) incubated radioactive arachidonic acid with washed human platelets and found that it was rapidly and almost exclusively converted to three, more polar oxygenated products. The molecular structure of these products was subsequently determined by mass spectrometry. One of the compounds was identified as a 20-carbon 12-hydroxy-fatty acid (HETE) which apparently had been produced in a novel lipoxygenase reaction. Previous to this work, only a lipoxygenase catalysing the incorporation of oxygen at the 11 position had been recognized. A second product was a 17-carbon 12-hydroxy-fatty acid (HHT). This compound had previously been identified as a minor side product of prostaglandin biosynthesis by microsomes of sheep seminal vesicles, and is believed to be formed by fragmentation of the prostaglandin intermediate PGG_2 with the concomitant formation of malondialdehyde. The third product detected was a novel, hemi-acetal compound (PHD). This compound is presumed to be formed by the incorporation of a molecule of water into the intermediate, PGG_2.

It was shown that the presence of aspirin or indomethacin prevented the conversion of radioactive arachidonic acid into the prostaglandin metabolites, PHD and HHT, but increased the formation of the non-prostaglandin metabolite, HETE. This may suggest that, when prostaglandin synthesis in platelets is blocked, the novel lipoxygenase is capable of rapidly removing any free arachidonic acid. However, it also was found that another prostaglandin synthetase inhibitor, the acetylenic compound 5, 8, 11, 14-eicosatetraynoic acid (ETYA), prevented not only the formation of PHD and HHT, but also the formation of HETE (Hamberg & Samuelsson 1974).

In our own laboratory, we have confirmed that radioactive arachidonic acid is rapidly converted into oxygenated products by washed human platelets. However, when submicromolar amounts of arachidonic acid are incubated with platelets in plasma, the only reaction detected is a fairly slow incorporation of radioactivity into platelet phospholipids, probably occurring via an acyl transferase. When a much higher concentration (1 mM) of arachidonic acid is incubated with platelets in plasma, a small conversion into primary prostaglandins, PHD and, presumably, hydroxy-fatty acids does occur. Fig. 3 shows the relative conversion rates of arachidonic acid into PHD, PGE_2, PGG_2, PGH_2 and $PGF_2\alpha$ under these conditions.

Surprisingly, in these experiments by Hamberg & Samuelsson (1974), and ourselves, little radioactivity was detected in any of the stable prostaglandins (PGE_2, PGD_2 or $PGF_2\alpha$). Since the platelets can readily produce the intermediate prostaglandins, the small amounts of PGE_2 and $PGF_2\alpha$ that are formed might result simply from spontaneous breakdown of these intermediates (Hamberg & Samuelsson 1973; Nugteren & Hazelhof 1973; Willis et al. 1974).

An alternative scheme for the oxygenase activity of platelets is shown in Fig. 4. This mechanism is highly speculative and is based on a hypothesis by others of the mechanism of prostaglandin synthesis in seminal vesicle preparations (Smith & Lands 1972). In this mechanism it is proposed that, in one stage of the reaction, 11-hydroperoxy-5, 8, 12, 14-eicosatetraenoic acid is produced and reacts with oxygen to form a tetroxide. In a second stage of the reaction, this tetroxide interacts with substrate arachidonic acid on the enzyme surface to produce the reactive intermediate (I). This intermediate may dissociate to 12-hydroperoxy-5, 8, 10, 14-eicosatetraenoic, the precursor of HETE, or to the 11-hydroperoxy-5, 8, 12, 14-eicosatetraenoic acid, the precursor of PGG_2. The object of introducing this scheme is to point out the possibility that both PGG_2 and HETE might be produced from a single reactive intermediate (I) and that at this time there are still some aspects of prostaglandin

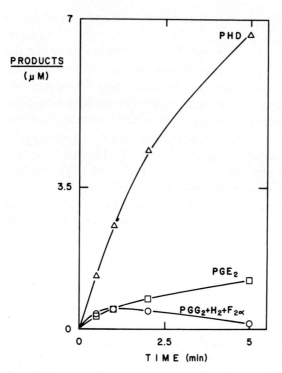

FIG. 3. Transformations of arachidonic acid by human platelets (3.6×10^9/ml) in EDTA plasma. Samples incubated with 1 mM [1-^{14}C]arachidonic acid were decanted into ethanolic stannous chloride at different times. After column chromatography, material in the PGF fraction (PGF$_2\alpha$, PGG$_2$ + PGH$_2$) was quantitated by radioimmunoassay (Smith *et al.* 1974*a*). Material in the PGE fraction was resolved into PHD and PGE$_2$ by thin layer chromatography using benzene, dioxane, acetic acid: 60:35:2 and the compounds were assayed for radioactivity in a liquid scintillation counter.

formation that are not fully understood. If the scheme is correct, it would suggest that aspirin and indomethacin act by favouring the formation of 12-hydroperoxy-5, 8, 10, 14-eicosatetraenoic acid at an intermediate stage in prostaglandin biosynthesis.

ENDOGENOUS ARACHIDONIC ACID—TRANSFORMATION BY THROMBIN

That PGE$_2$ and PGF$_2\alpha$ are produced when platelets are treated with thrombin, was detected by the sensitive but limited technique of biological assay (Smith & Willis 1970). Our knowledge of this process has been greatly advanced by the use of mass spectrometry.

In recent experiments by Hamberg *et al.* (1974*b*), techniques were developed

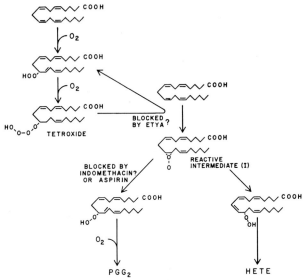

FIG. 4. A novel scheme of platelet oxygenase activity based on the hypothesis of Smith & Lands (1972).

to quantitatively determine the three major metabolites of arachidonic acid formed by washed human platelets, namely HETE, PHD and HHT. It was demonstrated that the stimulation of platelets with thrombin produced microgram amounts of these compounds and one hundred times less of the stable prostaglandins. These results indicate that micromolar amounts of endogenous arachidonic acid are converted to prostaglandin endoperoxides when platelets are stimulated with thrombin. On the other hand, platelets from subjects who had ingested aspirin two hours previously only produced trace amounts of the prostaglandin metabolites in response to thrombin, while the production of HETE was stimulated about three-fold.

When the phospholipids of platelets are labelled with arachidonic acid, as happens in plasma (see above) and then the platelets are washed and treated with thrombin, radioactive products chromatographically similar to HETE, HHT and PHD are produced (Bills & Silver 1975). Arachidonic acid comprises about 18% of the total fatty acids in platelet phospholipids (Marcus *et al.* 1969) and is, therefore, in plentiful supply for the production of prostaglandin endoperoxides.

ENDOGENOUS ARACHIDONIC ACID—A PRECURSOR OF MALONDIALDEHYDE

Fragmentation of the prostaglandin intermediate PGG$_2$ would be expected to produce HHT and malondialdehyde in equimolar amounts. It was shown some time ago (Okuma *et al.* 1971) that malondialdehyde is produced when washed platelets are treated with thrombin. Recent studies showing that this is prevented by aspirin (Hamberg *et al.* 1974*b*; Stuart *et al.* 1975) suggest that under these conditions malondialdehyde, like PHD and HHT, is a metabolite of platelet prostaglandin synthesis. Although it was originally reported that malondialdehyde is not formed in platelet-rich plasma (Okuma *et al.* 1971) we have re-examined this question and have demonstrated that malondialdehyde can be formed during aggregation in platelet-rich plasma in response to ADP, adrenaline, collagen or thrombin. Supporting the studies already mentioned (Hamberg *et al.* 1974*b*), about one hundred times more malondialdehyde was produced than PGE_2 (Ingerman *et al.* 1975).

IMPLICATIONS OF PROSTAGLANDIN FORMATION IN PLATELET AGGREGATION AND THE RELEASE REACTION

Neither aspirin nor indomethacin influence platelet shape change, primary aggregation or the release reaction induced by thrombin. Therefore, it seems unlikely that these effects are mediated by prostaglandin formation. On the other hand, aspirin does inhibit irreversible or second-wave aggregation and the associated release reaction induced by agents such as collagen, ADP or adrenaline (see Smith & Macfarlane 1974). Therefore, it does seem possible that these effects are mediated by prostaglandin formation.

Initial experiments showed that small amounts of PGE_2 and $PGF_{2\alpha}$ were formed during the second wave of platelet aggregation induced by adrenaline and early during collagen-induced aggregation. This suggested that prostaglandin formation by human platelets was associated with the platelet release reaction (Smith *et al.* 1973). Further support for this idea came with the demonstration that, when the platelets of subjects who had ingested aspirin or indomethacin were examined, there was a good correlation between the persistence of inhibition of second-wave aggregation and the persistence of inhibition of prostaglandin formation (Kocsis *et al.* 1973).

PROSTAGLANDIN ENDOPEROXIDES INDUCE AGGREGATION

Evidence recently was presented that the prostaglandin endoperoxides may be produced during irreversible aggregation in plasma in response to arachidonic acid, collagen or adrenaline. Again there appeared to be an association with the platelet release reaction (Smith *et al.* 1974*a*). Both Hamberg *et al.* (1974*a*) and Willis *et al.* (1974) reported that PGH_2 is formed by platelets in response to thrombin. It was demonstrated somewhat earlier that a short-lived platelet aggregating factor, designated LASS, is produced when arachidonic acid is incubated with sheep vesicular gland preparations (Willis & Kuhn 1973). Subsequently, it was shown that LASS also develops when platelet preparations were used as the enzyme source. LASS was partially isolated by thin layer chromatography and it was suggested that it was identical to a prostaglandin cyclic endoperoxide intermediate (Willis 1974). In 1974, the structures of the prostaglandin intermediates PGG_2 and PGH_2 were published and it was reported that both of these compounds, in submicromolar concentrations, induce the aggregation of human platelets (Hamberg et al. 1974a). These findings have since been extended by Willis et al. (1974).

FACTORS INVOLVED IN IRREVERSIBLE AGGREGATION

Although prostaglandin endoperoxides have been reported to cause irreversible aggregation there is good evidence that ADP is also necessary. 'Storage pool deficient' platelets, which release little ADP, have the capacity to produce LASS (Gerrard et al. 1974) and do produce prostaglandins in response to collagen (Willis & Weiss 1973). However these platelets do not aggregate irreversibly (Pareti et al. 1974). When aspirin-treated normal platelets and 'storage-pool deficient' platelets are mixed in equal proportions they aggregate irreversibly in response to collagen, although neither does so alone (White & Witkop 1972). It appears that the combination of prostaglandin formation and extracellular ADP is necessary for irreversible aggregation. A second piece of evidence is that ADP enhances aggregation induced by a prostaglandin endoperoxide (Willis et al. 1974) and that arachidonic acid enhances aggregation induced by ADP (Silver et al. 1973).

We have found further evidence of cooperativity between prostaglandin formation and ADP in recent studies with gel-filtered human platelets. These platelets do not aggregate in response to ADP, adrenaline or low concentrations of arachidonic acid alone, unless fibrinogen or plasma is added to the platelet suspending medium. However, the combination of adrenaline or ADP with arachidonic acid produces strong aggregation in the absence of fibrinogen (Fig. 5). Prostaglandin formation is probably involved in this cooperativity because no aggregation occurs when indomethacin is added before the arachidonic acid (Fig. 5). On the other hand, this inhibition does not occur when indomethacin and then adrenaline are added after arachidonic acid, presumably when the endoperoxide has already been formed. In preliminary experiments, we have found that little release of platelet 5-hydroxytryptamine (5HT) occurs with arachidonic acid alone, in concentrations of 100 μM or less. Considerable

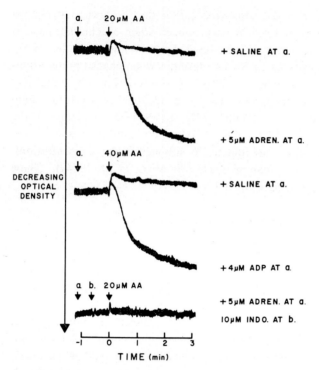

FIG. 5. Aggregation of human gel-filtered platelets suspended in calcium-free Tyrode's solution containing 2 mM-Mg^{2+} and 0.2% albumin but no fibrinogen, showing cooperativity between added adrenaline or ADP and arachidonic acid (AA) in inducing aggregation.

release of 5HT does occur during the irreversible aggregation that is promoted by the addition of ADP, adrenaline or plasma.

These results further demonstrate the complexities of irreversible aggregation in platelet-rich plasma. Apart from the seven factors accepted to be involved in primary aggregation, namely rate of stirring, temperature, pH, divalent cation concentration, presence of fibrinogen, metabolically active platelets and the aggregating agent, at least two additional factors now appear to be involved in secondary aggregation, namely extracellular ADP and prostaglandin formation. Considering how little we know about the way in which each of these factors influences platelet function *in vitro*, it obviously is going to take many years before we truly understand platelet function *in vivo*.

ACKNOWLEDGEMENTS

This work was supported in part by grants HL-14 890 and HL-6374 from the National Institutes of Health.

References

BERGSTRÖM, S., RYHAGE, R., SAMUELSSON, B. & SJÖVALL, J. (1963) The structures of prosta-glandin E_1, $F_{1\alpha}$ and $F_{1\beta}$. J. Biol. Chem. 238, 3555-3564

BERGSTRÖM, S., DANIELSSON, H. & SAMUELSSON, B. (1964) The enzymatic formation of prostaglandin E_2 from arachidonic acid. Biochim. Biophys. Acta 90, 207-210

BILLS, T. K. & SILVER, M. J. (1975) Phosphatidylcholine is the primary source of arachidonic acid utilized by prostaglandin synthetase. Fed. Proc. 34, 790 (abstr.)

GERRARD, J. M., WHITE, J. G., RAO, G. H. R., KRIVIT, W. & WITKOP, C. J. (1974) Labile aggregation stimulating substance (LASS) in the interaction of Hermansky-Pudlak (HP) and aspirin platelets. Circulation 50, no. 4, Suppl. III, 290 (abstr.)

HAMBERG, M. & SAMUELSSON, B. (1973) Detection and isolation of an endoperoxide inter-mediate in prostaglandin biosynthesis. Proc. Natl. Acad. Sci. U.S.A. 70, 899-903

HAMBERG, M. & SAMUELSSON, B. (1974) Prostaglandin endoperoxides. Novel transformations of arachidonic acid in human platelets. Proc. Natl. Acad. Sci. U.S.A. 71, 3400-3404

HAMBERG, M., SVENSSON, J., WAKABAYASHI, T. & SAMUELSSON, B. (1974a) Isolation and structure of two prostaglandin endoperoxides that cause platelet aggregation. Proc. Natl. Acad. Sci. U.S.A. 71, 345-349

HAMBERG, M., SVENSSON, J. & SAMUELSSON, B. (1974b) Prostaglandin endoperoxides. A new concept concerning the mode of action and release of prostaglandins. Proc. Natl. Acad. Sci. U.S.A. 71, 3824-3828

INGERMAN, C. M., SMITH, J. B. & SILVER, M. J. (1975) Malondialdehyde formation in platelet-rich plasma. Fed. Proc. 34, 289 (abstr.)

KLOEZE, J. (1967) in Prostaglandins (Bergström, S. & Samuelsson, B., eds.) (Proc. IInd Nobel Symp.), pp. 241-252, Interscience Publishers, London

KOCSIS, J. J., HERNANDOVICH, J., SILVER, M. J., SMITH, J. B. & INGERMAN, C. (1973) Duration of inhibition of platelet prostaglandin formation and aggregation by ingested aspirin or indomethacin. Prostaglandins 3, 141-144

MARCUS, A. J., ULLMAN, H. L. & SAFIER, L. B. (1969) Lipid composition of subcellular particles of human blood platelets. J. Lipid Res. 10, 108-114

MILLS, D. C. B. & MACFARLANE, D. E. (1974) Stimulation of the adenylate cyclase of human platelets by prostaglandin D_2. Thromb. Res. 5, 401-412

NUGTEREN, D. H. & HAZELHOF, E. (1973) Isolation and properties of intermediates in pros-taglandin biosynthesis. Biochim. Biophys. Acta 326, 448-461

OKUMA, M., STEINER, M. & BALDINI, M. G. (1971) Studies on lipid peroxides in platelets. II. Effect of aggregating agents and platelet antibody. J. Lab. Clin. Med. 77, 728-742

PARETI, F. I., DAY, H. J. & MILLS, D. C. B. (1974) Nucleotide and serotonin metabolism in platelets with defective secondary aggregation. Blood 44, 789-800

SEKHAR, N. C. (1970) Effect of eight prostaglandins on platelet aggregation. J. Med. Chem. 13, 39-44

SILVER, M. J., SMITH, J. B., INGERMAN, C. & KOCSIS, J. J. (1973) Arachidonic acid-induced human platelet aggregation and prostaglandin formation. Prostaglandins 4, 863-875

SMITH, J. B. & MACFARLANE, D. E. (1974) in Prostaglandins, vol. 2 (Ramwell, P., ed.), pp. 293-343, Plenum Press, New York

SMITH, J. B. & WILLIS, A. L. (1970) Formation and release of prostaglandins by platelets in response to thrombin. Br. J. Pharmacol. 40, 545P

SMITH, J. B. & WILLIS, A. L. (1971) Aspirin selectively inhibits prostaglandin production in human platelets. Nature New Biol. 231, 235-237

SMITH, J. B., INGERMAN, C., KOCSIS, J. J. & SILVER, M. J. (1973) Formation of prostaglandins during the aggregation of human blood platelets. J. Clin. Invest. 52, 965-969

SMITH, J. B., INGERMAN, C., KOCSIS, J. J. & SILVER, M. J. (1974a) Formation of an inter-mediate in prostaglandin biosynthesis and its association with the platelet release reaction. J. Clin. Invest. 53, 1468-1472

SMITH, J. B., SILVER, M. J., INGERMAN, C. M. & KOCSIS, J. J. (1974b) Prostaglandin D$_2$
    inhibits the aggregation of human platelets. *Thromb. Res. 5*, 291-299
SMITH, W. L. & LANDS, W. E. M. (1972) Oxygenation of polyunsaturated fatty acids during
    prostaglandin synthesis by sheep vesicular gland. *Biochemistry 11*, 3276-3285
STUART, M. J., MURPHY, S. & OSKI, F. A. (1975) A simple nonradioisotope technic for the
    determination of platelet life-span. *N. Engl. J. Med. 292*, 1310-1313
VAN DORP, D. A., BEERTHUIS, R. K., NUGTEREN, D. M. & VONKEMAN, H. (1964) The bio-
    synthesis of prostaglandins. *Biochim. Biophys. Acta 90*, 204-207
VANE, J. R. (1971) Inhibition of prostaglandin synthesis as a mechanism of action for aspirin-
    like drugs. *Nature New Biol. 231*, 232-235
WHITE, J. G. & WITKOP, C. J. (1972) Effects of normal and aspirin platelets on defective
    secondary aggregation in the Hermansky-Pudlak syndrome. *Am. J. Pathol. 68*, 57-66
WILLIS, A. L. (1974) Isolation of a chemical trigger for thrombosis. *Prostaglandins 5*, 1-25
WILLIS, A. L. & KUHN, D. C. (1973) A new potential mediator of arterial thrombosis whose
    biosynthesis is inhibited by aspirin. *Prostaglandins 4*, 127-129
WILLIS, A. L. & WEISS, H. J. (1973) A congenital defect in platelet prostaglandin production
    associated with impaired hemostasis in storage pool disease. *Prostaglandins 4*, 783-794
WILLIS, A. L., VANE, F. M., KUHN, D. C., SCOTT, C. G. & PETRIN, M. (1974) An endoperoxide
    aggregator (LASS), formed in platelets in response to thrombotic stimuli—purification,
    identification and unique biological significance. *Prostaglandins 8*, 453-508

Discussion

Haslam: Are the cyclic endoperoxides extracellular or intracellular messengers? Where are their receptors, if such entities exist?

Smith: Our knowledge of the activity of the endoperoxides is far too limited for me to answer these questions. However, we do know that whereas the endoperoxides dissolved in saline spontaneously break down to stable prostaglandins and the 17-carbon monohydroxy fatty acid HHT (Nugteren & Hazelhof 1973), the endoperoxides produced by platelets yield an additional product, the hemiacetal compound PHD (Hamberg *et al.* 1974a). This indicates that the platelets are metabolizing the endoperoxides, and presumably this is an intracellular event. On the other hand, the small amounts of endoperoxide that transiently accumulate during platelet aggregation seem to be outside the platelets (Smith *et al.* 1974; Hamberg *et al.* 1974b).

Marcus: Many years ago, when we were studying the fatty acids in platelets and platelet membranes, we were impressed by the relatively large amounts of arachidonic acid in platelet phosphatides (Marcus *et al.* 1962, 1969). Hamberg & Samuelsson (1974) have mentioned the possibility that upon treatment with thrombin, a limited pool of free arachidonic acid in platelets becomes available to the prostaglandin synthetase system. Would you care to comment on this concept? Is there any information on the intracellular source of arachidonic acid for prostaglandin synthesis? Is it a lipid from the membrane, the granules, or the cytosol?

Smith: Some recent work by Bills & Silver (1975) suggests that the primary source of the arachidonic acid is phosphatidylcholine, but obviously much more work needs to be done to answer these questions.

Marcus: This is surprising, since platelet phosphatidylcholine (lecithin) has much less arachidonic acid than platelet phosphatidylethanolamine, phosphatidylserine or phosphatidylinositol.

Mills: Imipramine and chlorpromazine can inhibit the release reaction and irreversible aggregation. Have you looked at the effects of other tricyclic antidepressant drugs on the synthesis of prostaglandins in platelets?

Smith: We have not worked with chlorpromazine or the tricyclic anti-depressant drugs. However, Panaganamala and co-workers (1974) have reported that chlorpromazine abolishes arachidonic acid-induced platelet aggregation, and Lee (1974) has shown that chlorpromazine and various tricyclic antidepressants inhibit prostaglandin biosynthesis in a cell-free system.

Marcus: Is chlorpromazine an anti-oxidant?

Smith: Yes, it is believed to work by scavenging hydroxyl ion free radicals.

Marcus: Working with unsaturated fatty acids *in vitro* always presents problems of interpretation of experimental results. Lipid peroxides can damage cell membranes and produce phenomena *in vitro* which may not occur *in vivo* because of natural defence mechanisms against lipid peroxides. In a brilliant series of experiments Hamberg & Samuelsson (1974) have shown that prostaglandin endoperoxides may play a role as regulators of cell function. Arachidonic acid was first converted to endoperoxides, which were then rapidly transformed mainly into non-prostaglandin metabolites. This rapid conversion could also be interpreted as a defence mechanism against the endoperoxides whose toxicity for platelets is manifested by membrane damage and aggregation.

Smith: I agree that the question of 'non-specific' lipid peroxidation presents a great problem. However, the work of Hamberg & Samuelsson (1974) shows that aspirin and indomethacin do not block the oxidation of arachidonic acid *per se*, but rather divert the route of oxidation away from the prostaglandins. This tends to support the idea that prostaglandins are mediators of irreversible aggregation.

Marcus: The experiments on aspirin inhibition of the fatty acid cyclo-oxygenase are very impressive (Hamberg *et al.* 1974*a*) and lend credence to the concept that prostaglandins are important mediators of platelet function. However, aspirin is a weak anti-aggregant, and I personally doubt its effectiveness as an anti-thrombotic agent.

Smith: The problem is that prostaglandin formation depends on lipid peroxidation. It has been shown that with certain preparations of prostaglandin synthetase from seminal vesicles, the formation of hydroperoxide is obligatory for prostaglandin formation (Smith & Lands 1972); so you can see this is a circular argument.

Marcus: Here we come to the crux of the problem. Can we correlate *in vitro* aerobic events which are related to peroxidative changes with *in vivo* phenomena that culminate in haemostasis or thrombosis? Are lipid peroxides immediately inactivated *in vivo*? Perhaps a thrombotic diathesis represents a situation *in vivo* wherein the mechanism for inactivating lipid peroxides breaks down.

Mustard: I think we ought to question the use of the term 'irreversible aggregation'. There is no evidence that true irreversible aggregation is produced by any physiological aggregating agent unless fibrin is formed to bind the platelets together. It is a dangerous misnomer which can confuse the interpretation of platelet function in different systems. The suspension system you are using is probably based on our observations that washed human platelets will show a primary and secondary wave of aggregation upon the addition of ADP if they are suspended in a medium containing fibrinogen and magnesium but no added calcium (Mustard *et al.* 1975). If calcium is included in the system the secondary wave does not occur. Also, if citrate is added to a suspension of washed human platelets in a medium containing calcium and magnesium, ADP-induced secondary aggregation is observed.

If blood is taken into hirudin or heparin and ADP is added to the platelet-rich plasma, secondary aggregation does not occur. If you add citrate, it does. It seems possible, therefore, that since the ADP-induced secondary phase in suspensions of washed human platelets or citrated platelet-rich plasma can be blocked with aspirin, it may be due to the formation of endoperoxide.

In view of this, do you observe the arachidonic acid or ADP effect if calcium is added to your suspending medium?

Smith: Yes. Calcium makes no difference.

Mustard: Have you examined whether the secondary wave of aggregation, which is fully inhibited with aspirin, is due to endoperoxide production?

Smith: We have not done that.

Born: Is there no added fibrinogen in the system (Fig. 5, p. 216), even though arachidonic acid has an effect?

Smith: None is added.

Mustard: Presumably arachidonic acid will induce aggregation with washed human platelets without added fibrinogen because arachidonic acid induces the reaction which includes the release of platelet fibrinogen. Both thrombin and collagen will cause aggregation of washed human platelets without added fibrinogen.

Smith: In our experiments using gel-filtered platelets prelabelled with

[^{14}C]5-hydroxytryptamine we saw very little release of radioactivity with arachidonic acid alone, but much more release in the presence of adrenaline. This could fit in with your idea.

Mustard: The effect of arachidonic acid and collagen on thrombin-degranu-lated rabbit platelets is of interest. As I indicated earlier (pp. 96, 202), these platelets have discharged their amine storage granules yet they still show a normal aggregation response to ADP in the presence of added fibrinogen (Reimers *et al.* 1973). These platelets will also undergo a shape change and aggregation in response to collagen and they show a normal response to the ionophore A23187 (that is, shape change and aggregation) (Kinlough-Rathbone *et al.* 1975). The addition of arachidonic acid to a suspension of thrombin-degranulated rabbit platelets induced shape change and some aggregation. If these thrombin-degranulated platelets are mixed with aspirin-treated washed rabbit platelets and arachidonic acid is added, there is extensive aggregation. The addition of collagen to the mixture of thrombin-degranulated and aspirin-treated platelets also leads to extensive aggregation. Possibly the collagen interacts with the thrombin-degranulated platelets to lead to the formation of endoperoxide, which causes the aggregation and release reaction in the aspirin-treated normal platelets.

It seems that the endoperoxide can form when platelets adhere to collagen; endoperoxide formation can also be activated, with *human* platelets, by bringing the platelets together in a magnesium, no calcium, system. This may relate to the crucial point raised by Dr Lüscher—the importance of surface–surface contact. Have you any evidence on the effect of surface–surface contact in terms of, say, activating a phospholipase?

Smith: I suspect that contact may be a stimulus for the formation of prostaglandins, but I have no evidence for this in platelets. Piper & Vane (1971) have summarized what is known about the stimuli for prostaglandin formation by different cells throughout the body. The only unifying factor seems to be what they call a 'disturbance of the cell membranes'.

Mills: I do agree with the importance of Dr Mustard's point that the biphasic aggregation of platelets is just a citrate artifact. This is not to say that the things Dr Smith is talking about are not relevant to certain situations, particu-larly the situation with collagen. Collagen-induced release is not an artifact of citrate, as it occurs in heparinized plasma. I would at the same time take issue with the statement that one should abandon the term 'irreversible aggregation'. It is an irreversible phenomenon in that the platelets cannot do the same things, because they have lost the constituents that they originally had.

Born: That is an important point. We have also been looking at what happens to platelets after they have been through the sequence of plasma coagulation and fibrinolysis. Those platelets have apparently normal membrane transport functions but they have, of course, lost some intracellular organelles; and it is not yet certain whether these can be reconstituted.

Smith: Dr Mills' point about collagen may also apply to adrenaline; we have obtained biphasic aggregation with adrenaline in heparinized plasma. So, perhaps the citrate artifact applies only to ADP.

Mustard: If you can obtain this effect of adrenaline in hirudin-plasma, I will believe it! Heparin has effects on platelet aggregation which can vary with the batch of heparin.

Mills: Dr Smith mentioned that we have evidence for two different prostaglandin receptors on the platelet. Fig. 1 shows the accumulation of radioactive cyclic AMP in platelets after a single addition of either PGD_1 or PGE_1, and either PGD_2 or PGE_2. The concentrations were for D_2 and E_1, 0.5 μM; and for D_1 and E_2, 100 times higher (50 μM). We have observed repeatedly that

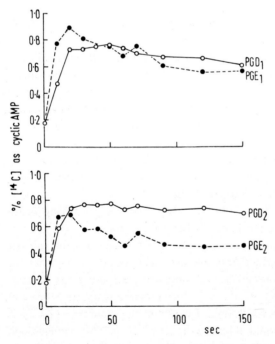

FIG. 1 (Mills). Effects of D and E prostaglandins on the accumulation of cyclic AMP in platelets previously labelled by incubation with [^{14}C]adenine. *Upper figure*: PGD_1 (50 μM) or PGE_1 (0.5 μM). *Lower figure*: PGD_2 (0.5 μM) or PGE_2 (50 μM). Prostaglandins were added at zero time to a bulk incubation from which subsamples were removed and assayed at the times indicated.

the D prostaglandins seem to stimulate incorporation of radioactivity into cyclic AMP more slowly, and the peak levels persist for rather longer.

Haslam: Was a phosphodiesterase inhibitor present in this experiment?

Mills: No.

Haslam: Then your results suggest that a secondary component of the action of D prostaglandins might be to cause an inhibition of a cyclic AMP phosphodiesterase, or alternatively the difference between D and E prostaglandins could be explained by a potentiation of a phosphodiesterase by the latter.

Mills: Yes. In the former case, however, we would expect D type prostaglandins to enhance the response to E prostaglandins; which they do not.

Born: There are pharmacological considerations in these possible differences; the molecules are extremely alike, but it might be due to subtle differences in diffusional access?

Mills: Yes, but I don't know how one could examine that.

White: I notice a trend to by-pass the complicated chemistry of prostaglandins and to concentrate only on malondialdehyde. I wonder what your views are on that, Dr Smith?

Smith: At the moment, it seems reasonable to assume that malondialdehyde is a by-product of prostaglandin formation and, since it is much easier to measure than the prostaglandins or the other prostaglandin metabolites, it appears to be a useful marker. Hamberg *et al.* (1974*a*) have reported that aspirin inhibits the formation of malondialdehyde by platelets, and Stuart *et al.* (1975) have shown that this effect persists if the aspirin is taken orally. This, of course, correlates with the well-known persistence of the effects of aspirin on platelet aggregation and platelet prostaglandin formation.

References

BILLS, T. K. & SILVER, M. J. (1975) Phosphatidylcholine is the primary source of arachidonic acid utilized by prostaglandin synthetase. *Fed. Proc. 34*, 790 (abstr.)

HAMBERG, M. & SAMUELSSON, B. (1974) Prostaglandin endoperoxides. Novel transformations of arachidonic acid in human platelets. *Proc. Natl. Acad. Sci. U.S.A. 71*, 3400-3404

HAMBERG, M. SVENSSON, J. & SAMUELSSON, B. (1974*a*) Prostaglandin endoperoxides. A new concept concerning the mode of action and release of prostaglandins. *Proc. Natl. Acad. Sci. U.S.A. 71*, 3824-3828

HAMBERG, M., SVENSSON, J., WAKABAYSHI, T. & SAMUELSSON, B. (1974*b*) Isolation and structure of two prostaglandin endoperoxides that cause platelet aggregation. *Proc. Natl. Acad. Sci. U.S.A. 71*, 345-349

KINLOUGH-RATHBONE, R. L., CHAHIL, A. & MUSTARD, J. F. (1975) Effect of A23,187 on thrombin-degranulated washed rabbit platelets. *Fed. Proc. 34*, 855 (abstr.)

LEE, R. E. (1973) The influence of psychotropic drugs on prostaglandin biosynthesis. *Prostaglandins 5*, 63-68

MARCUS, A. J., ULLMAN, H. L., SAFIER, L. B. & BALLARD, H. S. (1962) Platelet phosphatides:

their fatty acid and aldehyde composition and activity in different clotting systems. *J. Clin. Invest. 41*, 2198-2212

MARCUS, A. J., ULLMAN, H. L. & SAFIER, L. B. (1969) Lipid composition of subcellular particles of human blood platelets. *J. Lipid Res. 10*, 108-114

MUSTARD, J. F., PERRY, D. W., KINLOUGH-RATHBONE, R. L. & PACKHAM, M. A. (1975) Factors responsible for ADP-induced release reaction of human platelets. *Am. J. Physiol. 228*, 1757-1765

NUGTEREN, D. H. & HAZELHOF, E. (1973) Isolation and properties of intermediates in prostaglandin biosynthesis. *Biochim. Biophys. Acta 326*, 448-461

PANAGANAMALA, R. V., SHARMA, H. M., SPRECHER, H., GREER, J. C. & CORNWELL, D. G. (1974) A suggested role for hydrogen peroxide in the biosynthesis of prostaglandins. *Prostaglandins 8*, 3-11

PIPER, P. & VANE, J. (1971) The release of prostaglandins from lung and other tissues. *Ann. N.Y. Acad. Sci. 180*, 363-385

REIMERS, H. J., PACKHAM, M. A., KINLOUGH-RATHBONE, R. L. & MUSTARD, J. F. (1973) Effect of repeated treatment of rabbit platelets with low concentrations of thrombin on their function, metabolism and survival. *Br. J. Haematol. 25*, 675-689

SMITH, J. B., INGERMAN, C., KOCSIS, J. J. & SILVER, M. J. (1974) Formation of an intermediate in prostaglandin biosynthesis and its association with the platelet release reaction. *J. Clin. Invest. 53*, 1468-1472

SMITH, W. L. & LANDS, W. E. M. (1972) Oxygenation of polyunsaturated fatty acids during prostaglandin synthesis by sheep vesicular gland. *Biochemistry 11*, 3276-3285

STUART, M. J., MURPHY, S. & OSKI, F. A. (1975) A simple nonradioisotope technic for the determination of platelet life-span. *N. Engl. J. Med. 292*, 1310-1313

Significance of glucose and glycogen metabolism for platelet function

W. SCHNEIDER and A. R. L. GEAR

Medizinische Universitätsklinik und Poliklinik, Homburg/Saar, Germany, and Department of Biochemistry, The University of Virginia, Charlottesville, USA

Abstract Platelet functions in haemostasis require a source of energy, which is provided by both glycolysis and oxidative phosphorylation. Several investigations have emphasized a predominant role for glucose as a substrate and the dependence of platelet function on glycogen as an energy store. This dependence is not surprising as platelets are contractile cells, and their functions depend on contractile mechanisms. Contractile cells, however, require efficient glycogenolysis and glucose metabolism for their functions in spite of their capacity for oxidative phosphorylation.

Accordingly, the glycogen content of human blood platelets is fairly high and resembles that of human muscle cells. Glycogen can be mobilized in two different ways:

(1) By the cyclic AMP-dependent enzyme cascade for phosphorylase activation and glycogen synthetase inhibition. This is a protein kinase-mediated phosphorylation which results in covalent modification of the enzymes. The reaction, however, involves not only enzymes of glycogen metabolism but also other enzymes and proteins, such as membrane proteins. Thus, activation of the protein kinase system by cyclic AMP leads to changes in membrane permeability and reactivity, and therefore probably results in an inhibition of platelet function.

(2) Calcium ions at a concentration of about 10^{-6}M are able directly to activate phosphorylase b kinase. Such an ion concentration is exactly what is needed to induce the contractile mechanisms in blood platelets, and provide them with energy. This activation mechanism is independent of the protein kinase system, which is stimulated by cyclic AMP, and is, therefore, not accompanied by a decrease in glycogen synthetase activity.

From a metabolic point of view, 'resting' platelets are similar to cells showing density-dependent inhibition of growth, whereas aggregating cells display some metabolic features characteristic of stimulated and transformed cells. Thus, the inducing mechanism for platelet aggregation in haemostasis might resemble the general reaction pattern of a stimulated cell, modified by the absence of a nucleus and the inability to proliferate.

Blood platelets contain mitochondria, and exhibit Pasteur and Crabtree effects, demonstrating their dependence on the efficiency of oxidative phosphorylation, at least in the 'resting state' (review: Mustard & Packham 1970; Gross & Schneider 1971). On the other hand, investigations with inhibitors of glycolysis and respiration (Mürer 1969) showed that both oxidative phosphorylation and glycolysis contribute to the energy needed for platelet functions. This conclusion has been generally accepted. However, in spite of this, since Lüscher (1956) first described the importance of glucose as a factor for retraction, several findings have emphasized the predominant role of glucose as a substrate for platelet function (Doery et al. 1970). Later on, Kinlough-Rathbone et al. (1972) reported that platelets, resuspended in a solution free of glucose, lose their sensitivity to aggregation induced by different stimuli. Added glucose restores platelet sensitivity only if no antimycin is added. These results indicate that glucose as a substrate is able to restore the platelet response to release-inducing stimuli only if complete glucose oxidation is allowed.

Besides glucose, glycogen is important as an energy store for platelet function (Weber & Unger 1964; Scott 1967; Karpatkin & Charmatz 1970). The special role of glucose and glycogen metabolism in platelet function is not surprising if we remember that platelets are contractile cells. Aggregation and retraction, as well as the earlier phases of aggregation such as shape changes and pseudopod formation, are 'unthinkable without the activation and/or relaxation of a contractile mechanism' (Lüscher et al. 1972). Contractile cells, however, depend on glycogen as the most important cytoplasmic energy source. That is why the ability of muscle cells to perform prolonged and heavy exercise is directly proportional to the initial glycogen concentration (Hultman 1967). In contrast to muscle cells, platelets do not possess phosphocreatine as an additional high energy reserve and, therefore, depend critically on glycogen as a potential energy source.

RESULTS AND DISCUSSION

In line with the above discussion, the glycogen content of human blood platelets is fairly high. The values given in the literature depend on the estimation technique. Drastic treatment, such as boiling with potassium hydroxide and ethanol precipitation, gave values ranging from 23.6 (Seitz 1965), to 28.4 (Löhr et al. 1961) to 56.8 µmol glucose equivalents per 10^{11} platelets (Scott 1967). However, when we used a sensitive fluorometric assay (Passonneau 1970) we were able to measure a glycogen content of 98.5 ± 15.5 ($\bar{x} \pm$ s.d., $N = 26$) µmol glucose equivalents per 10^{11} platelets. This glycogen content of human blood platelets is similar to that of human muscle cells (Keul *et al.* 1972).

The sensitive fluorometric estimation enabled us to study the influence of some substances which are known to activate glycogen metabolism in skeletal muscle. Of particular interest were dibutyryl adenosine $3':5'$-cyclic monophosphate (dibutyryl cyclic AMP), prostaglandin E_1 (PGE_1) and adenosine. These compounds stimulate glycogenolysis in skeletal muscle by activating the classic cyclic AMP-dependent enzyme cascade. Since platelet function depends on the glycogen content (Weber & Unger 1964; Scott 1967), a decrease in glycogen caused by the activation of phosphorylase via a cyclic AMP-dependent mechanism might be one explanation for the inhibitory effect of cyclic AMP on platelet function (Salzman 1972).

Experimentally we have shown (Schneider 1974) that adenosine (10^{-4}M), dibutyryl cyclic AMP (10^{-3}M) and PGE_1 (10^{-7} to 10^{-6}M), in concentrations known to inhibit platelet functions, all led to a significant decrease in platelet glycogen content. The values obtained after 20 to 30 minutes were about 50% of the initial values. It is beyond doubt that this effect results from an increased amount of total phosphorylase and phosphorylase *a* (E.C. 2. 4. 1. 1) activated by a cyclic AMP-dependent protein kinase (E.C. 2. 7. 1. 37). This platelet enzyme was first described by Marquis *et al.* (1971). Accordingly, the ratio of phosphorylase *a* to total phosphorylase increased from about 30% to 60% (Schneider 1974) under the influence of 10^{-3}M-dibutyryl cyclic AMP, which inhibits platelet function completely. Activity became normal again within 20 to 30 minutes. Since then, we have shown that the amount of phosphorylase *a* in very carefully prepared and unstimulated platelets is 13.3 $\pm$ 7.5% ($\tilde{x}$ $\pm$ S.D., $N = 10$), with a range of 3.4 – 29.1% (Gear & Schneider 1975). This low value for resting platelets is in accordance with the findings of Scott (1967) and has important metabolic consequences. Karpatkin & Langer (1969) and Deisseroth *et al.* (1970) found no change in the amount of phosphorylase *a* under the influence of different stimuli. This result was probably obtained because their phosphorylase *a* activity of about 50% was already much elevated. Our values, however, correspond more to those obtained from skeletal muscle.

In spite of opposite effects on platelet function, comparison of glycogen levels in human blood platelets inhibited by dibutyryl cyclic AMP, as well as in platelets aggregated by ADP, revealed the same pattern of decreased glycogen (Schneider 1974). The lowered content of glycogen cannot be the reason for the inhibition by dibutyryl cyclic AMP since aggregation by ADP caused a similar fall in glycogen. This conclusion is further confirmed by the fact that glycogen decreases slowly but continuously, reaching its lowest point after 20–30 minutes, whereas functional inhibition occurs within seconds. Furthermore, since activation of the cyclic AMP-dependent enzyme cascade causes both phosphorylase activation and inhibition of platelet function, the phosphorylase activation seen during aggregation must be independent of the protein kinase system. This observation is supported by the fact that aggregating agents cause a decrease in adenylate cyclase activity even though glycogenolysis is stimulated during aggregation (Deisseroth et al. 1970; Mills & Smith 1972; Salzman et al. 1972; Haslam, this volume, pp. 121–144). Consequently, an independent mechanism for phosphorylase activation must exist during normal aggregation. In line with this it is known that the phosphorylase kinase of skeletal muscle can be activated by levels of calcium ions as low as 10^{-6}M (Fischer et al. 1971; Krebs et al. 1971; Sacktor et al. 1974). These concentrations are very similar to those which trigger the contractile mechanisms of muscle fibres.

Since the phosphorylase of platelets is similar to the muscle enzyme (Scott 1968), it was interesting to evaluate whether platelet phosphorylase kinase could be activated by the same low concentrations of calcium ions as observed for the skeletal muscle enzyme. For this purpose, phosphorylase activity after activation of phosphorylase kinase was assayed in the direction of glycogen synthesis using the isotopic filter paper technique described by Gilboe et al. (1972). The ratio of phosphorylase a and total phosphorylase was measured with and without 3 mM-AMP. For testing phosphorylase b kinase from human blood platelets, a crude extract, freed of nucleotides by gel filtration, was used. The activity of this enzyme was then measured against commercially available phosphorylase b as substrate (Gear & Schneider 1975). Using calcium-EGTA buffers according to Portzehl et al. (1964), we were able to show that even calcium concentrations of 0.3 μM were able to stimulate phosphorylase b kinase. The activation constant of the enzyme proved to be just below 1 μM, which is in the same range as that reported for skeletal muscle. It is interesting that this concentration which activates platelet phosphorylase b kinase can also trigger the contractile mechanism of human blood platelets (Cohen 1974).

For comparison of the two different activation mechanisms of phosphorylase, phosphorylase a content was measured after aggregation of platelets by 10^{-5}M-ADP and inhibition of platelet function by 10^{-3}M-dibutyryl cyclic AMP in platelet-rich plasma. The percentage of phosphorylase a in the controls was 10.4%. It was increased by ADP-induced aggregation to 31.4%. On the other hand, inhibition by dibutyryl cyclic AMP resulted in an increase to 35.9%. This experiment demonstrates that approximately the same degree of phosphorylase activation and, hence, the same pattern of glycogen decrease, was reached in both cases.

To ensure that this activation is the result of different metabolic pathways, we compared the effects of the cyclic AMP-dependent enzyme cascade on both phosphorylase and glycogen synthetase activities. For this purpose, glycogen synthetase activity was estimated by an isotopic filter paper method, using UDP-[^{14}C]glucose as a substrate according to Thomas et al. (1968). By addition of glucose-6-phosphate, the amount of the phosphorylated, but inactive D-form, was determined. If aggregation by ADP leads to phosphorylase activation independent of the cyclic AMP-dependent protein kinase pathway, the relative amount of the active form (glycogen synthetase I) should remain constant. In contrast to this, the inhibition of aggregation caused by dibutyryl cyclic AMP should lower the percentage of the active, or non-phosphorylated glycogen synthetase. This was the case in our experiments: ADP-induced aggregation (10^{-5}M) had no effect on the amount of glycogen synthetase I ($35.2 \pm 5.8\%$) when compared with the controls ($32.3 \pm 4.4\%$) whereas inhibition by dibutyryl cyclic AMP resulted in a significant decrease ($19.5 \pm 6.0\%$). Thus, our findings support the hypothesis that glycogen synthetase is not phosphorylated during aggregation. Hence, the glycogen mobilization occurring during aggregation is independent of the cyclic AMP-dependent enzyme cascade. This result is consistent with the finding by Scott (1967) that glycogen synthesis remained active during platelet aggregation. Since ADP by itself has no influence on phosphorylase activity, our findings lead to the hypothesis that release of calcium during aggregation initiates glycogen breakdown by direct stimulation of phosphorylase kinase. Thus, the release of calcium simultaneously triggers the platelet contractile processes and the necessary energy from glycogenolysis. However, the question still remains as to the immediate source of this calcium. It might come from the membranes, the tubular system, the mitochondria or other granules, which are known to accumulate significant amounts of this ion. Furthermore, the initiation of the actual changes in intracellular calcium concentration is uncertain. A reasonable explanation might be that a primary event involves disturbance of the platelet membrane.

However, our findings do not explain the inhibition of platelet function under the influence of substances which increase the intracellular content of cyclic AMP. To gather further information, we investigated some effects of dibutyryl cyclic AMP on glucose metabolism. In contrast to these effects, the metabolic changes during aggregation are well documented. It has been shown that glycogenolysis and glycolytic flow rates are stimulated (McElroy et al. 1971). At the same time the ATP content of the platelets decreases during ADP-induced aggregation (Holmsen 1965).

For further studies, human blood platelets in citrated platelet-rich plasma were incubated for 60 minutes at 37 °C with 10^{-3}M-dibutyryl cyclic AMP.

During the incubation period, glucose decarboxylation was measured by trapping the labelled $^{14}CO_2$, and the incorporation of labelled glucose into glycogen was estimated by the filter paper technique (Gilboe *et al.* 1972). At the beginning and at the end of the incubation period, the glucose content was measured enzymically in perchloric acid extracts. Our results show that the incorporation of glucose into glycogen is reduced. This finding is not unexpected since we have already shown that cyclic AMP activates phosphorylase while inhibiting glycogen synthetase, and it helps us to rationalize the previously mentioned decrease in glycogen. At the same time glucose consumption was found to be significantly reduced. At first we interpreted these findings as a reduced glycolytic flow rate, thus explaining the inhibition induced by dibutyryl cyclic AMP. This would be in accordance with the results reported by Zieve & Schmukler (1971). They observed a reduced production of lactate after adding cyclic AMP to platelet homogenates. However, a comparison between the decrease in glycogen content and the decrease in glucose consumption revealed that the two parameters were equivalent to each other. There was thus no decrease in the glycolytic flow rate but a decrease in glucose *uptake* which corresponded to the glucose released from glycogen.

The possibility of an increase in glucose-6-phosphate which might inhibit hexokinase and glucose uptake was considered. On the other hand, this became unlikely since we found a decrease in both glycogen content and turnover. Also, glucose-6-phosphate should activate glycogen synthetase. Direct estimation of the glucose-6-phosphate content in platelets revealed no significant difference between dibutyryl cyclic AMP and control preparations. An alternative might be an increased activity of glucose-6-phosphatase. Recently, a rise in the activity of this enzyme under the influence of dibutyryl cyclic AMP has been described for human liver (Schwartz *et al.* 1974). It takes, however, about 24 hours to reach its peak activity. Activation can be prevented by inhibition of protein and nucleic acid synthesis. Therefore, a similar mechanism for blood platelets seems to be unlikely.

Finally, an actual inhibition of glucose uptake through the plasma membrane might explain the reduced glucose consumption caused by dibutyryl cyclic AMP. McDonagh *et al.* (1968) reported that the glucose penetration into human blood platelets is very slow compared to other hexoses and pentoses and might therefore be a limiting factor. Using the Millipore filtration technique and [6-^{14}C]glucose as an indicator for glucose uptake through the platelet membrane we were able to demonstrate that all agents which increase intracellular cyclic AMP content, immediately cause a reduced glucose uptake. ADP, however, results in an increase in glucose uptake. These findings parallel those of McElroy *et al.* (1971), who observed increased glucose decarboxylation during aggregation and shape changes. However, they noted an inhibition of glucose decarboxylation under the influence of inhibitors of aggregation and shape changes, such as dibutyryl cyclic AMP, adenosine and PGE_1. These results indicate that the dibutyryl cyclic AMP, adenosine and PGE_1-induced metabolic events—that is, a decrease in both glycogen content and glucose uptake—are probably caused by alterations of the platelet membrane (Chang & Cuatrecasas 1974). In the case of these inhibitors, which activate the cyclic AMP-dependent protein kinase system, we can assume that membrane phosphorylation modifies membrane permeability. Recently Booyse et al. (1973) described changes in the membrane permeability of human blood platelets which were induced by phosphorylation of membrane proteins via the cyclic AMP-dependent protein kinase system.

CONCLUSIONS

When all the information about platelet metabolism is summarized, 'resting' platelets seem to be similar to cells showing a density-dependent inhibition of growth, as for example reduced membrane permeability, high cell content of cyclic AMP and low tendency to aggregation (Pollack & Hough 1974). This opinion is confirmed by the findings of Karpatkin et al. (1970), who reported a higher rate of glycogen synthesis in platelet suspensions containing lower concentrations of platelets. This indicates a decrease in cyclic AMP and, thus, a shift of the equilibrium between glycogen synthetase and phosphorylase towards glycogen synthesis. With higher platelet concentrations the decrease of glycogen synthesis probably results from an increase in phosphorylase a activity. This, in turn, must be the result of increased cyclic AMP concentration. Therefore, the haemorrhagic disorder in thrombocythaemia (review: Marcus & Zucker 1965) could correspond to density-induced growth control of non-proliferating cells.

A stimulated cell, however, passes from the stage of density-dependent inhibition of growth to a phase of increased membrane permeability, decreased cyclic AMP content, loss of density control and increased tendency to aggregate (Bannai & Sheppard 1974). Initial effects seem to involve surface changes in membrane permeability. These, in turn, cause changes in metabolic flow rates and cyclic AMP content. From a metabolic point of view this phase of growth stimulation and cell transformation is similar to the condition of blood platelets during induction of aggregation. Therefore, the functional behaviour of blood platelets in haemostasis might follow a general pattern of a stimulated cell (Born 1972), modified by the loss of the nucleus and the inability to proliferate.

ACKNOWLEDGEMENTS

This work was supported by the Deutsche Forschungsgemeinschaft. The skilful technical assistance of Frau G. Kaiser and Frl. G. Scheuer was much appreciated. Dr Brunnberg, Upjohn G.m.b.H., Heppenheim/Germany, kindly supplied the PGE_1. A. R. L. Gear is in receipt of an NIH Research Career Development Award (IKO4 HL 70759-01).

References

BANNAI, S. & SHEPPARD, J. R. (1974) Cyclic AMP, ATP and cell contact. *Nature (Lond.)* 250, 62-64

BOOYSE, F. M., GUILIANI, D., MARR, J. J. & RAFELSON, M. E. (1973) Cyclic adenosine 3′,5′-monophosphate dependent protein kinase of human platelets: membrane phosphorylation and regulation of platelet function. *Ser. Haematol.* 6, 3, 351-366

BORN, G. V. R. (1962) Current ideas on the mechanism of platelet aggregation. *Ann. N.Y. Acad. Sci. 201*, 4-12

COHEN, I. (1974) Contractile regulation of human blood platelets. *Abstr. Internat. Symp. on Blood Platelets*, Istanbul, 1974, p. 21

CHANG, K.-J. & CUATRECASAS, P. (1974) Adenosine triphosphate-dependent inhibition of insulin-stimulated glucose transport in fat cells. *J. Biol. Chem. 249*, 3170-3180

DEISSEROTH, A., WOLFE, S. M. & SHULMAN, N. R. (1970) Platelet phosphorylase activity in the presence of activators and inhibitors of aggregation. *Biochem. Biophys. Res. Commun. 39*, 551-557

DOERY, J. C. C., HIRSH, J. & COOPER, I. (1970) Energy metabolism in human platelets: interrelationship between glycolysis and oxidative metabolism. *Blood 36*, 159-168

FISCHER, E. H., HEILMEYER, L. M. G. & HASCKE, R. H. (1971) Phosphorylase and the control of glycogen degradation. In *Current Topics in Cellular Regulation* (Horecker, B. L. & Stadtman, E. R., eds.), vol. A, pp. 211-251, Academic Press, New York & London

GEAR, A. R. L. & SCHNEIDER, W. (1975) Control of platelet glycogenolysis: activation of phosphorylase kinase by calcium. *Biochim. Biophys. Acta 392*, 111-120

GILBOE, D. P., LARSON, K. L. & NUTTAL, F. Q. (1972) Radioactive method for the assay of glycogen phosphorylase. *Analyt. Biochem. 47*, 20-27

GROSS, R. & SCHNEIDER, W. (1971) Energy metabolism. In *The Circulating Platelet* (Johnson, S. A., ed.), pp. 123-188, Academic Press, New York & London

HASLAM, R. J. (1975) This volume, pp. 121-144

HOLMSEN, H. (1965) Changes in the radioactivity of P^{32}-labelled acid-soluble organophosphates in blood platelets during collagen- and adenosine diphosphate-induced platelet aggregation. *Scand. J. Clin. Lab. Invest. 17*, 537-548

HULTMAN, E. (1967) Studies on muscle metabolism of glycogen and active phosphate in man with special reference to exercise and diet. *Scand. J. Clin. Lab. Invest. 19*, Suppl. 94, 1-63

KARPATKIN, S. & LANGER, R. M. (1969) Human platelet phosphorylase. *Biochim. Biophys. Acta 185*, 350-359

KARPATKIN, S. & CHARMATZ, A. (1970) Heterogeneity of human platelets. III. Glycogen metabolism in platelets of different sizes. *Br. J. Haematol. 19*, 135-143

KEUL, J., DOLL, E. & KAPPLER, D. (1972) *Energy Metabolism of Human Muscle*, University Press, Baltimore

KINLOUGH-RATHBONE, R. L., PACKHAM, M. A. & MUSTARD, J. F. (1972) The effect of glucose on the platelet response to release-inducing stimuli. *J. Lab. Clin. Med. 80*, 247-255

KREBS, E. G. (1971) Protein kinases. In *Current Topics in Cellular Regulation* (Horecker, B. L. & Stadtman, E. R., eds.), vol. 5, pp. 99-133, Academic Press, New York & London

LÖHR, G. W., WALLER, H. D. & GROSS, R. (1961) Beziehungen zwischen Plättchenstoffwechsel und Retraktion des Blutgerinnsels unter besonderer Berücksichtigung der Thrombopathie Glanzmann-Naegeli. *Dtsch. Med. Wochenschr. 86*, 897-950

LÜSCHER, E. F. (1956) Glukose als Cofaktor bei der Retraktion des Blutgerinnsels. *Experientia 12*, 294

LÜSCHER, E. F., PROBST, E. & BETTEX-GALLAND, M. (1972) Thrombosthenin: structure and function. *Ann. N.Y. Acad. Sci. 201*, 122-130

MARCUS, A. J. & ZUCKER, M. B. (1965) *The Physiology of Blood Platelets*, pp. 82-86, Grune & Stratton, New York

MARQUIS, N. R., VIGDAHL, R. L. & TAVORMINA, P. A. (1971) Cyclic AMP-dependent platelet protein kinase. *Fed. Proc. 30*, 423Abs

MCDONAGH, R. P., BURNS, H. J., DELAIMI, K. E. & FAUST, R. C. (1968) Sugar penetration into human blood platelets. *J. Cell. Physiol. 72*, 77-80

MCELROY, F. A., KINLOUGH-RATHBONE, R. L., ARDLIE, H. G., PACKHAM, M. A. & MUSTARD, J. F. (1971) The effect of aggregating agents on oxidative metabolism of rabbit platelets. *Biochim. Biophys. Acta 253*, 64-77

MILLS, D. C. B. & SMITH, J. B. (1972) The control of platelet responsiveness by agents that influence cyclic AMP metabolism. *Ann. N.Y. Acad. Sci. 201*, 391-399

MUSTARD, J. F. & PACKHAM, M. A. (1970) Factors influencing platelet function: adhesion, release and aggregation. *Pharmacol. Rev. 22*, 97-187

MÜRER, E. H. (1969) Clot retraction and energy metabolism of platelets. Effect and mechanism of inhibitors. *Biochim. Biophys. Acta 172*, 266-276

PASSONNEAU, J. V. (1970) Fluorometrische Bestimmung mit Phosphorylase a. In *Methoden der enzymatischen Analyse*, vol. 2 (Bergmeyer, H. U., ed.), pp. 1095-1099, Verlag Chemie, Weinheim/Bergstrasse

POLLACK, R. E. & HOUGH, P. V. C. (1974) The cell surface and malignant transformation. *Ann. Rev. Med. 25*, 431-446

PORTZEHL, H., CALDWELL, P. C. & RÜEGG, J. C. (1964) The dependence of contraction and relaxation of muscle fibres from the crab Maia Squinado on the internal concentration of free calcium ions. *Biochim. Biophys. Acta 79*, 581-591

SACKTOR, B., WU, N. C. & LESCURE, O. (1974) Regulation of muscle phosphorylase b kinase activity by inorganic phosphate and calcium ions. *Biochem. J. 137*, 535-542

SALZMAN, E. W. (1972) Cyclic AMP and platelet function. *N. Engl. J. Med. 286*, 358-363

SALZMAN, E. W., KENSLER, P. C. & LEVINE, L. (1972) Cyclic 3′,5′-adenosine monophosphate in human blood platelets. IV. Regulatory role of cyclic AMP in platelet function. *Ann. N.Y. Acad. Sci. 201*, 61-71

SCHNEIDER, W. (1974) Regulation of energy metabolism in human blood platelets by cyclic AMP. In *Platelets, Production, Function, Transfusion and Storage* (Baldini, M. G. & Ebbe, S., eds.), Grune & Stratton, New York

SCHWARTZ, A. L., RÄIHÄ, N. C. R. & RALL, T. W. (1974) Effect of dibutyryl cyclic AMP on glucose-6-phosphatase activity in human fetal liver explants. *Biochim. Biophys. Acta 343*, 500-509

SCOTT, R. B. (1967) Activation of glycogen phosphorylase in blood platelets. *Blood 30*, 321-330

SCOTT, R. B. (1968) The role of glycogen in blood cells. *N. Engl. J. Med. 278*, 1436-1439

SEITZ, I. F. (1965) Biochemistry of normal and leukemic leukocytes, thrombocytes, and bone marrow cells. *Adv. Cancer Res. 9*, 303-410

THOMAS, J. A., SCHLENDER, K. K. & LARNER, J. (1968) A rapid filter paper assay for UDP-glucose-glycogen-glycosyl-transferase, including an improved biosynthesis of UDP-^{14}C-glucose. *Analyt. Biochem. 25*, 486-499

WEBER, E. & UNGER, W. (1964) Über Veränderungen des Glykogengehaltes in Blutplättchen während der Gerinnung. *Biochem. Pharmacol. 13*, 23-30

ZIEVE, P. D. & SCHMUKLER, M. (1971) The effect of cyclic AMP on glycogenolysis and glycolysis in human platelets. *Biochim. Biophys. Acta 252*, 280-284

Discussion

Cohen: Dr Schneider, you rightly mentioned the question of calcium concentration, which in the micromolar range (10^{-6}M) induced glycogenolysis and glycolysis. On the other hand, in the concentration range of 0.5×10^{-3}M to 10^{-3}M, calcium inhibits glycolysis in the enolase step and causes uncoupling of oxidative phosphorylation and pronounced morphological changes in membrane structures (Wainio 1970). This is probably why, once release occurs, calcium is extruded and the platelet commits suicide.

Schneider: Do you think that even during the release reaction, millimolar concentrations of calcium are reached within the cell? As far as I know, if all the calcium of a cell were equally distributed one would not reach millimolar concentrations. One might come close to 10^{-4}M.

Cohen: In the microenvironment of the platelet, when all the calcium is released, you may have a transitory millimolar concentration.

Mills: The calcium concentration in platelets would be between 20 and 30 mM if it were evenly distributed throughout the cell water.

Haslam: Surely, most of this calcium never gains access to the cytoplasm? It is extracellular after release. The calcium concentration within the platelet will then be in the micromolar range, similar to that Dr Schneider has been using.

Feinberg: Using the spectral shift of intraplatelet murexide to Ca–murexide we estimate that the addition of ADP (10^{-5}M) to platelets in plasma induces a redistribution of about 20-30 μmoles of calcium.

Schneider: As a matter of fact, Dr Cohen, one can easily demonstrate that glycolysis is even stimulated during aggregation and the release reaction. Therefore, an inhibitory effect of calcium ions on energy metabolism during aggregation and release is unlikely (for review see Gross & Schneider 1971).

Cohen: I agree that in the first step you would have an increase in glycolysis, but once release occurs, there are profound alterations in the plasma membrane.

Born: Is it not true, as Dr Mustard said, that the cell does not commit suicide with the release reaction? It is a specific function in which particular constituents are released by a mechanism analogous to exocytosis. The remainder of the cell seems to remain structurally and functionally intact; that is certain from what our results on membrane function suggest.

Mustard: This point must be emphasized. The use of the term 'irreversible aggregation', or death of the cell, in relation to the release reaction, is a fundamental error. The platelet is an extremely hardy structure. As I have emphasized, you can stimulate rabbit platelets with release-inducing stimuli *in vitro*, recover them, put them back into a rabbit's circulation, and they show normal survival (Reimers *et al.* 1973). Also we could not show, in pigs, that thrombin infusions cause irreversible aggregation and damage to platelets (Mustard *et al.* 1966). The concept that the platelet release reaction is associated with the destruction or irreversible aggregation of platelets is fundamentally wrong.

Cohen: Even at high concentrations of thrombin?

Mustard: Yes; with suspensions of washed platelets, at thrombin concentrations of 5 to 10 units/ml, you can release the amine storage granules contents, recover the platelets and demonstrate a normal aggregation response to ADP and a normal platelet survival when the platelets are infused into a rabbit's circulation.

Born: We have recently established that three active transports through platelet membranes, namely those for 5-hydroxytryptamine (5HT), potassium and adenosine, have normal initial velocities in platelets recovered from plasma that had been clotted with thrombin and lysed by activation of plasminogen with streptokinase (Zuzel *et al.* 1976).

Holmsen: I wonder whether the inhibition of glucose uptake by adenosine could be due to a competition between glucose and the ribose moiety of adenosine for the sugar carrier system. Platelets take up adenosine by two mechanisms, one with a low K_m and one with a high K_m (Sixma *et al.* 1973). The low K_m system is completely inhibited by papaverine. Did you attribute the inhibition of glucose uptake to adenosine-induced formation of cyclic AMP?

Schneider: Yes, because we found the same or an even more pronounced effect with prostaglandin E_1.

Holmsen: If I am not mistaken, the high K_m system can be inhibited by phlorizin, indicating that this system is specific for the sugar moiety of adenosine. You used rather high concentrations of adenosine, so most of it was transported by the high K_m system. Do you think adenosine and glucose are competing for the same transport system?

Schneider: We used phlorizin too, and in fact there was no increase in glucose uptake during ADP-induced aggregation. Basic glucose uptake, however, was elevated, by comparison with the controls. We saw this effect again when using deoxyglucose as an inhibitor of glucose uptake. Therefore, the inhibition of the glycolytic flow rate might lead to an unspecific increase in membrane permeability.

Born: Could it be that if the membrane is perturbed there is a passive, diffusional inflow of glucose? I cannot remember if that is, so for red cells or other cells.

Schneider: This is probably a very important point. In parallel with glucose uptake we measured the uptake of inorganic phosphate and found a quite similar pattern: phosphate uptake is inhibited by substances which increase the intracellular cyclic AMP content or turnover. As the glycolytic flow rate, however, is regulated by inorganic phosphate, this finding might be relevant to the regulation of energy metabolism in blood platelets. In fact, if ADP is added there is an increase in the uptake of inorganic phosphate. Therefore, the changes in glucose uptake during aggregation by ADP or during inhibition of aggregation by cyclic AMP could result from unspecific changes in membrane permeability and seemingly do not only concern the glucose transport mechanisms. The findings on sodium uptake reported by Dr Feinberg (p. 203) would fit very well into this scheme.

Pletscher: What kind of uptake is that? Is it a carrier-mediated uptake? Is it an uptake similar to that of glucose in muscle cells? And is it insulin-dependent?

Schneider: We were not able to show any effect of insulin on glucose transport in human blood platelets. We would have liked to do so, because Chang & Cuatrecasas (1974) have shown that the insulin-stimulated but not the basal rate of glucose uptake can be inhibited by membrane phosphorylation in fat cells and our first idea was that this could be the same in human blood platelets.

Pletscher: Have you ever studied platelets from a diabetic animal?

Schneider: No, we haven't.

White: Can platelets restore glycogen from amino acids by glyconeogenesis?

Schneider: Yes. This was described by Karpatkin *et al.* (1970).

Detwiler: Dr Schneider, when you measure glucose uptake using [6-^{14}C]-glucose, the assumption is that you are not losing ^{14}C as CO_2; but what about loss as lactate?

Schneider: We haven't measured lactate because our incubation period was only one minute and the amount of platelets very small. We therefore assumed that the production of lactate must be negligible.

Detwiler: If glucose uptake is levelling off with time, could that simply mean that you are reaching a steady-state?

Schneider: Yes, probably. But if a significant amount of lactate were formed, this would leave the cell during Millipore filtration and should reduce our uptake values.

Detwiler: But glucose in the medium could be taken up continuously and excreted as lactate. Several years ago I did some studies of substrates, products and intermediates of glycolysis (Detwiler & Zivkovic 1970). The striking fact to me was that essentially all the glycogen or glucose used could be accounted for as lactate, even in the presence of very active respiration. That didn't seem reasonable, so I have looked carefully at other people's data and I consistently find that where [^{14}C]glucose is used and data are given for the production of

[^{14}C]lactate and $^{14}CO_2$, lactate production is 10^2–10^3 times greater than CO_2 production. So I question whether the conversion of glucose to CO_2 ever means anything. The real question is how much labelled lactate has been formed.

Schneider: You are right; we have to do this control, and measure [^{14}C]lactate. But as we found an increase in the uptake of glucose during aggregation by ADP, the loss of radioactivity via lactate cannot be too important; and particularly because lactate production is stimulated during aggregation.

Detwiler: I agree. Your subsequent results would suggest that you had a valid measurement. But you would not disagree that glucose or glycogen do not appreciably go to CO_2? Have you looked at this question?

Schneider: We have measured the production of $^{14}CO_2$ from [6-^{14}C]glucose. Within one hour this was so extremely low that there should be no decarboxylation during our incubation period of one minute in these experiments. If, however, a certain amount of radioactivity is lost via lactate we should get almost no increase in glucose uptake in ADP-induced aggregation, as ADP would stimulate lactate production and we should lose even more. Therefore, I think our experiments with ADP are inconsistent with such an explanation. But you are right; we have to examine it.

Haslam: A point that may be relevant to this discussion is that muscle extensively utilizes circulating free fatty acids. We should, therefore, consider these as a possible major source of acetyl coenzyme A in the platelet.

In view of Dr Schneider's elegant demonstration of the activation of platelet phosphorylase kinase by calcium, is it possible that calcium, in addition to having a direct effect on platelet troponin, may initiate the phosphorylation of this troponin by phosphorylase kinase, as has been suggested for skeletal muscle (Stull *et al.* 1972)?

Adelstein: Although troponin from skeletal muscle can be phosphorylated by phosphorylase kinase it has not been shown that this phosphorylation affects muscle contraction. However, in a recent paper England (1975) showed that the effect of adrenaline in increasing the contraction of a perfused rat heart was correlated with increasing phosphorylation of the inhibitory component troponin I.

It would be of interest to know if either platelet myosin or platelet troponin (assuming it can be purified) could serve as a substrate for platelet phosphorylase kinase.

Holmsen: I wondered about the breakdown of glycogen. You mentioned phosphorylase. What about enzymes that break the 1,6 bond? Are they present in platelets?

Schneider: I think so, but I have no experience in this field.

Holmsen: If there is not, do you think that glycogen is never completely broken down, and that there always is a limit dextran left?

Schneider: Probably. One always ends up with 30–40% of the initial amount of glycogen. Even an increase in prostaglandin E_1 concentration or very large amounts of dibutyryl cyclic AMP do not lower these final levels further. And I think these results correspond to the findings reported by Scott (1967).

Born: That seems biochemically curious. Could it be a non-attackable form of glycogen?

Mills: It's a limit dextran containing 1,6 glycosidic bonds.

References

CHANG, K.-J. & CUATRECASAS, P. (1974) Adenosine triphosphate-dependent inhibition of insulin-stimulated glucose transport in fat cells. Possible role of membrane phosphorylation. *J. Biol. Chem. 249*, 3170-3180

DETWILER, T. C. & ZIVKOVIC, R. V. (1970) Control of energy metabolism in platelets. A comparison of aerobic and anaerobic metabolism in washed rat platelets. *Biochim. Biophys. Acta 197*, 117-126

ENGLAND, P. J. (1975) Correlation between contraction and phosphorylation of the inhibitory subunit of troponin in perfused rat heart. *FEBS Lett. 50*, 57-60

GROSS, R. & SCHNEIDER, W. (1971) Energy metabolism. In *The Circulating Platelet* (Johnson, S. A., ed.), pp. 123-188, Academic Press, New York

KARPATKIN, S., CHARMATZ, A. & LANGER, R. M. (1970) Glycogenesis and glyconeogenesis in human blood platelets. Incorporation of glucose, pyruvate, and citrate into platelet glycogen; glycogen synthetase and fructose-1,6-diphosphatase activity. *J. Clin. Invest. 49*, 140-149

MUSTARD, J. F., ROWSELL, H. C. & MURPHY, E. A. (1966) Platelet economy (platelet survival and turnover). *Br. J. Haematol. 12*, 1-24

REIMERS, H. J., PACKHAM, M. A., KINLOUGH-RATHBONE, R. L. & MUSTARD, J. F. (1973) Effect of repeated treatment of rabbit platelets with low concentrations of thrombin on their function, metabolism and survival. *Br. J. Haematol. 25*, 675-689

SCOTT, R. B. (1967) Activation of glycogen phosphorylase in blood platelets. *Blood 30*, 321-330

SIXMA, J. J., TRIESCHNIGG, A. M. C. & HOLMSEN, H. (1973) Adenosine uptake in intact human blood platelets. *IVth International Congress on Thrombosis and Haemostasis*, Vienna, abstr. 357

STULL, J. T., BROSTROM, C. O. & KREBS, E. G. (1972) Phosphorylation of the inhibitor component of troponin by phosphorylase kinase. *J. Biol. Chem. 247*, 5272-5274

WAINIO, W. W. (1970) Energy conservation. In *The Mammalian Mitochondrial Respiratory Chain* (Wainio, W. W., ed.), pp. 331-350, Academic Press, New York & London

ZUZEL, M. IRVING, W. & BORN, G. V. R. (1976) Membrane transports of platelets present in plasma during clotting and lysis. In *Proceedings of the Vth Congress of the International Society of Thrombosis and Haemostasis*, Paris *(Thromb. Diath. Haemorrh.)* (Biggs, R., ed.), in press

Elemental composition of platelet dense bodies

R. J. SKAER

Department of Haematological Medicine, University of Cambridge

Abstract Mineral elements present in the dense bodies of human platelets have been detected by quantitative microprobe analysis. Sections of frozen-dried platelets and also whole mounts of air-dried, atropinized platelets have been used. The only elements detectable in the dense bodies are calcium and phosphorus. The ratios of the peaks of these two elements vary slightly between individuals but correspond approximately to an atomic ratio of just over 3 phosphorus atoms to 2 calcium atoms. This changes to a new constant ratio of just over 1 phosphorus atom to 1 calcium atom when dried platelets are extracted with lipid solvents. If certain assumptions are made, the absolute quantities of calcium and of phosphorus compounds in dense bodies can be calculated. From 1.99–2.61 mg Ca/g dry weight of platelets are found in the dense bodies. This is within the published range for total platelet calcium. Microprobe analyses of platelet cytoplasm show there is very little calcium in platelets except in dense bodies.

The presence of up to 5 mg phospholipid in the dense bodies of 10^{11} platelets is deduced and its existence discussed in relation to platelet factor 3. The stability of dense bodies is dependent on the presence of calcium. Dense bodies dissolve from platelets fixed in the absence of calcium and do not reappear if the platelet is stained with osmium tetroxide after fixation. The significance of these findings is discussed.

The production of an irreversible aggregate of platelets is dependent on the release reaction. To investigate the control of this release and its consequences, one needs quantitative information about the substances released. Most of these substances are contained in platelet dense bodies—a type of cytoplasmic granule that is both heavy and electron dense (White 1970). Dense bodies are known to contain large amounts of ATP (Baker *et al.* 1959), 5-hydroxytryptamine (5HT; serotonin) (Davis & White 1968) and ADP (Mills *et al.* 1968). Both the latter substances can themselves provoke or enhance the release reaction (Holmsen *et al.* 1969*b*).

239

There is a large but variable quantity of calcium in platelets (Cousin & Caen 1964). On aggregation up to 88 % of the total calcium is released (Mürer 1969). White (1969a, 1971) has claimed that calcium is present in dense bodies, since the time course of its release coincides with the release reaction, and platelet calcium does not exchange with extracellular ^{45}Ca (Mürer & Holme 1970).

We have used electron-probe analysis to investigate the mineral elements present in dense bodies (Skaer et al. 1974). This has provided direct evidence that large amounts of both calcium and phosphorus are present in dense bodies in a fixed ratio to each other. We now find that apart from these two mineral elements there are no elements heavier than sodium present in dense bodies. Their electron density must be due to these two elements alone. In this paper I want to discuss the extent to which we can get quantitative information about the composition of dense bodies from the P:Ca ratios obtained from the microprobe. This knowledge of the composition of dense bodies influences our understanding of their stability under a variety of conditions. Finally I shall discuss how quantitative knowledge of the substances present in dense bodies highlights features of the release reaction and its control.

MATERIALS AND METHODS

The technique of microprobe analysis has been described elsewhere (Skaer et al. 1974). We have used an AEI EMMA-4 transmission electron microscope which is equipped with a minilens that focuses the beam on the specimen to a spot approximately 150 nm in diameter. This spot is smaller than most dense bodies, which have diameters of up to 320 nm. The elements in the irradiated part of the specimen give off X-rays whose energies and number are measured in a Kevex Si Li detector. The number of pulses are recorded against energy, giving peaks at energies corresponding to the elements in the specimen. To obtain a quantitative estimate of an element present in the specimen we subtract the background irradiation from the total integral counts under the peak corresponding to that element.

Normal human platelets were prepared for microanalysis in two ways:

1. *Frozen-dried* in platelet-rich plasma, then embedded in Spurr resin and sectioned as described in Skaer et al. (1974).

2. *Air-dried*. Heparinized platelet-rich plasma was placed on hydrophobic, carbon-coated grids for 10 seconds. The grid was then blotted dry. Atropine at a final concentration of 0.04 mg/ml was added to most samples to prevent the release reaction (White 1969b). Microprobe analysis showed this treatment did not influence the composition of dense bodies.

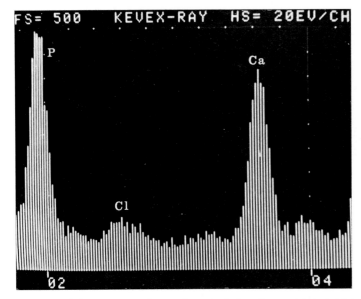

FIG. 1. Emission spectrum from a dense body in a frozen-dried platelet, sectioned on a dry knife edge and flattened mechanically. (From Skaer *et al.* 1974. Reproduced by kind permission of the Company of Biologists Ltd.)

RESULTS AND DISCUSSION

Phosphorus: calcium ratio

A fixed ratio of 1.15 (s.E. $\pm$ 0.04, $n = 18$) between phosphorus and calcium has already been found in the dense bodies of frozen-dried, sectioned platelets (Fig. 1) (Skaer *et al.* 1974). With air-dried platelets, we find this ratio varies slightly between individuals from a P:Ca ratio of 1.301 $\pm$ 0.038 ($n = 12$) to 1.094 $\pm$ 0.048 ($n = 14$) (Fig. 2). There is no consistent difference in ratio between large and small dense bodies, nor between those spherical and tadpole-shaped, nor between very dense and fairly dense.

In order to calculate the absolute quantities of compounds in the dense bodies one needs one compound or class of compounds whose absolute quantity is known. The other components can then be calculated from their ratio to this known compound.

The quantity of adenine nucleotides given off in the release reaction is known and was therefore chosen as the basis for the calculations. Adenine nucleotides contribute a significant proportion to the phosphorus peak recorded in the microprobe. It is likely, however, that the phosphorus compounds in dense

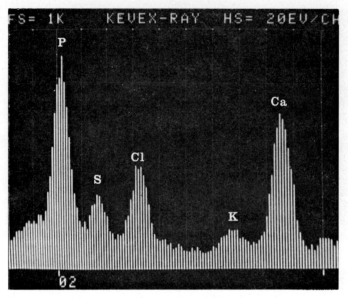

FIG. 2. Emission spectrum from a dense body. Whole mount of an air-dried platelet.

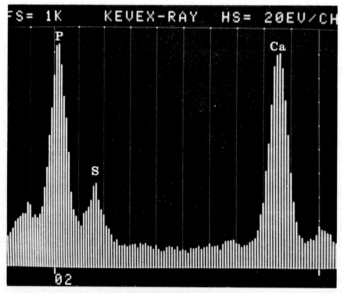

FIG. 3. Emission spectrum from a dense body. Whole mount of a desiccated platelet extracted for 16 min with dry 2:1 chloroform/methanol.

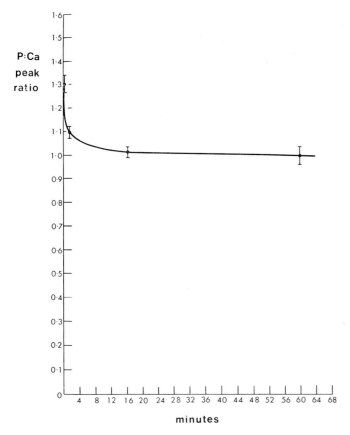

FIG. 4. Graph showing the change in P: Ca peak ratio of dense bodies with time of extraction with dry 2:1 chloroform/methanol.

bodies are not only the adenine nucleotides but also phospholipid (Skaer *et al.* 1974). In order to find the peak count for phosphorus that corresponds to the adenine nucleotides, any phospholipid present must first be removed. We have done this by extracting desiccated platelets with dry 2:1 chloroform/methanol containing molecular sieve 4A drying agent. This dissolves most phospholipid without affecting the adenine nucleotides.

Desiccated air-dried platelets were treated with chloroform/methanol for periods between one minute and one hour and the P:Ca ratio of the dense bodies was measured. The ratio falls rapidly from 1.301 ± 0.038 ($n = 12$) until after 15 minutes it reaches a new constant value (Figs. 3 & 4) of 1.014 ± 0.022 ($n = 12$).

At this stage in the calculations we make two fairly basic assumptions. First, that the phosphorus peak after chloroform/methanol extraction is due solely to ATP and ADP and, secondly, that the adenine nucleotides liberated during the release reaction come from the dense bodies alone. This latter assumption is supported by the results of Holmsen *et al.* (1969*a*) who incubated platelets for two hours at 37 °C with ^{14}C-labelled adenosine or adenine. Although the metabolic adenine nucleotides were strongly labelled, those given off by the release reaction were virtually unlabelled and therefore presumably sequestered in dense bodies. Non-specific leakage of adenine nucleotides is cancelled out by subtracting the control figures from the test.

The virtual lack of radioactivity released shows also that there is no general increase in leakiness to adenine nucleotides during the release reaction.

They find that collagen releases up to 1.605×10^{-6}M-ATP/10^{11} platelets and 2.76×10^{-6}M-ADP/10^{11} platelets and that thrombin releases 3.6×10^{-6}M-ATP/ 10^{11} platelets and 5.7×10^{-6}M-ADP/10^{11} platelets. The figures given by Mills & Thomas (1969) lie between those given by Holmsen *et al.* and have in fact been used for our calculations. Mills & Thomas' figures are 2.8×10^{-6}M-ATP and 3.6×10^{-6}M-ADP per 10^{11} platelets.

We must now transpose the peak ratios we have measured into atomic ratios. This can be done by using the microprobe on test compounds of calcium and phosphorus which have different atomic ratios. We have used tribasic calcium phosphate with 2P:3Ca, calcium glycerophosphate with 1P:1Ca and dicalcium ATP with 3P:2Ca. The resulting graph of peak ratio against atomic ratio is a straight line passing through the origin (Fig. 5).

The calculation is now fairly straightforward. By applying Avogadro's number, 6.02×10^{23}, to Mills & Thomas' figures we can calculate how many molecules of ATP and ADP are present in dense bodies. From this we obtain the total number of atoms of phosphorus present and from the atomic ratios we have already obtained we can estimate the number of calcium atoms.

Taking the peak ratio of 1.014 from chloroform/methanol extracted platelets, the result of this calculation is 1.99 mg Ca/g dry wt. Blood from another donor whose chloroform/methanol extracted platelets had a peak P:Ca ratio of 0.768 gives a figure of 2.61 mg Ca/g dry weight.

Cousin & Caen (1964) found the total calcium in platelets was 1.23–3.9 mg Ca/g dry wt. The fact that our figures for the calcium in dense bodies lies within the range given for platelet total calcium agrees with our observation that when the microprobe spot is on the cytoplasm of platelets and not on a dense body we only rarely get a significant reading for calcium (Fig. 6).

The fact that extraction with chloroform/methanol alters the P:Ca ratio so much is rather surprising and suggests that a large amount of a phosphorus compound soluble in lipid solvents is present in dense bodies. If we assume

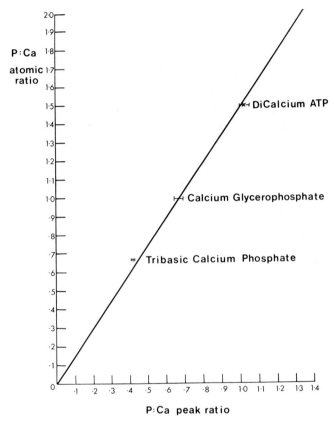

FIG. 5. Graph relating P:Ca peak ratios to P:Ca atomic ratios. The standards used to construct the graph are phosphorus, calcium compounds of known composition.

this compound to be a typical phospholipid with a molecular weight of 814—that of sphingomyelin—we can calculate from the P:Ca ratios before and after extraction how much of such a phospholipid is present. The steps in the calculation are the same as for calcium. The quantities we find are 3.6–5 mg phospholipid/10^{11} platelets, depending on the P:Ca ratios we use. This quantity is substantially more than would be present just in a bimolecular lipid membrane round the granule. These large amounts of phospholipid may be significant in view of the argument that the phospholipid platelet factor 3 may be localized in dense bodies (Skaer *et al.* 1974). It further suggests that the two categories of platelet granule Bessis (1973) calls dense bodies and phospholipid droplets may well be the same. White (1968) has made a similar claim, though very tentatively.

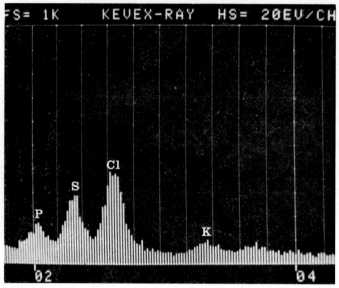

FIG. 6. Emission spectrum from the cytoplasm of a platelet. Whole mount of an air-dried platelet. Notice the large chlorine peak and the absence of a calcium peak.

Other elements

The microprobe shows that no elements heavier than sodium apart from calcium and phosphorus are present in dense bodies. The small potassium peak in probes of dense bodies from air-dried platelets (Fig. 2) is almost certainly cytoplasmic for it is absent from frozen-dried, sectioned, dense bodies (Fig. 1). Emission due to any heavy metal elements such as copper has been shown to be from the grid and its holder by the use of palladium grids mounted in a titanium specimen holder (Skaer *et al.* 1974). Chlorine is not present in dense bodies, although it occurs in spectra from both frozen-dried, sectioned dense bodies and also those that have been air-dried. In the sectioned material the chlorine is in the embedding resin (Skaer *et al.* 1974) and in the air-dried material it is cytoplasmic chlorine superimposed on the dense bodies. This is demonstrated by the absence of a fixed ratio between chlorine and phosphorus or calcium. It is also demonstrated by the surprising fact that the chlorine in the cytoplasm of desiccated platelets is completely soluble in dry 2:1 chloroform/methanol (Fig. 7). When the chlorine is completely removed from the cytoplasm no chlorine signal is obtained from the dense bodies. It seems unlikely that chlorine should be in this odd form in both cytoplasm and dense bodies. Chlorine in the cytoplasm of desiccated red cells is unaffected by dry chloroform/methanol.

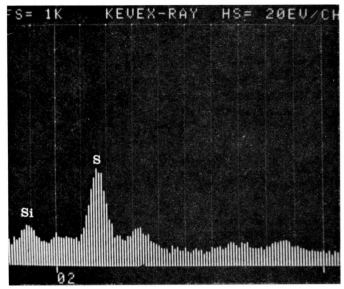

FIG. 7. Emission spectrum from the cytoplasm of a platelet. Whole mount of a desiccated specimen extracted for 1 min with dry 2:1 chloroform/methanol. The chlorine peak has nearly gone.

Stability of dense bodies

We have found that if we rigorously exclude calcium ions from our glutar-aldehyde fixative solutions the dense bodies lose their electron density and disappear. Their electron density, however, is retained if we fix in glutaraldehyde in a non-chelating buffer such as Hepes and add 1.25 mM-calcium chloride to the fixative (Skaer *et al.* 1974). We now find that if calcium is leached out during fixation other constituents of dense bodies are also lost. Fig. 8 shows a normal air-dried platelet showing dense bodies. Fig. 9 shows a platelet that has lost its calcium during fixation. Even though it has been treated with osmium tetroxide, no dense bodies can be seen. It is known that there are substances in dense bodies, such as phospholipid and 5HT, that would be expected to react with osmium tetroxide after glutaraldehyde fixation (Tranzer *et al.* 1966). In fact the platelet in Fig. 9 has been processed by a common preparative technique used by many electron microscopists. *Citrated* platelet-rich plasma was fixed for one hour at room temperature in 3% EM grade glutaraldehyde in 0.1 M-*phosphate buffer*, then washed in *phosphate buffer overnight* at 4 °C, then treated for one hour in 1% *osmium tetroxide in cacodylate buffer*. In this schedule the processes given in italics might almost have been designed specifically to remove calcium. In fact many people see dense bodies

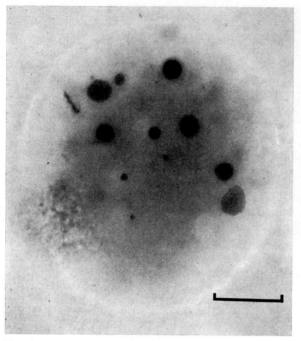

FIG. 8. Unstained, air-dried, whole mount of a platelet × 18750. The scale mark is 1 μm. The dense bodies are clearly visible.

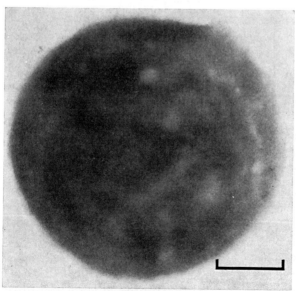

FIG. 9. Whole mount of a platelet, fixed as described in the text in glutaraldehyde and osmium tetroxide × 18750. The scale mark is 1 μm. No dense bodies are visible.

in standard preparations for the electron microscope only because they have unwittingly added calcium as a contaminant of commercial glutaraldehyde (Oschman & Wall 1972) or because they have misidentified overstained lysosomes. These remarks about the importance of calcium to the stability of dense bodies probably also apply to homogenized dense bodies which are commonly isolated in chelating agents such as EDTA.

These observations on the importance of calcium for the stability of dense bodies might seem at first sight to be incompatible with the results obtained by Berneis *et al.* (1970). They found that mixtures of 5HT or other biogenic amines with ATP formed long-chain polymers in the presence of a small amount of calcium; large amounts of ionized calcium, however, broke up the polymers.

In the case of dense bodies it seems likely that the large amount of calcium contained in them is not in an ionized form (Skaer *et al.* 1974), in spite of the fact that ionized calcium in the fixative helps to preserve them. However, a reasonable level of ionized calcium in the external medium will prevent dissociation of non-ionized calcium in the dense bodies.

The release reaction

Estimates of the amounts of substances present in dense bodies should help with a quantitative understanding of the effects of the release reaction. Applying this to calcium, if all the calcium present in dense bodies were liberated during the release reaction the calcium concentration of the serum would increase by 0.25 mg Ca/100 ml of plasma (assuming a normal frequency of 450 000 platelets/μl of plasma). This change in calcium concentration should be detectable with present techniques and yet it has not been reported. Published figures give the same quantity of calcium in plasma as in serum—that is, after the release reaction (McLean & Hastings 1935; Lumb 1963; Bauditz 1967). This might simply mean that in the preparation of platelet-free plasma for analysis, the release reaction has been triggered by centrifugation (O'Brien & Woodhouse 1968). Alternatively the figures may be genuine and the calcium trapped at high concentration between the aggregated platelets, or even possibly taken up again by the platelets after the release reaction. Bygdeman & Stjärne (1971) found no significant uptake of ionized $^{45}Ca^{2+}$ during and slightly after the release reaction. Calcium in dense bodies, however, may not be ionized (Skaer *et al.* 1974) and may therefore behave differently.

I should like to finish by discussing briefly what effect all these substances have on the growth and stability of the platelet aggregate. It is a juvenile characteristic to ask a question to which one does not know the answer, but I should like to end by doing just that. Is it coincidental that at least two of the substances contained in dense bodies and liberated in the release reaction, ADP and 5HT, are released in quantities that can provoke or enhance the release reaction? In other words, can the release reaction be regarded as a system with positive feedback in relation both to completion of the release reaction in each individual platelet, and also to recruitment of new platelets to the aggregate? A consequence of this would be that the release reaction would always go to completion, and the production of the irreversible platelet clot would be essentially the same process as the production of the initial reversible clump, but carried out for a longer time and with the reactants at higher concentration. This is not what is observed. At the level of the individual platelet one can often find a few remaining dense bodies in platelets that have undergone secondary aggregation in response to an initial stimulus that was less than optimum. Moreover, up to a certain limit, the stronger the stimulus for the release reaction, the more 5HT is released (Sneddon 1972). This graded release is presumably a graded release of dense bodies. At the level of recruitment, the quantity of ADP that can be released by platelets is very high. With platelets at the normal circulating frequency in blood of 2.5×10^{11} per litre the quantity of ADP that could be liberated from dense bodies is 9 μM. Hardisty *et al.* (1970) found the threshold for the release reaction is 0.2–1.4 μM. Thus in blood there is at least 6.5 times as much ADP that can be released from the platelets as will trigger the release reaction. With aggregated platelets the local concentration will be much higher. Moreover, unless the presence of citrate in plasma drastically affects plasma ADPase, the half-life of ADP in plasma is relatively long—8–12 minutes (Holmsen *et al.* 1969a)—compared with the speed of the release reaction. It is true that dense bodies also release ATP—an antagonist of the release reaction (Born 1972). This is released, however, in lower concentration than ADP and with a shorter half-life (3–5 minutes, Holmsen *et al.* 1969a). Nevertheless platelets are apparently not normally recruited exponentially to the growing clot. The effects would be disastrous.

It may be that platelets change their susceptibility and response to ADP after their first exposure to it. Moreover, the conditions under which ADP is presented by the release reaction are different from an initial stimulus with ADP. The differences associated with the production of an irreversible clot are ATP, phospholipid and calcium—all in high concentration and with calcium, possibly, in a special form.

ACKNOWLEDGEMENTS

I am most grateful to Dr Patricia D. Peters who operated the EMMA-4 and to Mr J. P. Emmines who prepared the specimens. Dr H. le B. Skaer made valuable comments on the manuscript; Dr A. D. Bangham gave helpful advice on the area occupied by phospholipid films. This work was financed by the Leukaemia Research Fund in the laboratory of Professor F. G. J. Hayhoe. Funds for instrumentation and research on the microanalyser were provided by the British Science Research Council.

References

BAKER, R. V., BLASCHKO, H. & BORN, G. V. R. (1959) The isolation from blood platelets of particles containing 5-hydroxytryptamine and adenosine triphosphate. *J. Physiol. (Lond.)* *149*, 55P

BAUDITZ, W. (1967) Der Plasmacalciumwert beim Menschen und seine Altersabhängigkeit. *Z. Gesamte Exp. Med. 142*, 9-21

BERNEIS, K. H., PLETSCHER, A. & DA PRADA, M. (1970) Phase separation in solutions of noradrenaline and adenosine triphosphate: influence of bivalent cations and drugs. *Br. J. Pharmacol. Chemother. 39*, 382-389

BESSIS, M. (1973) *Living Blood Cells and their Ultrastructure*, pp. 387-388, Springer-Verlag, Berlin, Heidelberg & New York

BORN, G. V. R. (1972) The functional physiology of blood platelets. In *Platelet Function and Thrombosis. A Review of Methods* (Mannucci, P. M. & Gorini, S., eds.), pp. 3-22, Plenum Press, New York & London

BYGDEMAN, S. & STJÄRNE, L. (1971) Calcium uptake and collagen-induced platelet release reaction. *Scand. J. Haematol. 8*, 183-188

COUSIN, C. & CAEN, J. (1964) Dosage du magnésium et du calcium dans les plaquettes sanguines humaines. *Rev. Fr. Etud. Clin. Biol. 9*, 520-523

DAVIS, R. B. & WHITE, J. G. (1968) Localisation of 5-hydroxytryptamine in blood platelets: a radioautographic and ultrastructural study. *Br. J. Haematol. 15*, 93-99

HARDISTY, R. M., HITTON, R. A., MONTGOMERY, D., RICKARD, S. & TREBILCOCK, H. (1970) Secondary platelet aggregation: a quantitative study. *Br. J. Haematol. 19*, 307-320

HOLMSEN, H., DAY, H. J. & STORM, E. (1996a) Adenine nucleotide metabolism of blood platelets. VI. Subcellular localisation of nucleotide pools with different functions in the platelet release reaction. *Biochim. Biophys. Acta 186*, 254-266

HOLMSEN, H., DAY, H. J. & STORMORKEN, O. (1969b) The blood platelet release reaction. *Scand. J. Haematol.* Suppl. 8, 3-26

LUMB, G. A. (1963) Determination of ionic calcium in serum. *Clin. Chim. Acta 8*, 33-38

McLEAN, F. C. & HASTINGS, A. B. (1935) Clinical estimation and significance of calcium-ion concentrations in the blood. *Am. J. Med. Sci. 189*, 601-613

MILLS, D. C. B. & THOMAS, D. P. (1969) Blood platelet nucleotides in man and other species. *Nature (Lond.) 222*, 991-992

MILLS, D. C. B., ROBB, I. A. & ROBERTS, G. C. K. (1968) The release of nucleotides, 5-hydroxytryptamine and enzymes from human blood platelets during aggregation. *J. Physiol. (Lond.) 195*, 715-729

MÜRER, E. H. (1969) Thrombin induced release of calcium from blood platelets. *Science (Wash. D.C.) 166*, 623

MÜRER, E. H. & HOLME, R. (1970) A study of the release of calcium from human blood platelets and its inhibition by metabolic inhibitors, N-ethylmaleimide and aspirin. *Biochim. Biophys. Acta 222*, 197-205

O'BRIEN, J. R. & WOODHOUSE, M. A. (1968) Platelets: their size, shape and stickiness *in vitro*: degranulation and propinquity. *Exp. Biol. Med. 3*, 90-102

OSCHMAN, J. L. & WALL, B. J. (1972) Calcium binding to intestinal membranes. *J. Cell Biol.* 55, 58-73

SKAER, R. J., PETERS, P. D. & EMMINES, J. P. (1974) The localisation of calcium and phosphorus in human platelets. *J. Cell Sci.* 15, 679-692

SNEDDON, J. M. (1972) Divalent cations and the blood platelet release reaction. *Nature New Biol.* 236, 103-104

TRANZER, J. P., DA PRADA, M. & PLETSCHER, A. (1966) Ultrastructural localisation of 5-hydroxytryptamine in blood platelets. *Nature (Lond.)* 212, 1574-1575

WHITE, J. G. (1968) The origin of dense bodies in the surface coat of negatively stained platelets. *Scand. J. Haematol.* 5, 371-382

WHITE, J. G. (1969a) The dense bodies of human platelets: inherent electron opacity of the serotonin storage particles. *Blood* 33, 598-606

WHITE, J. G. (1969b) Effects of atropine on platelet structure and function. *Scand. J. Haematol.* 6, 236-245

WHITE, J. G. (1970) Origin and function of platelet dense bodies. *Ser. Haematol.* 3, 17-46

WHITE, J. G. (1971) Platelet morphology. In *The Circulating Platelet* (Johnson, S. A., ed.), pp. 45-121, Academic Press, New York & London

Discussion

Born: I believe you have also shown calcium spots on the surface of platelets?

Skaer: Yes. We find calcium spots on the surface of human platelets fixed in glutaraldehyde containing 1.25 mM-calcium (Skaer *et al.* 1974). If we leave calcium out the spots are not visible. We are worried, however, because we don't see them in frozen–dried platelets. One possibility is that there is a phosphatase in the membrane that is not instantly destroyed by fixation and releases inorganic phosphate in the presence of calcium, and so calcium phosphate is deposited as spots at the site of the enzyme.

Born: Are they physiological or artifactual?

Skaer: The concentration of calcium in the fixative when we see these spots is the normal level of ionized calcium in the blood. On the other hand, fixation would seem to be necessary to show up the spots in unstained platelets. As we don't see the spots in frozen–dried material, they may be artifacts of fixation.

Crawford: I have two questions on the technique, Dr Skaer. You give 150 nm as the size of the microprobe spot. What would you estimate as the actual resolving power of the procedure?

Skaer: The resolution for viewing objects is very much the same as with a normal transmission electron microscope; the size of the spot for analysis is about 150 nm.

Crawford: I had wondered whether you saw any heterogeneity in the population of dense bodies, which might suggest refilling or repletion of the granules. Also, have you had any opportunity of looking at platelets from patients with carcinoid tumours where the 5-hydroxytryptamine levels may be as much as three times higher than normal, or cord blood where the platelet 5HT concentration is quite low but, in our experience, both the ATP and the calcium content are apparently normal?

Skaer: I haven't looked at either of those situations; they would certainly be interesting. There are differences in the appearance of dense bodies—some have a pale halo round a dense centre, and so on; but we haven't found any differences in the ratios that could be interpreted as refilling or formation.

Hardisty: Can you distinguish with certainty between the least dense of the dense bodies and the α-granules?

Skaer: Yes, we can.

Pletscher: I am glad to see that you have found, with a different technique from ours, what are essentially similar results! We have isolated the granules, and have them in a very pure form and have analysed their constituents (see pp. 261-279). We work mainly with rabbit and guinea pig platelets and, as we heard earlier from Dr Mustard, there are species differences in the cations. Guinea pig and rabbit platelets contain mainly magnesium, whereas human platelets have almost exclusively calcium.

In rabbit 5HT organelles we found 0.55M bivalent cations and 0.75M nucleotides, which would give a ratio of about four atoms of phosphorus to about one bivalent cation, which is calcium plus magnesium. So we agree that there are large amounts of bivalent cations.

As to the form in which these metals occur, I agree that they cannot be in an ionized form, because together with the other constituents the concentration would be such that the 5HT organelles would explode, for osmotic reasons. There are some clues here from nuclear magnetic resonance spectroscopy and also from ultracentrifugation experiments. It has been shown that bivalent cations, in contrast to monovalent cations, cause the rings of nucleotides to stack vertically and as one adds calcium or magnesium in rising concentrations to an ATP solution the molecular weight increases. This may be the reason why this calcium is not present in free (un-ionized) form and it may also explain why, in eliminating the calcium, you also get rid of the ATP, because of disaggregation.

We have found another clear effect. In a solution of ATP and 5HT one gets a higher molecular weight than one would expect on the basis of the single components. If one adds bivalent cations the molecular weight goes up even more; however, if one exceeds a critical concentration of bivalent cations the molecular weight decreases again. The increase is probably due to intermolecular interaction between 5HT and ATP, probably by electrostatic and Van der Waals forces. If the calcium concentration becomes too high there might be competition between 5HT, which has a positively charged NH_3^+

group, and Ca^{2+}. This might displace 5HT from the aggregates, which would lead to a decrease in the molecular weight.

On the electron density of the granules, this is not due to calcium in our fixation method. We fix in glutaraldehyde and osmium tetroxide. Only then do we see these highly dense bodies. You say that the density is due to calcium, Dr Skaer, but how does one explain the following finding: after treatment with reserpine, the electron density of the 5HT organelles disappears and so does their 5HT. If one incubates such platelets in a 5HT solution, the electron-dense organelles reappear. Furthermore, in guinea pig platelets there are very few dense bodies. However, if one isolates them, as I shall describe later (pp. 261-279), one gets very nice organelles that are not electron-dense, except for the occasional granule which has a dense core. This agrees with the low 5HT content of the guinea pig platelet (10–20 times less than in the rabbit platelet). The calcium content is about the same as that of rabbit platelets. After incubation of guinea pig platelets in 5HT many of these electron-dense organelles appear. This happens with human platelets too.

Holmsen: Firstly, I have a comment that may have a bearing on Dr Pletscher's comments. Some years ago we speculated whether the inherent opacity of the dense granules was due to dense packing of Ca, ATP and ADP. We had estimated the concentration of these substances in the granules of human platelets to be at least 53, 58 and 184 mM, respectively (Holmsen & Day 1971). The nucleotides and $CaCl_2$ were mixed together in these proportions and a heavy precipitate formed that was washed and then examined electron micro-scopically by Dr J. G. White. No electron density was found whether whole mounts, glutaraldehyde fixed or osmium tetroxide post-fixed, were used.

Secondly, I have a comment for Dr Skaer. You assumed that ATP and ADP are the main phosphorus compounds in the dense granules. I think there is a third major source, inorganic pyrophosphate. It has been established that human platelets contain up to 3 µmol $PP_i/10^{11}$ cells, most of which is releasable with thrombin. Patients with storage pool disorder have platelets that are almost devoid of dense granules, and these cells have markedly decreased levels of PP_i (Silcox *et al.* 1973). This strongly suggests that PP_i is a constituent of the dense granules.

Pletscher: Only some of the platelet organelles capable of storing 5HT appear electron-dense with our fixation method—those that are filled with 5HT. However, there are others with little 5HT content but capable of storing the amine if it enters the platelet. All these organelles contain nucleotides. Therefore it might be more appropriate to call the organelles capable of storing 5HT 'nucleotide organelles'. It just happens that in rabbits almost all the bodies are dense, because all of them are filled with 5HT, whereas in humans and guinea pigs the majority are not dense (by our fixation technique), because of their small content of 5HT. According to the amount of 5HT which enters them they can be more or less filled, and be denser or less dense. This may also cause some individual variation. There are many nucleotide bodies in every platelet which cannot be seen in the electron microscope but if one supplies exogenous 5HT, they become dense because they contain ATP.

Sneddon: Dr Skaer, when you use this technique you identify the area under the probe by photography, and the area appears electron-dense by the staining methods you employ. However, as Dr Pletscher has indicated, the electron-dense granules in human platelets are few in number but can be increased by 'loading' the platelets with 5HT. Your results would indicate that calcium is only present in high concentrations in granules exhibiting electron density; therefore are your platelets maximally loaded with 5HT? If they are not, one would expect to find '5HT empty' granules which presumably contain both ATP and Ca^{2+} but little or no 5HT, giving a Ca^{2+} value similar to that of the electron-dense granules. Also, if the platelets are loaded with 5HT to increase the electron density of the granules, does the probe register the presence of Ca^{2+} in the 'new' electron-dense granules?

Skaer: The platelets we analyse are completely unstained and are also unfixed. 5-Hydroxytryptamine does not itself make platelet dense bodies electron-dense in the unstained state; but it can make the dense bodies osmiophilic. Perhaps one should call dense bodies that have been treated with osmium 'super-dense bodies', then! It is in this condition that Professor Pletscher and many other electron microscopists observe them. Different degrees of osmiophilia after glutaraldehyde fixation may mean different amounts of 5HT in dense bodies. As our fixation experiments reported here have shown, however, it may also mean differing degrees of dense-body degradation due to loss of calcium through the normal preparative procedures. When calcium goes, almost all the other contents of dense bodies go too.

Since we analyse 'native' unaltered dense bodies, and all the elements in 5HT are lighter than sodium, our microprobe results give no information about 5HT and its distribution.

We don't believe there are 'nucleotide bodies' that are not intrinsically electron dense. We have made many hundreds of microprobe analyses on regions of platelet cytoplasm that are free of visible dense bodies. The phosphorus peaks one obtains from these regions are not accompanied by a significant calcium peak and are probably due to 'phospholipid'; for such phosphorus peaks are completely absent from platelets that have been extracted with chloroform/methanol. For platelets treated with lipid solvents every phosphorus peak is associated with a calcium peak and comes from a body that is electron dense. Thus we claim that by using unfixed, unstained platelets we can see all the bodies that contain substantial amounts of stored ATP and ADP; we see them because they also always contain large amounts of calcium, and this makes them electron-dense.

Sneddon: Could it be that there is something else in a dense body, whether or not it is 5HT which makes it electron-dense, that perhaps also increases or alters the Ca^{2+} so that it is easier to pick up? I would have thought you must find calcium elsewhere in the cytoplasm in addition to the dense bodies.

Skaer: The energy dispersive analysis we have used will reveal any element that contributes to electron density. Calcium is not very electron-dense but it is present in such large amounts in dense bodies that they are opaque to electrons. The microprobe will detect calcium in whatever form it is present, provided it is in sufficient concentration. Calcium is clearly present elsewhere in platelets, but in much smaller amounts than in the dense bodies.

Sneddon: By your calculations, if you have a 5HT-loaded platelet, would you expect a greater value for your calcium concentration than you would in a reserpinized platelet?

Skaer: I would like to look at reserpinized platelets with this technique, to see what we find in terms of calcium: phosphorus ratios.

Pletscher: It is clear that there is a difference in fixation technique here. Dr Skaer's bodies are dense because of their calcium content, whereas ours show their high density because of the presence of 5HT.

White: What are the lower limits of your measurement of calcium? You said there is no calcium in the cytoplasm but does this mean that if there were a calcium flux across to some contractile apparatus you wouldn't be able to measure it, by this method?

Skaer: At present we can only detect stores of calcium, not calcium fluxes. There are, however, various ways of obtaining greater sensitivity. For dense bodies we have used a standard counting time of 40 seconds; if one probed a spot in the cytoplasm for rather longer than that one would get a slightly larger peak for calcium in the cytoplasm.

Born: In muscle the concentration of free calcium in the cytoplasm is believed to be about 10^{-8}M. If this rose a little during calcium release to, say, double, or even up to 10 times, would you be able to measure the increase?

Skaer: It would be very difficult. So far as I know no one has been able, by using the microprobe, even to show calcium stored in the sarcoplasmic reticulum of muscle (Yarom *et al.* 1974).

Cohen: You have presented good evidence about the localization of calcium not only in the dense bodies, but also in the plasma membrane and in membranous structures lining the open canalicular system, with very nice electron micrographs. Would it be too presumptuous or too early to propose that there are two pools of calcium and, using Dr Holmsen's terminology for adenosine nucleotides, to suggest that there may be a metabolic pool of calcium and a storage pool? The storage pool would be located in the dense bodies and the metabolic pool in membrane structures. Professor Lüscher has shown electron micrographs of the membranous structure of the dense tubular system associated with the plasma membrane. This system, as Professor Lüscher proposed, could be the equivalent of the muscle sarcoplasmic reticulum and could function as a calcium reservoir. This calcium could be made available to actomyosin sites. Is this a feasible model?

Skaer: It is very likely that the calcium we find on plasma membranes has come from outside the platelet and been deposited on the membranes during fixation, but I think the microprobe could well solve the question of whether it is the surface membranes or the open canalicular system or the closed dense tubular system that contains the major part of the calcium as a store, apart from the dense bodies.

Detwiler: We were interested in identifying a metabolic pool of calcium and we have used antimonate to localize calcium (Sato *et al.* 1975). Unfortunately there are complications, primarily because the fixatives that retain calcium abolish most of the fine structure. What we expected was a membrane source. What we found was calcium in the nucleoid of the α-granule; within 5 or 10 seconds after adding thrombin, it was gone. This suggests a possible functional role.

Cohen: Didn't Dr Shepro find pyroantimonate deposits only after thrombin treatment (Robblee *et al.* 1973)? This would be contrary to your findings.

Shepro: The procedure for localizing calcium by potassium pyroantimonate (in the glutaraldehyde fixative) and electron microscopy must be viewed conservatively, since the pyroantimonate precipitate may contain cations other than calcium. Dr Lois Robblee in our laboratory showed that in thrombin-treated platelets the precipitates are located primarily near the surface of the plasma membrane and apparently in close association with fibrin. Precipitates were also seen intracellularly, near the granules. In the controls, precipitates were few and only extracellular. When platelets were washed with a medium containing EGTA before the glutaraldehyde–pyroantimonate was added, the number of precipitates was markedly reduced. However, as I say, the presence or absence of precipitates shown with this technique can be interpreted in several ways (Robblee *et al.* 1973).

Crawford: Dr Skaer, is the procedure sufficiently non-destructive to allow you to do some autoradiography after, say, pre-loading with ^{45}Ca or [^{3}H]5HT? Perhaps you could then juxtapose the pictures to get evidence to support your localization.

Skaer: ^{45}Ca is very bad for autoradiography; you can probably localize [^{3}H]5HT to dense bodies. Davis & White (1968) have done that for rabbit platelets.

Born: The localization of [^{3}H]5HT was not very precise, unfortunately.

Mustard: You showed peaks for sulphur; the bulk of the sulphur, when you label platelets with ^{35}S, is in mucopolysaccharides (glycosaminoglycans). We have been interested for some time in the localization of this material. Some is on the membrane and I believe some is in granules (Riddell & Bier 1965; Packham *et al.* 1972). Did you detect much sulphur in the cytoplasm or in the granules?

Skaer: Yes; there is a fair bit in the cytoplasm, but probably very little in the dense bodies. The sulphur peaks in the pictures I showed are genuine, for an anticontaminator was used throughout this study. The peaks may well indicate that sulphur is in the cytoplasm above and below the dense bodies. We have tried to relate the size of the sulphur peak to that of the calcium and phosphorus peaks obtained from dense bodies. As we don't get a fixed ratio of S: Ca or S: P we assume the sulphur is in the cytoplasm and not in the dense bodies.

Mustard: When you label platelets with ^{35}S, remove much of the surface material with ADP and stimulate them with thrombin, ^{35}S-labelled mucopolysaccharide is released into the supernatant (Riddell & Bier 1965; Packham *et al.* 1972). In these experiments you can show that there is no lysis. Have you any evidence about the site of this releasable ^{35}S-labelled mucopolysaccharide?

Skaer: No. White (1971) has claimed that some is in the dense bodies, but we don't know.

Pletscher: In isolated dense bodies from rabbits and guinea pigs we measured the uronic acid and hexosamines (components of mucopolysaccharides). There are just traces—nothing like the amount of 5HT or nucleotides.

Marcus: Some time ago we were interested in trying to see whether the platelet membrane was characterized by the presence of a specific phospholipid or group of phospholipids (Marcus *et al.* 1969). The results were somewhat disappointing in that the phospholipid components of platelet subcellular compartments were amazingly similar. The phospholipids of platelet granules were qualitatively and quantitatively similar to those of the membranes. I was wondering whether you had partitioned your chloroform/methanol extracts with appropriate salts in order to remove non-lipid, phosphorus-containing compounds from the organic phase of the extract. Occasionally, if this is not done, such non-lipid compounds will increase the values obtained in lipid phosphorus determinations.

Skaer: No, we didn't do this. As we extract whole platelets with chloroform/methanol, partitioning the soluble material would tell one very little about what is localized where.

Marcus: You mentioned that the probe can detect copper, but that no copper was noted in the dense bodies. In some recent work we have extracted a lipid fraction from platelets which binds 5HT. The extract is in the aqueous portion of a partitioned tetrahydrofuran or chloroform/methanol extract, and it contains copper. Since the starting material for this work is whole platelets, we do not yet know the origin of this copper, but we have subsequently ascertained that at least part of whole platelet copper can be accounted for by the enzyme superoxide dismutase.

Pletscher: We find traces of copper in the granules by the atomic absorption method.

References

Davis, R. B. & White, J. G. (1968) Localisation of 5-hydroxytryptamine in blood platelets: a radioautographic and ultrastructural study. *Br. J. Haematol. 15*, 93-99

Holmsen, H. & Day, H. J. (1971) Adenine nucleotides and platelet function. *Ser. Haematol. 4*, 28-58

Marcus, A. J., Ullman, H. L. & Safier, L. B. (1969) Lipid composition of subcellular particles of human blood platelets. *J. Lipid Res. 10*, 108-114

Packham, M. A., Radojewski, A. M., Perry, D. W. & Mustard, J. F. (1972) Loss of platelet mucopolysaccharides during ADP-induced aggregation and release reaction. *Circulation 46*, Suppl. 2, 32

Riddell, P. E. & Bier, A. M. (1965) Electrophoresis of S^{35}-labelled material released from clumping platelets. *Nature (Lond.) 205*, 711-712

Robblee, L. S., Towle, C., Shepro, D. & Belamarich, F. A. (1973) Pyroantimonate localization of cations in thrombin-treated platelets. *Fed. Proc. 32*, 414Abs

Sato, T., Herman, L., Chandler, J., Stracher, A. & Detwiler, T. C. (1975) Localization of a thrombin-sensitive calcium pool in platelets. *J. Histochem. Cytochem. 23*, 103-106

Silcox, D. C., Jacobelli, S. & McCarty, D. J. (1973) Identification of inorganic pyrophosphate in human platelets and its release on stimulation with thrombin. *J. Clin. Invest. 52*, 1595-1604

Skaer, R. J., Peters, P. D. & Emmines, J. P. (1974) The localisation of calcium and phosphorus in human platelets. *J. Cell Sci. 15*, 679-692

White, J. G. (1971) Platelet morphology. In *The Circulating Platelet* (Johnson, S. A., ed.), pp. 45-121, Academic Press, New York & London

Yarom, R., Peters, P. D. & Hall, T. A. (1974) Effect of glutaraldehyde and urea embedding on intracellular ionic elements. X-ray microanalysis of skeletal muscle and myocardium. *J. Ultrastruct. Res. 49*, 405-418

The organelles storing
5-hydroxytryptamine in blood platelets

A. PLETSCHER and M. DA PRADA

Research Division, F. Hoffmann-La Roche & Co. Ltd, Basel, Switzerland

Abstract In blood platelets 5-hydroxytryptamine (5HT) is stored in specific organelles (storage vesicles) which also contain nucleotides such as adenosine 5′-triphosphate (ATP), bivalent cations, small amounts of soluble proteins, adenosine 3′:5′-cyclic monophosphate, and glycosaminoglycans. In rabbit platelets there seems to be some exchange between the nucleotides of the 5HT storage organelles and of the extravesicular metabolic pool. The 5HT concentration of the isolated organelles is higher in rabbits than in man and guinea pigs. Accordingly, in rabbits platelets show more dense bodies, and the isolated 5HT organelles exhibit larger and more numerous dense osmiophilic cores than in man and guinea pigs. This intravesicular storage of 5HT is due to interaction of the amine with the nucleotides and possibly bivalent cations, whereby electrostatic and Van der Waals' forces are involved. No specific 5HT uptake at the vesicular membrane level has been observed up to now, although this membrane contains a Mg^{2+}-dependent ATPase. Nevertheless, intact isolated 5HT organelles discriminate between various amines in their uptake. Several basic compounds which release 5HT from the platelets specifically accumulate in the 5HT vesicles. Some are preferentially localized in the membrane (reserpine, chlorpromazine), others in the interior of the organelles (tyramine, chloroquine, mepacrine). Reserpine and mepacrine, respectively, can be used as tools for determining the platelet half-life and for observing the 5HT storage organelles in platelets *in vivo* by fluorescence microscopy.

Blood platelets of various species, double fixed with glutaraldehyde–osmium tetroxide, show on electron microscopy specific subcellular organelles 1000-2000 Å (100-200 nm) in diameter (Da Prada *et al.* 1971, 1972*d*; Tranzer *et al.* 1966). They exhibit a highly osmiophilic core which is surrounded by a single membrane (Fig. 1). These organelles, distinctly different from other subcellular platelet structures such as α-granules, mitochondria and glycogen particles, have been clearly demonstrated to be the storage sites for 5-hydroxytryptamine (5HT vesicles, dense bodies) (Tranzer *et al.* 1966; Bak *et al.* 1967; Da Prada *et al.* 1967). Evidence exists that the 5HT storage organelles are already

261

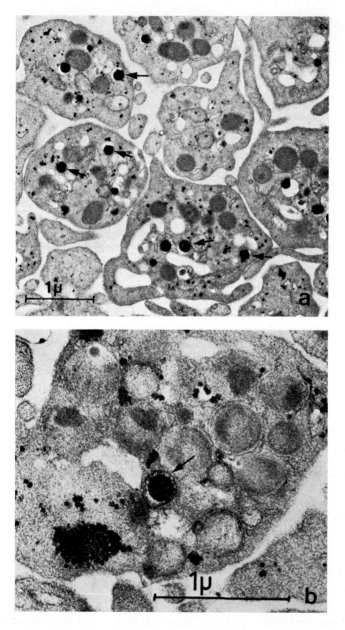

FIG. 1. Electron micrographs of isolated platelets with dense bodies (= 5-hydroxytryptamine organelles) (arrows). *a*, rabbit; *b*, man. (Photographs by J. P. Tranzer.)

preformed in the megakaryocytes, the stem cells of the blood platelets. These organelles do not yet contain high amounts of 5HT. Therefore, in the mega-karyocytes never or only rarely do vesicles with an osmiophilic content occur. However, after loading the animals with 5HT (e.g. by intraperitoneal injection), many highly osmiophilic organelles morphologically identical to the dense bodies in the mature platelets appear in the megakaryocytes (Tranzer et al. 1972).

The 5HT storage organelles of platelets can be isolated in a highly purified form by ultracentrifugation of platelet homogenates in a continuous Urografin density gradient (Da Prada & Pletscher 1968). This paper deals with the biochemical and physicochemical characteristics of these organelles.

CONTENTS OF ORGANELLES

5-Hydroxytryptamine

For the measurement of the composition of the vesicular contents the isolated 5HT organelles have been lysed by repeated freezing and thawing in distilled water and the vesicular membranes removed by ultracentrifugation. Table 1 indicates (in nmoles per μg protein) that the 5HT content in different species varies, being high in rabbits and relatively low in man and guinea pigs. Since the vesicular concentration of adenosine 5′-triphosphate (ATP) varies less than that of 5HT (Table 1), the molar ratios 5HT/ATP vary greatly between rabbits, guinea pigs and man, amounting to 2.3, 0.06 and 0.13,

TABLE 1

Soluble components present in the 5-hydroxytryptamine (5HT) organelles of various species

Constituent	Rabbit	Guinea pig	Man
5HT	21.0 ± 1.7	0.6 ± 0.2	0.25 ± 0.05
Histamine	9.0 ± 0.1	traces	traces
ATP	9.1 ± 0.1	11.1 ± 0.0	1.9 ± 0.4
ADP	1.9 ± 0.1	5.9 ± 0.2	
GTP	2.1 ± 0.2	1.9 ± 0.5	
UTP	0.7 ± 0.0	1.0 ± 0.2	
Cyclic AMP	$2.5 ± 0.6 × 10^{-3}$		
Uronic acid	0.01	none	
Hexosamines	0.26	0.04	
Ca^{2+}	2.1	1.5	
Mg^{2+}	8.4	9.8	

The values are averages, some given with s.e.m., and are indicated in nmol/μg total protein.

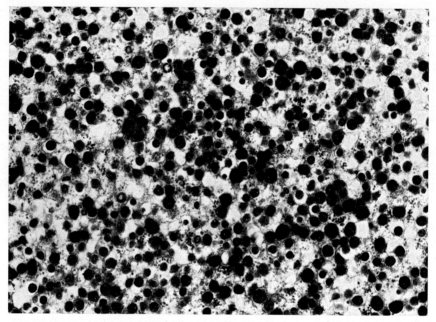

Fig. 2. Electron micrograph of isolated 5-hydroxytryptamine organelles of rabbit platelets. × 18000. (Photograph by J. P. Tranzer.)

respectively (Pletscher *et al.* 1969, 1974; Da Prada & Pletscher 1968; Da Prada *et al.* 1971, 1972*d*).

The species differences in the vesicular 5HT content also appear with electron microscopy since, as already shown, the electron density of the 5HT organelles depends on their 5HT concentration. In fact, the majority of the organelles of rabbits are highly osmiophilic (Fig. 2), whereas a great proportion of those of guinea pigs and of man look empty or only partially filled (Fig. 3). However, in spite of the relatively low 5HT content and osmiophily, the guinea pig and human 5HT organelles must be considered as storage sites of 5HT since their amine concentration (in nmoles per μg protein) was found to be more than 100 times greater than that of any other subcellular platelet fraction (Fig. 4) (Da Prada *et al.* 1967, 1971, 1972*d*; Pletscher *et al.* 1969).

These findings indicate that the 5HT storage organelles, especially of man and guinea pigs, are not fully saturated with 5HT. In fact, after treatment of guinea pigs with large doses of 5HT (intraperitoneally) or after incubation of isolated human platelets in plasma containing 5HT, the content of this amine in the isolated platelets and their storage organelles was at least 10 times higher than in untreated animals. In addition, the dense bodies in the platelets

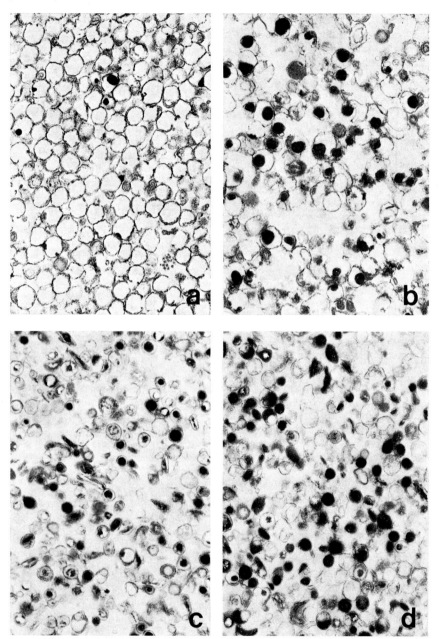

Fig. 3. Electron micrographs of isolated 5-hydroxytryptamine (5HT) organelles of blood platelets. *a*. normal guinea pig; *b*, guinea pig pretreated with four intraperitoneal injections each of 100 mg/kg 5HT (as creatinine sulphate) at intervals of 8 hours. The organelles were isolated 8 hours after the last injection; *c*, human, normal; d, human, after incubation of the platelets for 1 hour at 37 °C in plasma containing 500 μg 5HT/ml (as creatinine sulphate). *a* and *b*: × 28 000; *c* and *d*: × 18 000. (Da Prada *et al.* 1971, 1972*d*, with permission of *The Journal of Physiology* and *Experientia*.)

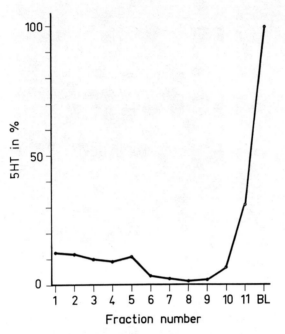

Fᴉɢ. 4. Distribution of endogenous 5-hydroxytryptamine (5HT) in various subcellular
fractions of human platelets. The values have been calculated in nmol 5HT/μg protein and
are indicated as percentages of the value found in the bottom layer (BL = 100%) containing
the 5HT organelles. Fractions 6 and 8 contain the α-granules and mitochondria, respectively.
Typical experiment. (Da Prada *et al*. 1972*d*, with permission of *Experientia*.)

became more numerous, and in the isolated 5HT storage organelles the number
of dense cores was markedly increased (Fig. 3) (Da Prada *et al*. 1971, 1972*d*).

Nucleotides

The 5HT storage organelles of various species (rabbit, guinea pig and man)
contain considerable concentrations of nucleotides. In rabbits and guinea pigs,
ATP has the highest share, but substantial amounts of adenosine 5'-diphosphate
(ADP) and guanosine 5'-triphosphate (GTP) as well as minor quantities of
uridine 5'-triphosphate (UTP) have also been found (Table 1) (Da Prada &
Pletscher 1970*a*; Goetz *et al*. 1971; Pletscher *et al*. 1974).

The origin of the nucleotides in the storage organelles is not yet clear.
Evidence exists that they are already present in the precursor organelles of the
megakaryocytes before they contain substantial amounts of 5HT (Tranzer
et al. 1972). Therefore, the possibility has to be considered that the nucleotides

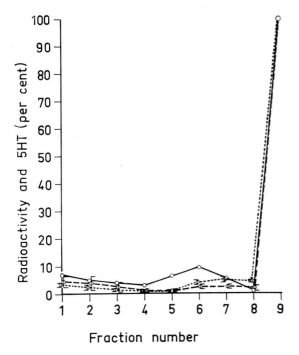

Fraction number

Fig. 5. Subcellular distribution of [^{14}C]triphosphonucleotides in rabbit platelets incubated in modified Tyrode solution at 37 °C for 2 hours with 0.5 g/ml [^{14}C]adenosine and [^{14}C]guanosine, respectively. The radioactivity as well as the endogenous 5-hydroxytryptamine (5HT) were calculated in µg/µg protein and are indicated as percentages of the respective values found in the organelles. Fraction 9 consists of the 5HT storage organelles. – – – –, [^{14}C]adenosine 5′-triphosphate (average with s.e. of 3 experiments); ⎯⎯⎯, [^{14}C]guanosine 5′-triphosphate (1 experiment); . . . . ., endogenous 5HT (average with s.e. of 3 experiments). (Da Prada & Pletscher 1970*b*, with permission of Pergamon Press Ltd.)

are incorporated into the organelles at the same time as the latter are formed in the megakaryocytes.

The problem of the turnover of the nucleotides in the storage organelles of platelets is not yet settled. Isolated 5HT organelles of blood platelets suspended *in vitro* did not take up labelled ATP nor form this nucleotide from precursors like adenine or adenosine. When, however, intact platelets of rabbits were incubated for two hours with radioactive adenine, adenosine or guanine and guanosine, labelled ATP (about 1 % of the total vesicular nucleotides) or GTP respectively accumulated in the 5HT storage organelles (Fig. 5) (Da Prada & Pletscher 1970*b*). This finding may indicate that the nucleotides stored in the 5HT organelles of blood platelets show some exchange with the nucleotides of the metabolic pool (extravesicular nucleotides), at least in the rabbit. Human platelets incubated with radioactive adenosine did not seem to accumulate any radioactivity in the releasable (vesicular) pool (Holmsen *et al.* 1969). Therefore, the pool of stored nucleotides in human platelets has been considered to be rather stable. Whether this will still be true when the fraction of pure 5HT storage organelles instead of the crude particulate fraction is measured for radioactivity remains to be investigated.

The 5HT storage vesicles of rabbit and guinea pig platelets also contain adenosine 3′:5′-cyclic monophosphate (cyclic AMP). The concentration of this nucleotide per μg protein in these organelles has been found to be about 4000 times less than that of ATP, but up to more than 100 times higher than the content of cyclic AMP in whole platelets and the other subcellular particulate fractions. No measurable adenylate cyclase activity could be detected in the isolated storage organelles or their membranes, whereas in the cytoplasmic membrane the enzyme was present (Da Prada *et al.* 1972*b*). It is conceivable that inactivation by storage of cyclic AMP in 5HT vesicles and its release from these organelles may participate in the regulation of the biological activity of the nucleotide in platelets.

Other constituents

The content of water-soluble proteins in the 5HT storage vesicles, in contrast to that in adrenal chromaffin granules, is very low. In rabbit organelles it amounts to about 0.01 g/ml, i.e. about 2 % of the vesicular content of ATP plus 5HT (0.22 + 0.25 g/ml respectively) (Pletscher *et al.* 1974). It is therefore unlikely that intravesicular proteins play a major role in the storage of 5HT in the organelles.

In addition, bivalent metals are present in the storage vesicles. In 5HT organelles of rabbit and guinea pig platelets, the molar concentration of Mg^{2+} has been found to be 4 and 6 times respectively that of Ca^{2+} and to be of the same order as the molar ATP content (Table 1, p. 263). Bivalent cations may have importance in the intravesicular storage of 5HT, since *in vitro* the aggregation of the amine with ATP is influenced by these ions (see below). The exact role of the bivalent metals in the 5HT storage organelles *in vivo* remains, however, to be demonstrated. It is possible that part of the bivalent cations are bound to proteins of the membrane. Furthermore, whole platelets of man, in contrast to those of rabbits and guinea pigs, contain more Ca^{2+} than Mg^{2+}. Therefore, Ca^{2+} may be the predominant bivalent metal ion in human 5HT organelles.

The finding of some uronic acid and hexosamines in 5HT storage organelles indicates the presence of traces of glycosaminoglycans. However, their amount is probably far too small for them to play a role in the vesicular storage of 5HT and other amines (Table 1, p. 263) (Da Prada *et al.* 1972*a*).

Finally, the 5HT storage vesicles may also contain endogenous amines other than 5HT. Thus, the storage organelles of rabbits show a rather high concentration of histamine (Table 1) (Da Prada *et al.* 1967) which is much larger than that in the other subcellular structures. Other species, such as guinea pigs, rats and man, seem to contain at best small amounts of histamine in their storage organelles.

Intermolecular interaction

The concentration of the major constituents (i.e. 5HT and ATP) of the storage organelles of platelets expressed in weight per volume was found to be rather high, especially in rabbits. Based on approximate measurements, made by two different methods, of the volumes of the 5HT organelles of rabbit platelets, this concentration amounted to values as high as 22 and 25 g%, respectively (Pletscher *et al.* 1969; Goetz *et al.* 1971). Provided the two constituents were present in monomolecular form, the osmotic pressure would be of such order that the stability of the organelles in physiological media, such as cytoplasm, Tyrode solution and plasma, could not be explained. Therefore, an intermolecular interaction between the low molecular weight compounds in the organelles is likely to occur.

Nuclear magnetic resonance and ultraviolet spectroscopy of aqueous solutions containing 5HT and ATP indicated the existence of intermolecular binding between these two constituents. The principal bond seems to be an ionic interaction between the side-chain amino group of 5HT and the negatively charged phosphate groups of ATP. In addition, it has been claimed that the adenine and indole rings form mixed stacks held together by weak intermolecular forces (Nogrady *et al.* 1972). Analytical ultracentrifugation experiments confirmed and extended these findings. Thus, the apparent average molecular weights of aqueous solutions of 5HT and ATP were rather high and markedly increased (up to 10 000) with rising concentration (Fig. 6) and decreasing temperature (Berneis *et al.* 1969*a*). The apparent average molecular weights also depended on the molecular ratios of amine to ATP, reaching maximal values at a ratio of about 2. This ratio corresponds to that occurring in 5HT organelles of rabbit platelets. When ATP was substituted by GTP, the apparent average molecular weights were even higher, whereas solutions of ADP + 5HT or UTP + 5HT showed about the same as or lower molecular weights respectively than corresponding solutions of ATP + 5HT (Da Prada & Pletscher 1970*a*; Berneis *et al.* 1970, 1971). Addition of small amounts of bivalent cations (e.g.

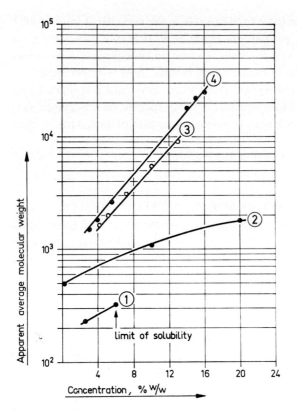

FIG. 6. Dependence of apparent average molecular weight on concentration (percentage by weight). Curve 1, 5-hydroxytryptamine (5HT) oxalate; 2, adenosine 5′-triphosphate (ATP); 3, 5HT oxalate + ATP, molar ratio 2 (pH about 2) and (middle point) 5HT chloride + ATP, molar ratio 2 (pH adjusted to 6); 4, fluid from 5HT organelles (pH about 6). (Berneis *et al.* 1969*a*, copyright 1969 by the American Association for the Advancement of Science.)

Ca^{2+} or Mg^{2+}) to a given solution with 5HT + ATP enhanced its apparent average molecular weight, whereas with high amounts of bivalent metal ions this enhancement was reversed. Monovalent cations (K^+ and Na^+) had no marked effect (Berneis *et al.* 1969*b*).

The dilute contents of the 5HT organelles (obtained by osmotic shock of the organelles followed by removal of the vesicular membranes by centrifugation) also yielded high apparent average molecular weights on analytical ultracentrifugation. These, too, increased with rising concentration of the vesicular fluid (Fig. 6) and decreasing temperature (Berneis *et al.* 1969*a*).

The above mentioned findings indicate that in the 5HT organelles 5HT and ATP are probably held together by intermolecular forces, in which bivalent cations may be involved. The forces may be different in nature, e.g. electro-static (interaction between NH_2 group of 5HT and phosphate groups of ATP) and of the Van der Waals' type (formation of 'clusters' of 5HT/ATP 'mono-mers'). Intravesicular binding to ATP of the 5HT that has penetrated through the membrane of the storage vesicles is probably a reason for the accumulation of the amine in these organelles against an apparent 5HT concentration gradient between organelles and cytoplasm. Interaction between 5HT and ATP also explains why the 5HT storage vesicles, despite their high content of low molecular weight compounds, show osmotic stability in physiological media. Finally, the increased aggregation between 5HT and ATP with dimin-ishing temperature may be connected with the fact that the isolated 5HT storage organelles lose less 5HT at $0\,°C–4\,°C$ than at $37\,°C$.

The importance of the interaction between ATP and monoamines for their storage was also shown by experiments with a microdiffusion system consisting of two chambers separated by an artificial membrane with low permeability to ATP, but freely permeable to the amines. In this system monoamines such as 5HT originally present in equal concentration in both chambers markedly accumulated (against an apparent concentration gradient) in the chamber to which ATP had been added. Furthermore, a decrease in temperature enhanced this accumulation, probably through increased aggregation of the solutes in the ATP-containing chamber (Da Prada *et al.* 1975*a*).

MEMBRANE

Like other membranes, such as those of adrenal chromaffin granules, the membranes of 5HT organelles contain various phospholipids. The phos-pholipid pattern of the membranes of these two organelles is similar with the exception that 5HT vesicular membranes do not contain lysophosphatidyl-choline (Table 2). The significance of this finding is not known. It has been suggested that lysophosphatidylcholine might be involved in the process of exocytosis of catecholamines in adrenal medulla. However, the absence of lysophosphatidylcholine in membranes of 5HT vesicles is not a strong argu-ment against the release of 5HT from these organelles by exocytosis, since the phospholipid may be formed only during the secretion process (Da Prada *et al.* 1972*c*).

With regard to the proteins little is known. Membranes of isolated 5HT organelles of rabbits showed ATPase activity which depended on the presence of Mg^{2+} and differed from the ATPase of the cytoplasmic platelet membrane, which is activated by Ca^{2+}, K^+ and Na^+. The Mg^{2+}-activated ATPase of the vesicular membranes was inhibited by N-ethylmaleimide and somewhat by

TABLE 2

Content of phospholipids and cholesterol in membranes of bovine adrenal chromaffin granules and of 5-hydroxytryptamine (5HT) organelles of rabbit platelets

	Chromaffin granules		5HT organelles	
	mg/mg protein	% total phospholipids	mg/mg protein	% total phospholipids
Total phospholipids	1.29 ± 0.15		0.77 ± 0.03	
Phosphatidyl choline		26.3 ± 0.7		33.8 ± 0.9
Phosphatidyl ethanolamine		34.8 ± 1.1		31.9 ± 1.1
Lysophosphatidyl choline		17.4 ± 1.0		nil
Sphingomyelin		12.0 ± 0.6		17.1 ± 1.6
Phosphatidyl inositol		1.5 ± 0.4		2.5 ± 0.8
Phosphatidyl serine		8.9 ± 0.6		11.9 ± 1.2
Cholesterol	0.25 ± 0.03		0.15 ± 0.01	

The values are averages with S.E.M., each of 3–5 experiments. (Da Prada et al. 1972c.)

Na^+ and Ca^{2+} but not by ouabain (which inhibits the enzyme of the cytoplasmic membrane). The K_m values for ATP and Mg^{2+} were 0.3×10^{-3} M and 0.6×10^{-3} M respectively (Heinrich et al. 1972). In preliminary experiments no ATP/Mg^{2+}-dependent 5HT transport at the level of the membranes of the 5HT organelles could be detected. In contrast, chromaffin granular membranes of adrenal medulla, which also contain a Mg^{2+}-stimulated ATPase (though somewhat different from that in 5HT vesicular membranes), showed a marked uptake of various monoamines including 5HT in the presence of Mg^{2+} and ATP (Da Prada et al. 1975b). The possible role of the ATPase of the vesicular membranes in the transport of 5HT into the storage vesicles of platelets remains to be further investigated. It has also to be considered that the membrane ATPase of the 5HT storage organelles might be important for the formation of ADP from granular ATP, for example during the release reaction.

In the membranes of isolated 5HT organelles of rabbit platelets another protein, actin (thrombosthenin A), has recently been discovered with an immunofluorescent method using specific anti-actin antibodies derived from patients with chronic progressive hepatitis. Actin also occurred, however, in membranes of other subcellular particles, such as the α-granules, as well as in the cytoplasm (G. Gabbiani, M. Da Prada & A. Pletscher, submitted for publication). Nevertheless, it has to be considered that an actomyosin system associated with the 5HT vesicular membranes might be involved in the release reaction of platelets.

FOREIGN COMPOUNDS

After administration *in vivo* or addition to platelet suspensions, various basic compounds, e.g. monoamines and polycyclic drugs (reserpine, chlorpromazine, imipramine, mepacrine, chloroquine, etc.), showed marked accumulation in the 5HT organelles (Fig. 7) (Da Prada & Pletscher 1969a, b, submitted for publication). The concentration of these compounds in the 5HT vesicles was up to more than 100 times higher than that in the other particulate subcellular fractions. The localization of the foreign substances at the level of the 5HT

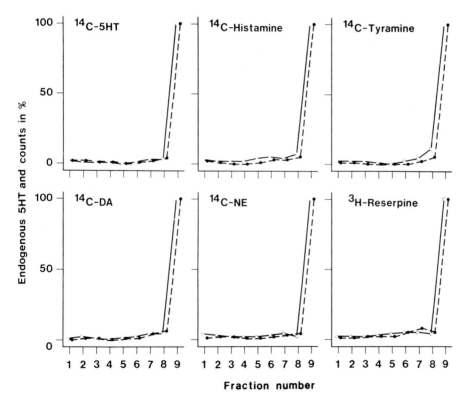

FIG. 7. Subcellular distribution of labelled biogenic amines and reserpine compared with the endogenous 5-hydroxytryptamine (5HT) in rabbit platelets. All labelled compounds were administered intraperitoneally, 5HT, histamine, dopamine (DA) and noradrenaline (norepinephrine, NE) 3 hours, tyramine 1 hour, and reserpine 16 hours befor isolation of the platelets. The results have been calculated as nmol/μg protein (endogenous 5HT) and counts/μg protein (labelled compounds). The values of the 5HT storage organelles (fraction 9) were taken as 100%. ————, labelled compounds; -----, endogenous 5HT. (For further information see Da Prada & Pletscher 1969a, b. Reproduced with permission of *Experientia*.)

organelles varied. Drugs like reserpine and chlorpromazine accumulated preferentially in the vesicular membrane, since after osmotic shock of the organelles and subsequent ultracentrifugation the drugs were localized in the membrane fraction at the bottom of the tube. In contrast, biogenic amines (e.g. 5HT, dopamine, noradrenaline, histamine and tyramine) and basic drugs like chloroquine and mepacrine seemed to be preferentially located in the interior of the organelles, since these compounds were mainly found in the supernatant after osmotic shock of the organelles. Imipramine probably accumulated in both the interior and the membranes of the organelles.

Little is known about the mechanism of accumulation of the foreign compounds in the organelles. Drugs like reserpine and chlorpromazine may be preferentially dissolved in the lipids of the vesicular membrane, or their positively charged basic moieties may bind by electrostatic forces to electronegative groups of the membrane proteins. Other basic substances, like biogenic amines, mepacrine and chloroquine, seem to interact chiefly with the negatively charged phosphate groups of the intravesicular ATP. Such interaction has indeed been shown in an artificial system using the above-mentioned microdiffusion chambers. Thus, the diffusion of mepacrine from one chamber into the other markedly decreased when the chamber to which the drug had been added was also supplemented with ATP.

Isolated 5HT organelles of rabbit platelets incubated in plasma discriminate between the various monoamines with regard to their uptake, which showed the following order: 5HT > dopamine > adrenaline > noradrenaline > tyramine = 5-hydroxydopamine = tryptamine > histamine (Table 3) (Da Prada & Pletscher 1969c). The reason for these differences is not known. It may be connected with a specific carrier system responsible for the transport of the amines through the vesicular membrane (for which no evidence exists as yet). In addition, differences in molecular shape and charges between the various amines influencing their penetration through the vesicular membrane or differences in their intravesicular interaction with ATP are possibly involved.

The above-mentioned drugs and amines (e.g. tyramine) which accumulate in the 5HT storage vesicles cause a decrease of the endogenous 5HT in platelets, as a result of liberation of the amine from the organelles. The mechanism of liberation of 5HT by the various compounds probably differs. The compounds that are mainly localized in the interior of the storage vesicles (e.g. biogenic amines and mepacrine) may displace the endogenous 5HT from its storage complex, for example by competitive interaction for the electronegative sites of the ATP. Compounds accumulating preferentially in the vesicular membrane (e.g. chlorpromazine and reserpine) may act at the membrane level.

TABLE 3

Uptake of radioactive amines by isolated 5-hydroxytryptamine (5HT) organelles incubated in plasma at 37 °C for 30 minutes

Amine		Number of expts	Uptake
	Tryptamine	3	10 ± 2
	5-Hydroxy-tryptamine	14	100 ± 9
	Tyramine	2	13 ± 3
	Dopamine	3	68 ± 2
	Histamine	3	2 ± 1
	Adrenaline	4	36 ± 4
	Noradrenaline	6	29 ± 3
	5-Hydroxy-dopamine	3	13 ± 1

Concentration of amines in incubation fluid, 0.57 μM. The values represent averages with s.e. and are expressed as percentages of the [^{14}C]5HT taken up by the organelles in the same experiment. Absolute uptake of [^{14}C]5HT in ng per ng endogenous 5HT: 0.91 ± 0.08 (14 experiments). (Da Prada & Pletscher 1969c.)

Chlorpromazine has been suggested to alter the structure of biological membranes (membrane fluidization) (Seeman 1972), possibly allowing the 5HT vesicular contents to be liberated. The exact mode of action of reserpine is unknown. Major damage to the 5HT storage vesicles or a liberation of 5HT by exocytosis induced by the drug is unlikely. Thus, density gradient centrifugation in Urografin (as mentioned above, p. 263) of homogenates of reserpinized rabbit platelets yielded a bottom layer consisting of virtually pure vesicles (Fig. 8) (Da Prada et al. 1968). These were similar in shape to the organelles obtained from normal platelets and still contained about 63% and

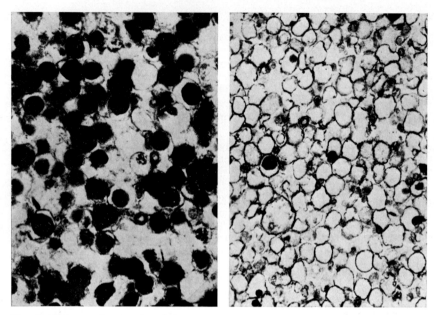

Fig. 8. Electron micrographs of the 5-hydroxytryptamine (5HT) organelles of the bottom layer obtained by density gradient centrifugation of homogenates of rabbit platelets. *Left*, normal animals; *right*, animals pretreated with 5 mg/kg reserpine intraperitoneally, 16 hours before isolation of platelets. (Da Prada *et al.* 1968, with permission of Pergamon Press Ltd.)

34% respectively of the original ATP and histamine. The organelles from reserpinized platelets, however, did not show significant amounts of 5HT (about 0.5% of the original content) and therefore looked empty on electron microscopy. Interestingly, one molecule of reserpine accumulated in the 5HT storage organelles corresponded to more than 30 000 molecules of 5HT liberated (Da Prada & Pletscher 1969a). A displacement mechanism, for example due to competition with 5HT, for the ATP in the vesicles is therefore not probable.

SUMMARY AND CONCLUSIONS

The storage of 5HT in the platelet organelles probably starts when the mature platelets, segregated from the megakaryocytes (containing precursor organelles rich in ATP), reach the circulating blood. The 5HT, which probably derives from the enterochromaffin system, is transported into the platelets by a specific mechanism located at the cytoplasmic membrane level (Pletscher 1968). Once within the platelets the amine is stored in the 5HT organelles (5HT vesicles) which, when loaded with sufficient amounts of 5HT, become electron-dense (dense bodies) on double fixation with glutaraldehyde–osmium tetroxide. In species like rabbit, the organelles probably take up more 5HT during the life-time of the platelets than in those of man and guinea pig. Accordingly, circulating platelets of rabbits contain more dense bodies than those of man and guinea pig. The vesicular storage is due to reversible inter-action (by electrostatic and Van der Waals' forces) of the amine with nucleotides, especially ATP and possibly bivalent cations. Up to now, no evidence exists that the vesicular membranes which contain a Mg^{2+}-dependent ATPase participate in the storage process. Various basic substances, such as aromatic amines and drugs, accumulate in the 5HT organelles, but the storage of 5HT is more efficient than that of other aromatic amines.

The 5HT stored in the organelles is liberated during the release reaction as well as by the basic compounds mentioned. Different mechanisms are re-sponsible for the liberation of the amine. Contractile proteins may play a role in the release reaction since actin has been found to be associated with the membrane of the storage organelles.

The nucleotides of the storage organelles seem to have a certain turnover in rabbits. Whether this is true also in man remains to be further elucidated. The possibility has to be considered that during the release reaction part of the vesicular ATP undergoes transformation into ADP as a result of the action of the ATPase present in the membranes of the organelles. Furthermore, the 5HT storage vesicles may participate in regulating the function of cyclic AMP in the platelets since this nucleotide, too, has been found to be accumulat-ed in these organelles.

Finally, some foreign basic substances which accumulate in the 5HT organ-elles provide tools for investigating the physiology and pathophysiology of platelets. Thus, labelled reserpine which has been shown to bind irreversibly to the membrane of 5HT storage vesicles as well as to other subcellular struc-tures can be used to determine the platelet half-life *in vivo* (Enna *et al.* 1975). Furthermore, the recent discovery of a marked accumulation of fluorescent compounds like mepacrine in the interior of the 5HT storage vesicles allows the visualization of these organelles by fluorescence microscopy and thus the study of the storage organelles in the intact platelets *in vivo*.

References

BAK, I. J., HASSLER, R., MAY, B. & WESTERMAN, E. (1967) Morphological and biochemical studies on the storage of serotonin and histamine in blood platelets of the rabbit. *Life Sci.* 6 (II), 1133-1146

BERNEIS, K. H., DA PRADA, M. & PLETSCHER, A. (1969a) Micelle formation between 5-hydroxytryptamine and adenosine triphosphate in platelet storage organelles. *Science (Wash. D.C.) 165*, 913-914

BERNEIS, K. H., PLETSCHER, A. & DA PRADA, M. (1969b) Metal-dependent aggregation of biogenic amines: a hypothesis for their storage and release. *Nature (Lond.) 224*, 281-283

BERNEIS, K. H., DA PRADA, M. & PLETSCHER, A. (1970) Metal-dependent aggregation of nucleotides with formation of biphasic liquid systems. *Biochim. Biophys. Acta 215*, 547-549

BERNEIS, K. H., DA PRADA, M. & PLETSCHER, A. (1971) A possible mechanism for uptake of biogenic amines by storage organelles: incorporation into nucleotide-metal aggregates. *Experientia 27*, 917-918

DA PRADA, M. & PLETSCHER, A. (1968) Isolated 5-hydroxytryptamine organelles of rabbit blood platelets: physiological properties and drug-induced changes. *Br. J. Pharmacol. 34*, 591-597

DA PRADA, M. & PLETSCHER, A. (1969a) Storage of exogenous monoamines and reserpine in 5-hydroxytryptamine organelles of blood platelets. *Eur. J. Pharmacol. 7*, 45-48

DA PRADA, M. & PLETSCHER, A. (1969b) Different localisation of reserpine and tyramine within the 5-hydroxytryptamine organelles of blood platelets. *Experientia 25*, 923-924

DA PRADA, M. & PLETSCHER, A. (1969c) Differential uptake of biogenic amines by isolated 5-hydroxytryptamine organelles of blood platelets. *Life Sci. 8* (I), 65-72

DA PRADA, M. & PLETSCHER, A. (1970a) Identification of guanosine-5'-triphosphate and uridine-5'-triphosphate in subcellular monoamine storage organelles. *Biochem. J. 119*, 117-119

DA PRADA, M. & PLETSCHER, A. (1970b) Synthesis and storage of nucleotides in blood platelets. *Life Sci. 9* (II), 1271-1282

DA PRADA, M., PLETSCHER, A., TRANZER, J. P. & KNUCHEL, H. (1967) Subcellular localisation of 5-hydroxytryptamine and histamine in blood platelets. *Nature (Lond.) 216*, 1315-1317

DA PRADA, M., PLETSCHER, A., TRANZER, J. P. & KNUCHEL, H. (1968) Action of reserpine on subcellular 5-hydroxytryptamine organelles of blood platelets. *Life Sci. 7* (I), 477-480

DA PRADA, M., PLETSCHER, A. & TRANZER, J. P. (1971) Storage of ATP and 5-hydroxytryptamine in blood platelets of guinea pigs. *J. Physiol. (Lond.) 217*, 679-688

DA PRADA, M., VON BERLEPSCH, K. & PLETSCHER, A. (1972a) Storage of biogenic amines in blood platelets and adrenal medulla: lack of evidence for direct involvement of glycosaminoglycans. *Naunyn-Schmiedeberg's Arch. Pharmacol. 275*, 315-322

DA PRADA, M., BURKARD, W. P. & PLETSCHER, A. (1972b) Cyclic AMP of blood platelets: accumulation in organelles storing 5-hydroxytryptamine and ATP. *Experientia 28*, 845-846

DA PRADA, M., PLETSCHER, A. & TRANZER, J. P. (1972c) Lipid composition of membranes of amine storage organelles. *Biochem. J. 127*, 681-683

DA PRADA, M., TRANZER, J. P. & PLETSCHER, A. (1972d) Storage of 5-hydroxytryptamine in human blood platelets. *Experientia 28*, 1328-1329

DA PRADA, M., OBRIST, R. & PLETSCHER, A. (1975a) Accumulation of acetylcholine and aromatic monoamines by interaction with adenosine-5'-triphosphate. *J. Pharm. Pharmacol. 27*, 649-651

DA PRADA, M., OBRIST, R. & PLETSCHER, A. (1975b) Discrimination of monoamine uptake by membranes of adrenal chromaffin granules. *Br. J. Pharmacol. 53*, 257-266

ENNA, S. J., DA PRADA, M. & PLETSCHER, A. (1975) Subcellular distribution of reserpine in blood platelets: evidence for multiple pools. *J. Pharmacol. Exp. Ther. 191*, 164-171

GOETZ, U., DA PRADA, M. & PLETSCHER, A. (1971) Adenine- guanine- and uridine-5'-phosphonucleotides in blood platelets and storage organelles of various species. *J. Pharmacol. Exp. Ther. 178*, 210-215

HEINRICH, P., DA PRADA, M. & PLETSCHER, A. (1972) Magnesium-dependent ATP-ase in membranes of 5-hydroxytryptamine storage organelles. *Biochem. Biophys. Res. Commun. 46*, 1769-1775

HOLMSEN, H., DAY, H. J. & STORM, E. (1969) Adenine nucleotide metabolism of blood platelets. VI. Subcellular localization of nucleotide pools with different functions in the platelet release reaction. *Biochim. Biophys. Acta 186*, 254-266

NOGRADY, T., HRDINA, P. D. & LING, G. M. (1972) Investigation into the association between serotonin and adenosine triphosphate in vitro by nuclear magnetic resonance and ultraviolet spectroscopy. *Mol. Pharmacol. 8*, 565-574

PLETSCHER, A. (1968) Metabolism, transfer and storage of 5-hydroxytryptamine in blood platelets. *Br. J. Pharmacol. 32*, 1-16

PLETSCHER, A., DA PRADA, M. & TRANZER, J. P. (1969) Transfer and storage of biogenic monoamines in subcellular organelles of blood platelets. In *Mechanisms of Synaptic Transmission* (Akert, K. & Waser, P. G., eds.) (*Progr. Brain Res.*, vol. 31), pp. 47-52, Elsevier, Amsterdam

PLETSCHER, A., DA PRADA, M., BERNEIS, K. H., STEFFEN, H., LÜTOLD, B. & WEDER, H. G. (1974) Molecular organisation of amine storage organelles of blood platelets and adrenal medulla. *Adv. Cytopharmacol. 2*, 257-264

SEEMAN, P. (1972) The membrane actions of anesthetics and tranquilizers. *Pharmacol. Rev. 24*, 583-655

TRANZER, J. P., DA PRADA, M. & PLETSCHER, A. (1966) Ultrastructural localisation of 5-hydroxytryptamine in blood platelets. *Nature (Lond.) 212*, 1574-1575

TRANZER, J. P., DA PRADA, M. & PLETSCHER, A. (1972) Storage of 5-hydroxytryptamine in megakaryocytes. *J. Cell Biol. 52*, 191-197

Discussion

Born: I wonder how the experiments were done in which you found various drugs in the granular layer. Is there a possibility of redistribution during preparation?

Pletscher: We checked that. We made homogenates of platelets from animals treated with the labelled drugs. The 5-hydroxytryptamine organelles were destroyed in the homogenates. To these homogenates we added normal platelets from which the 5HT organelles were isolated. There was no evidence of a major accumulation of the drugs in the isolated organelles.

Born: In your experiments with dopamine, might you get exactly the same distribution with other nucleoside phosphates or even with inorganic phosphate or pyrophosphate? In other words, how specific is this redistribution effect?

Pletscher: It can be done with ADP and ATP. I don't know if it would also work with pyrophosphate.

Skaer: Isn't it likely that drugs as soluble in lipids as chlorpromazine and imipramine will eventually end up in dense bodies, with their high 'phospholipid' content?

Born: That was what I was wondering, too. The initial distribution of such drugs is determined by numerous simultaneous rates; and their ultimate distribution by their lipid solubility. Paasonen and his co-workers showed that high concentrations of chlorpromazine and similar drugs can actually damage platelets (Paasonen 1964); presumably the sites of damage provide some indication of distribution.

Holmsen: Professor Pletscher, it worries me that you find 100% of your labelled ATP in the particulate fraction *only* in the dense granules. In human platelets that were labelled either with [^{14}C]adenine, [^{14}C]adenosine or [^{32}P]orthophosphate we (Holmsen *et al.* 1969) found 90–95% of the particle-bound, radioactive ATP and ADP in the membranes, mitochondria and α-granules, and only 5–10% in the dense granules. However, more than 90% of the total *platelet* nucleotide radioactivity was found in the soluble fraction.

Pletscher: I described a distribution in the particulate matter, not a concentration. I did not speak of the absolute amounts. We have calculated them, however. In the case of mepacrine, more than 85% is in the small granule fraction. Less chlorpromazine is found in granules, because there is a substantial amount in the cytosol. We have not done absolute measurements for the labelled ATP, only a relative one, in relation to the endogenous ATP of the organelles.

Holmsen: I feel it is unfair to express data from subcellular fractionation *only* in percentage distributions of substances among the *particulate* fractions. What is in the soluble fraction—and what are the recoveries?

Pletscher: Our recovery for 5HT organelles from rabbit platelets is of the order of 50%, which is not too bad for this type of isolation work. With regard to the ATP, after two hours' incubation with labelled precursors (adenine, adenosine) about 1% of the ATP in the granules is labelled, which is quite significant.

Holmsen: That is about what we find in the dense granules too. And about 1% of the total adenine nucleotide radioactivity is released during the release reaction (Holmsen *et al.* 1969). But how do you explain the fact that the granules pick up radioactivity when they are in the intact platelets, but refuse to do so after they are isolated?

Pletscher: I cannot explain it. The isolated organelle does not take up ATP. There must be a transport system which functions only *in vivo.* Subcellular structures like microtubules may therefore be important; but I don't know.

Born: That is still a particularly interesting puzzle. Where, in chromaffin granules as in the platelet granules, does the non-metabolic ATP come from?

Pletscher: I would say that pre-formed ATP is already present in the megakaryocyte and may be incorporated into the organelles at the moment of their formation.

Mustard: Reimers' studies (Reimers *et al.* 1975) confirm that Professor Pletscher is correct—there is an exchange between the cytoplasmic and granule ATP. Reimers labelled the platelet metabolic pool nucleotides either with

^{32}P or with [^{14}C]adenosine *in vitro*, washed the platelets and then incubated them in a tissue culture medium. By 18 hours the specific activity of the ATP released by thrombin stimulation was essentially the same as that of the ATP in the platelets before stimulation and that remaining in the platelets after stimulation. In these experiments there was less than 10% platelet lysis. To obtain these results, the ATP in the cytoplasmic pool and the granule pool of rabbit platelets has to be in equilibrium. There is, therefore, a slow exchange. If the rabbit platelets labelled *in vitro* are reinfused into the rabbit's circulation, they can be harvested several days later. The specific activities of the releasable nucleotides and the platelet nucleotides are the same. This exchange is affected by reserpine.

Reimers finds that the rate of exchange of 5HT is at least 300 times greater than the rate of transfer of ATP in rabbit platelets. This is interesting in terms of what is taking place. He has also been able to demonstrate a transfer of cytoplasmic ATP into the granules of human platelets (Reimers *et al.* 1975).

Born: That still leaves the question of what brings about the accumulation of ATP.

Pletscher: As I said, we think ATP is already present in the megakaryocyte. We have evidence for this but it is incomplete, because Dr Tranzer was working out a method before he died which was relatively specific for ATP. It is not fully worked out yet. In addition, if one injects rabbits with 5HT, dense-cored granules appear in the megakaryocytes. So the organelles are probably there but not yet filled with 5HT. Maybe these organelles incorporate nucleotides during their formation.

Holmsen: We have some evidence that supports this mechanism (Holmsen *et al.* 1975). When platelets take up 5HT, will it combine with the granule-stored, non-metabolic ATP or with the extragranular, metabolic ATP? To answer this question we incubated human platelets that had radioactive metabolic adenine nucleotides, with 5HT. Then these platelets were stimulated to release with various agents, and they released 3–4 times more 5HT than control platelets that had not been incubated with 5HT. However, the same amounts of ATP and ADP were released from both types of platelets, and with the same specific radioactivity. This indicates that 5HT combines with granule-located ATP and not with the extragranular pool of ATP.

Skaer: Professor Pletscher, am I right in assuming that you prepare the dense bodies at low temperature?

Pletscher: Yes. The preparation is done at 4 °C!

Skaer: I am sure low temperature helps to retain some 5HT in the dense bodies despite the use of chelating agents in the initial homogenization of the platelets.

Pletscher: How many dense bodies do you see in a human platelet?

Skaer: About eight, on average.

Pletscher: If we fill them with 5HT we see about the same number, after osmium staining.

Nachman: Professor Pletscher, your subcellular separations are the cleanest I have ever seen. While I understand the density separation of the dense granule, I have difficulty understanding the extremely clean separation of the granule that doesn't contain 5HT. Why is it still so dense?

Pletscher: We had great methodological difficulties; Dr Da Prada was experimenting for over a year and was successful only when he used Urografin density gradients. The granules that are empty of 5HT still contain most of their ATP and their bivalent cations. The mere absence of 5HT probably does not make too great a difference to the density of the granules.

Nachman: Is this complex of ATP and metal ions enough to give the granule that buoyant density? If one took liposomes and wrapped them round ATP and calcium, one wonders if they would come down with the same density.

Shepro: We are now comparing a platelet vesicle preparation that has high calcium uptake activity (Robblee *et al.* 1973*a*, *b*) with the original homogenate and with the granule fraction. Samples are centrifuged on a continuous sucrose gradient and fractions are measured for ^{45}Ca. Calcium binding or uptake is observed in the granule preparation, and a calcium-sensitive ATPase may be present (mitochondrial calcium uptake was not involved). One might question whether all of the granules are *fully packed* in the circulating platelet.

Pletscher: We have a recovery of about 50% of the granules and we found in the granular membranes an ATPase sensitive to Mg^{2+}, not to Ca^{2+}. How pure are your preparations? Have you looked at them electron microscopically?

Shepro: That is the key question. We talk about 'granules' as if they are a homogeneous group. I would imagine that the granules vary, and certainly data obtained from uptake/storage experiments will vary with procedures: washed or unwashed, Ca^{2+} concentration, sampling times, and so on.

Marcus: Although it may be related to the way the assays are done we have noted that the supernatants from platelet homogenates which were spun on a sucrose gradient contain a good deal of ATPase activity which is not inhibitable by reagents which affect the sodium-dependent, potassium-stimulated ATPase or the calcium-magnesium ATPase. We have also recently found that platelet homogenates contain a good deal of reductase activity.

Mills: When 5HT is accumulated by an ATP–bivalent metal ion chelate, what is the counter-ion which is displaced to preserve electrical neutrality in the granule?

Born: In the chromaffin granules of the bovine adrenal gland the counter-ion is catecholamine, mostly adrenaline; normally these granules contain almost no potassium. When the gland is stimulated and the adrenaline is released it is replaced stoichiometrically by potassium.

Pletscher: I do not know what the counter-ion is. In chromaffin granules 'monomers' are probably formed, with one ATP and three to four adrenaline and noradrenaline molecules, interacting by electrostatic forces, and by hydrogen-bonding. In addition these monomers seem to be aggregated by much weaker forces, for example of the Van der Waals type.

Mills: But there is a difference here. In the adrenal chromaffin granules there is a fixed stoichiometry between nucleotide and amine. In the platelet this stoichiometry is variable. My question is, what could the counter-ion be?

Pletscher: I agree; there are ATP-rich and amine-poor granules. With regard to the counter-ion, calcium and magnesium are present, in relatively high amounts. In their presence the ATP molecules aggregate, possibly by interaction of one bivalent cation with ATP molecules. Whether K^+ is also a counter-ion remains to be demonstrated. Proteins can probably be excluded because there is so little protein in the granules.

Holmsen: I find it unlikely that calcium can be displaced by 5HT. The Ca-ATP binding constant is about 10^5, whereas that of 5HT–ATP can hardly be more than 10^2.

Haslam: Surely one could approach this problem by measuring the release of, for example, potassium from platelets that have and have not been incubated with an excess of 5HT?

Born: That is an experiment that I have long planned to do; but Professor Pletscher could do it better because he has the granules pure. It cannot be done with whole platelets because the amount of potassium in their cytoplasm is large compared to that in the granules, so one would not be able to demonstrate any differences. But as between one fraction of pure granules containing little 5HT and another containing much more, it should be possible to demonstrate a stoichiometrically equivalent difference in the potassium, if that is indeed the counter-ion.

Shepro: My colleague, Frank Belamarich, has supervised a study on the comparative aspects of haemostasis in vertebrates and invertebrates. We have data which show that duck thrombocytes, which contain 5HT and are aggregated by the amine, will release 5HT after collagen stimulation, and nucleotides are *not* released during aggregation. Obviously, not all granules store 5HT and nucleotides in the same fashion (Belamarich *et al.* 1973; Stiller *et al.* 1975).

Crawford: Professor Pletscher, what proportion of the granules contain histamine?

Pletscher: This differs with different species. In the rabbit, the granules contain almost as much histamine as 5HT. In guinea pigs and probably man, very little histamine is present.

Feinberg: Since you have found a turnover of granule ATP and ADP, would you also expect a turnover of granule calcium?

Pletscher: I don't know. We have preliminary unexplained findings with calcium indicating that reserpine increases the influx of this cation into the platelets.

In connection with the accumulation of basic drugs in 5HT storage organelles, I would like to mention an interesting phenomenon that has recently been noticed in our laboratories by Dr H. P. Lorez and Dr M. Da Prada with platelets loaded with mepacrine. On observation with the fluorescence microscope such platelets showed fluorescent granular structures whose number corresponded to that of the dense bodies previously observed on electron microscopy. After intense irradiation with blue-violet light, platelets loaded with mepacrine started flashing; that is to say, their fluorescence markedly increased for a few seconds and then decreased again. Several flashes occurred successively in one platelet, their number (determined by microfluorimetric registration) being of the order of that of the 5HT storage organelles. These flashes were probably the consequence of a liberation of mepacrine from the organelles and may be due to a decrease in the fluorescence quenching of the liberated mepacrine.

Mustard: A film was made several years ago at Rockefeller University of stimulated granulocytes degranulating. The process resembled an exploding flashbulb. Your phenomenon seems to be similar.

Nachman: The difference is that the granulocyte explosion is occurring into a closed vacuole system, so that lysosomal enzymes do not get out into the cytoplasm. Here the cell is killing itself.

Pletscher: In our case the whole cell is illuminated, so I don't know if the fluorescent dye goes into the cytoplasm or in the cytoplasmic membrane or the canalicular system.

Born: The phenomenon you have discovered appears artifactual, in that thrombin clearly induces a different process, more akin to exocytosis.

Marcus: Is it conceivable that there is an oxidative change in the 5HT molecule, possibly involving the hydroxyl group, during uptake and transport? We rely on the ^{14}C label in the side-chain when we measure the uptake and release of 5HT. If one adds methylene blue to platelets, 5HT is released (Schick & Yu 1973). When Okuda & Nemerson (1968) studied platelet uptake of 5HT under nitrogen, it became suppressed, but ATP levels remained constant. We have not been able to measure changes in the hydroxyl group of 5HT in studies of its metabolism. Perhaps it is undergoing a change as it crosses the cell membrane, as in the case of iron, where ferric iron does not cross the cell membrane until it is converted to ferrous iron. Perhaps 5HT is modified during binding and then reconverted on the inner side of the membrane.

Crawford: The fluorimetric assays which depend upon more of the 5HT molecule do in general support the ^{14}C studies, in our experience.

Born: All our investigations depended on determining both intact 5HT with a specific bioassay for it and at the same time the radioactivity originating in the labelled molecule. This provided, of course, a measure of the extent to which 5HT was inactivated (see, for example, Born 1962).

Pletscher: We don't measure radioactivity only. We identify this radioactivity by paper chromatography and spectrofluoroscopy. So what we measure is really 5HT.

Born: There is one interesting point: we found that only one compound out of some thirty analogues of 5HT is taken up like 5HT itself all the way; that is, not only by the membrane transport but apparently also concentrated by the granules; and that is 5-hydroxy-α-methyltryptamine. With other substitutions all over the molecule, even after the removal of the 5-hydroxy group, many of the resulting analogues became bound with high affinities to the same membrane receptor(s) but not one was accumulated by the storage granule in the same way as 5HT (Born *et al.* 1972).

Marcus: This is an important observation.

Pletscher: There are several specificities in these transports; there is a specificity at the level of the external membrane and probably at the level of the granular membrane, and also inside the granules. These specificities are not necessarily congruent. Histamine is taken up poorly by the external membrane, but probably interacts vigorously with ATP within the granules.

Born: You proposed a model to explain the stoichiometric association of 5HT with nucleotides in the granules, in which the ATP molecules were stacked one above the other with the amine molecules intercalated, rather as others have proposed for the intercalation of various drugs in DNA (Waring 1975). A test of your model would be to find out how different substituents on the 5HT molecule would affect the possibility of fitting it adequately into such stacks. This could be done with molecular models.

Pletscher: The stacking model applies only for ATP alone. As soon as 5HT comes in, the vertical stacking is probably disrupted. We have another model now. According to this, one molecule of ATP interacts with two molecules of 5HT, probably by electrostatic and possibly other forces. These 'monomers' are then held together in a loose, reversible way by weaker forces, for example of the Van der Waals type.

Crawford: As I understood it, in the earlier analyses of the isolated catecholamine granules the molar ratio of amine to ATP seemed to be around 4:1. For this reason it was assumed that with four negative changes on the ATP polyphosphate chain, this represented the complex, holding the granule contents in an osmotically inactive state. However, I thought that with the more purified granule fractions the ratio was now revised to nearer 2:1 amine/ ATP?

Pletscher: We find a ratio of about four catecholamines to one ATP molecule.

Haslam: Hasn't it been claimed that in sympathetic nerves much of the noradrenaline is not bound to ATP?

Pletscher: In the splenic nerve it has been claimed that noradrenaline can be stored without ATP. We measured ATP in the total splenic nerve of calves and noticed that the ATP level was rather high immediately after quick removal of the nerve, but that the nucleotide content thereafter declined rather rapidly with time.

References

BELAMARICH, F. A., STILLER, R. A. & SHEPRO, D. (1973) The release reaction: is it a common mechanism in all types of hemostatic cells? *Ser. Haematol. 3*, 418-428

BORN, G. V. R. (1962) The fate of 5-hydroxytryptamine in a smooth muscle and in connective tissue. *J. Physiol. (Lond.) 161*, 160-174

BORN, G. V. R., JUENGJAROEN, K. & MICHAL, F. (1972) Relative activities on and uptake by human blood platelets of 5-hydroxytryptamine and several analogues. *Br. J. Pharmacol. 44*, 117-139

HOLMSEN, H., DAY, H. J. & STORM, E. (1969) Adenine nucleotide metabolism of blood platelets. VI. Subcellular localization of nucleotide pools with different functions in the platelet release reaction. *Biochim. Biophys. Acta 186*, 254-266

HOLMSEN, H., SETKOWSKY, C. A. & DAY, H. J. (1975) Possible association of newly absorbed serotonin with nonmetabolic, granula-located adenine nucleotides in human platelets. *Blood 45*, 413-416

OKUDA, M. & NEMERSON, Y. (1968) The influence of aerobic and anaerobic incubations on the uptake of serotonin by blood platelets. *Biochem. Pharmacol. 17*, 1473-1476

PAASONEN, M. K. (1964) On the mechanism of action of chlorpromazine in releasing 5-hydroxytryptamine from blood platelets *in vitro. Arch. Exp. Pathol. Pharmakol. 248*, 223-230

REIMERS, H. J., MUSTARD, J. F. & PACKHAM, M. A. (1975) Transfer of adenine nucleotides between the releasable and non-releasable compartments of rabbit blood platelets. *J. Cell Biol.* in press

ROBBLEE, L. S., SHEPRO, D. & BELAMARICH, F. A. (1973a) Calcium uptake and associated adenosine triphosphatase activity of isolated platelet membranes. *J. Gen. Physiol. 61*, 462-481

ROBBLEE, L. S., SHEPRO, D. & BELAMARICH, F. A. (1973b) The effect of thrombin and trypsin on calcium uptake by calf platelet membranes. *Microvasc. Res. 6*, 99-107

SCHICK, P. K. & YU, B. P. (1973) Methylene blue-induced serotonin release in human platelets. *J. Lab. Clin. Med. 82*, 546-553

STILLER, R. A., BELAMARICH, F. A. & SHEPRO, D. (1975) Aggregation and release in the thrombocytes of the duck. *Am. J. Physiol.* in press

WARING, M. (1975) Stacking interactions. *Chem. Ind. (Lond.)* February 1975, pp. 105-113

5-Hydroxytryptamine receptors
of platelets

G. V. R. BORN and F. MICHAL

Department of Pharmacology, University of Cambridge

Abstract Circulating platelets contain 5-hydroxytryptamine (5HT) in many mammals and so do thrombocytes in birds. The function of 5HT in these cells is still uncertain; but its significance has been increased by the recognition that platelets are similar to certain neurons in being (*i*) activated by 5HT and some related substances and (*ii*) able to accumulate 5HT.

In some species, including man, 5HT causes platelets to transform rapidly from smooth disks to spikey spheres which then aggregate. This activation is apparently mediated by a membrane receptor for 5HT. In other species, including the rabbit, platelets are not transformed or aggregated by 5HT which, however, potentiates the aggregating effect of other agents, e.g. adrenaline; these platelets too presumably have an activation receptor.

Platelets can accumulate 5HT apparently against high concentration gradients. However, an intracellular storage system for 5HT probably keeps its cytoplasmic concentration low. Accumulation at body temperature begins with non-diffusional transport of 5HT through the membrane. Near 0 °C the amine diffuses slowly into the platelets. At equilibrium, the intracellular 5HT concentration is proportional to the extracellular; but backward extrapolation indicates the existence of high-affinity binding sites for 5HT, presumably on the membrane, of the order of 10^3 per platelet. These sites may represent a transport receptor which may be part of a carrier for 5HT.

Are the activation and transport receptors identical or different? In platelets as in neurons, activation is inhibited more potently by methysergide than by imipramine, whereas the reverse is true for uptake. This would suggest the existence of two different 5HT receptors on platelets. However, the receptors have some properties in common. Thus, activation by 5HT as well as its uptake require external sodium; and both processes are accelerated after the enzymic incorporation of *N*-acetylneuraminic acid into the platelet membrane.

Since the discovery (Rand & Reid 1951) that blood platelets of many mammalian species including man contain 5-hydroxytryptamine (5HT) in comparatively high concentrations, much work has been done to find out how the

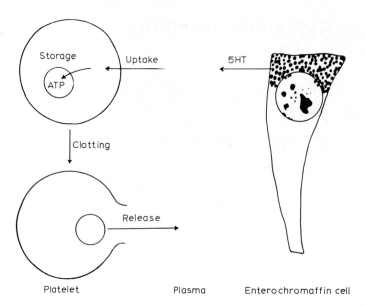

FIG. 1. Diagram made almost twenty years ago showing source and sink of platelet 5-hydroxytryptamine (5HT). No evidence obtained since then contradicts the propositions then made that platelet 5HT originates in the enterochromaffin cells of the intestinal mucosa; is taken up by platelets from the portal plasma and concentrated in their storage organelles in association with ATP; and is released during clotting. Two additional facts established subsequently are that release can occur also during platelet aggregation in the absence of clotting; and that the organelles release their contents by exocytosis rather than emerging intact.

amine comes to be there and what its biological function is (for reviews see Erspamer 1966; Pletscher 1968). The latter is still uncertain. As to the former, the evidence is that 5HT is accumulated by platelets during their life-time in the circulating blood. The only part of the circulation in which the blood plasma contains measurable amounts of 5HT is the portal, probably because of release of the amine from the enterochromaffin cells of the intestinal mucosa (Fig. 1). The evidence indicates that platelets have a mechanism for the active transport of 5HT through their outer membrane (Born & Gillson 1959) and another mechanism for accumulating 5HT in cytoplasmic organelles in association with ATP and divalent cations (Born 1958; Born et al. 1958; Baker et al. 1959; Tranzer et al. 1968; Pletscher et al. 1969). 5HT can also move slowly across the platelet membrane by passive diffusion, either in the cold (Born & Bricknell 1959) or after its release from the organelles by reserpine or by phenylalkylamines (Hughes & Brodie 1959).

When platelets are present in clotting plasma they lose some of their ATP

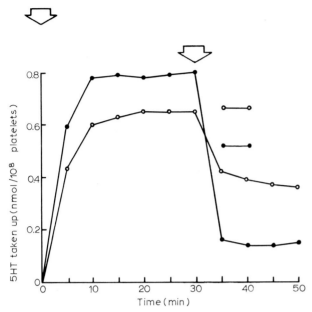

FIG. 2. Uptake and release by platelets of 5-hydroxytryptamine (5HT) added to human platelet-rich plasma which had (○—○) and had not (●—●) been clotted by thrombin (5 units/ml) and lysed by streptokinase (250 units/ml) added simultaneously (at the second arrow). Both control and clotted and lysed plasmas were incubated at 37 °C for 30 min before addition (at the first arrow) of 5HT labelled with ^{14}C at a concentration of 1 nmol/10^8 platelets. *Abscissa:* time (min). *Ordinate:* 5HT in platelets (nmol/10^8 platelets). (M. Zuzel & G. V. R. Born, unpublished results.)

and most of their 5HT at the same time (Born 1956, 1958), apparently in a specific release reaction which is induced by thrombin (Grette 1962). When streptokinase is added to citrated platelet-rich plasma at the same time as thrombin, a clot forms which is then rapidly lysed and most of the platelets are set free again singly. When radioactive 5HT is then added these serum platelets are still able to take it up at an initial velocity almost as great as that of control platelets in plasma which had not been made to clot (M. Zuzel & G. V. R. Born, unpublished 1975) (Fig. 2). This observation suggests that the outer membrane of the platelets retains the system which transports 5HT functionally intact in spite of the enzymic activities associated with the clotting and lysis of the surrounding plasma. That these enzymes do not damage the functional integrity of the platelets' outer membrane is also indicated by the persistence of adenosine transport at undiminished velocity (M. Zuzel & G. V. R. Born, unpublished 1975) and of an ouabain-sensitive movement of K^+ into the platelets (Zuzel et al. 1976).

5HT can aggregate the platelets of some mammalian species including man (Mitchell & Sharp 1964; Mills 1970) but not those of others, for example guinea pig and horse (Sinakos & Caen 1967). In at least one species of bird, the Aylesbury duck (*Anas platyrhynchos*), the circulating thrombocytes which are functionally analogous to mammalian platelets both contain 5HT and are aggregated by it, whether added or released from the cells themselves(Belamarich & Simoneit 1973). Reptiles, the evolutionary precursors of both birds and mammals, also possess nucleated thrombocytes. Whether they contain 5HT is still unknown for most species. The blood of the turtle (*Chrysemys scripta elegans*) contains 5HT but in the basophils, not in the thrombocytes; whether this 5HT is released during the haemostatic process appears to be unknown.

Apart from the question whether the 5HT of platelets has a regulatory role in their haemostatic function, there is increasing evidence of striking similarities in the involvement of 5HT with platelets on the one hand and with tryptamin-ergic neurons on the other (for review see Sneddon 1973). Both cell types are activated by the amine and possess mechanisms for its intracellular accumula-tion. Whether this is merely an example of economy in system design for completely different functions or whether the similarities imply something more is uncertain. Nevertheless, the similarities make the reactions of platelets to 5HT of interest not only for their own functional behaviour but also by pro-viding a model for a widely distributed type of neuron. The following analysis of the receptor actions of 5HT on platelets is likely, therefore, to be relevant also to nervous and perhaps also to other tissue.

5HT REACTING SITES FOR AGGREGATION AND FOR UPTAKE: ONE RECEPTOR OR TWO?

One of the most interesting questions, still unanswered, about 5HT receptors on platelets is whether those that mediate its aggregating effect are the same as or different from those which initiate its uptake. This question is still un-answered. We should like to discuss some recent observations of ours which bear on it, in the light of facts established earlier. These can be summarized as follows, first for aggregation and then for uptake.

Aggregation by 5HT differs in different mammals. In some, such as the cat, 5HT can elicit aggregation in two phases (White 1970) the second of which indicates the specific release of some platelet constituents, including 5HT itself, from intracellular organelles in which it is stored in association with adenine nucleotides. In others, including man, the velocity and extent of aggregation increase with 5HT concentration only up to a certain value (in man about 10 μM) and decrease with higher concentrations. These opposing effects of

5HT suggested that it has two different modes of molecular action on the platelet membrane. The phenomena were analysed very thoroughly (Baumgartner & Born 1968, 1969; Baumgartner 1969) and led to the hypothesis that 5HT produces its effects on aggregation by combining with specific membrane receptors identical with those concerned in its active uptake (Born & Gillson 1959; Born & Bricknell 1959). Aggregation and potentiation occur as long as a sufficient proportion of the receptors is free to react with molecules of 5HT. The platelets change shape when exposed to 5HT (Born 1970a), suggesting that its combination with the receptors induces structural changes in the platelet similar to those produced by ADP (Born 1965). The receptors transport 5HT through the membrane where the amine–receptor complex dissociates. After diffusing through the cytoplasm the amine is taken up into the storage organelles while the receptor returns free to react once more. As platelets accumulate 5HT the storage system becomes saturated (Born & Gillson 1959), but not as rapidly as aggregation is inhibited. With increasing saturation, 5HT in the platelets exchanges with 5HT in the medium at a rate similar to that of the active uptake. Because diffusion is much slower, this indicates that the transport system now moves 5HT across the membrane in both directions. If aggregation can only occur when the transport receptors return free, as the hypothesis proposed, their failure to do so would account for the self-inhibitory effect of 5HT.

There is increasing exchange of intracellular 5HT with that in the medium via the active transport system in the membrane (Born & Gillson 1959); in consequence a diminishing proportion of receptors return free to react. This saturation causes the inhibitory effect of 5HT on aggregation.

The hypothesis, therefore, made use of the specific mechanism by which platelets accumulate 5HT to account for its effects on aggregation. This accounted for several other observations. Thus, 5HT causes immediate aggregation of human platelets which consists of the first phase only. Furthermore, 5HT rapidly potentiates aggregation by adrenaline or ADP. The rapidity of the effects suggest its reaction with a receptor on the platelet surface and the simplest assumption is, of course, that the effects of 5HT on aggregation involve its reaction with the same receptors which mediate its uptake. Circumstantial support is the similarity in the concentration of 5HT (0.3–0.4 μM) at which uptake proceeds at half maximal velocity to that (about 0.5 μM) which causes half maximal velocity of aggregation.

Even the small difference could be explained by assuming that 5HT was already exerting a self-inhibitory effect on aggregation while its velocity was being measured because 5HT inhibits aggregation induced by itself as well as that induced by other agents including ADP, thrombin and adrenaline. The inhibition is both concentration- and time-dependent and appeared to have some features in common with inhibition by imipramine and chlorpromazine. These drugs have a 'stabilizing' effect on biological membranes (Seeman 1972). Another possible explanation of the inhibitory action of 5HT is, therefore, that it has a similar stabilizing effect on the platelet membrane. Such an effect on the membranes of other cells would incidentally explain some curious effects of 5HT, such as its potentiation of barbiturate hypnosis.

Determinations of the *uptake* of 5HT by platelets under conditions in which its active transport is abolished provided an estimate of the number of specific combining sites for 5HT on the platelet membrane (Born & Bricknell 1959). This was obtained by incubating citrated platelet-rich plasma at 0 °C with radioactive 5HT added at increasing concentrations. At equilibrium the concentration of 5HT in the platelet water was almost the same as that in the plasma, but the straight line relating the concentrations cut the y axis a little above the origin. This could be explained most simply by assuming the existence on the platelet membrane of high-affinity receptors for 5HT which became saturated at very low 5HT concentrations; and it was suggested that these receptors are part of the specific carrier mechanism responsible for transporting 5HT actively through the platelet membrane at 37 °C. The number of these receptors was calculated to be of the order of 10^4 per platelet. There is evidence that the platelet membrane has other receptors which are specific for ADP which number about 10^5 per platelet (Born 1965; Born & Feinberg 1975). If the number of ADP receptors is indeed one order of magnitude greater than the number of 5HT receptors, it would account for the approximately ten-fold difference in the concentrations of ADP (30–100 µM) and 5HT (5–10 µM) which cause maximum velocities of aggregation respectively for the two agents.

Several other observations also indicate some kind of functional relationship between the activating effect of 5HT on platelets and its active uptake by them. Thus, when 5HT is added to the platelet-rich plasma of rabbits in amounts that exceed the uptake capacity of the platelets, the velocity of aggregation produced by 5HT plus adrenaline (added merely to potentiate the effectiveness of 5HT) is progressively diminished and after some time completely inhibited. In contrast, 5HT added in smaller amounts which can be taken up completely produces only a transient inhibition of aggregation (Baumgartner 1969) (Fig. 3).

Not only uptake but also release of 5HT from the platelets can affect their aggregability reversibly. Reserpine causes the release of 5HT from the storage organelles in platelets *in vivo* and *in vitro* (Pletscher 1968). Most of the released 5HT gradually appears unchanged in the incubation medium. Now, it is known that adrenaline does not aggregate rabbit platelets but greatly potentiates the aggregating effect of 5HT. When adrenaline is added to platelet-rich rabbit

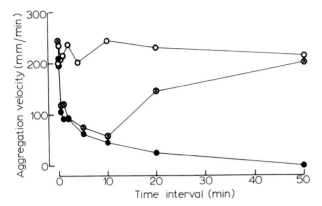

FIG. 3. Aggregation velocities of platelets in rabbit plasma produced by a mixture of 5-hydroxytryptamine (5HT) (5 μM) plus adrenaline (5 μM) at increasing time intervals after the addition of saline (○); 5 μM 5HT (⊗); or 50 μM 5HT (●) at time 0. The concentration of platelets in the plasma was 5.61×10^8/ml; the initial concentration of 5HT in the platelets was 5.3 nmol/10^8 platelets. Typical of three experiments. (From Baumgartner 1969; reproduced by permission of *The Journal of Physiology*.)

plasma after reserpine, there is no aggregation when the interval between the two additions is only a few seconds. As the interval is increased to several minutes adrenaline produces aggregation at increasing velocities; with still longer intervals the velocity decreases again (Baumgartner 1969). This aggregation is, presumably, caused by the synergistic actions of the added adrenaline and the released 5HT. Furthermore, rabbits treated with reserpine lose almost all the 5HT from their platelets. When these rabbits are then injected with 5HT the velocity at which their platelets can aggregate *in vitro* increases progressively (Baumgartner 1969). A reasonable explanation for these facts was that 5HT is progressively removed from the carrier system so that its capacity for transferring the amine through the platelet membrane increases, with a concomitant increase in aggregability. In accord with this was the slower increase in aggregation velocity when the breakdown of 5HT was decreased in the platelets by a monoamine oxidase inhibitor.

All the observations summarized so far are compatible with the simplest assumption of only one type of 5HT receptor on the platelet membrane. However, more recent evidence requires consideration of the possibility that there are two different receptors, one mediating uptake and the other aggregation. The main basis for this possibility is an analysis of the specificity of the reactions of platelets with 5HT through the use of seventeen analogues and of two potent antagonists to 5HT (Born *et al.* 1972). Most of the analogues used,

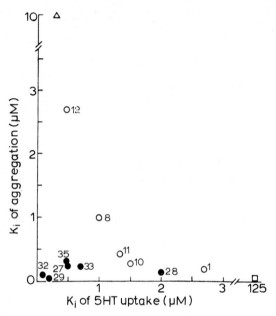

FIG. 4. Relationship between the inhibitory constants (K_i) for the inhibition of aggregation (*ordinate*) induced in human platelet-rich plasma by 5-hydroxytryptamine (5HT) and for the inhibition of 5HT uptake (*abscissa*). Analogues of 5HT (●) and analogues of tryptamine (○) are numbered as follows: 1 = tryptamine; 8 = *N'*-ethyltryptamine; 10 = *N'N'*-dimethyltryptamine; 11 = *N'N'*-diethyltryptamine; 12 = *N'N'*-dipropyltryptamine; 27 = 5-hydroxy-*N'N'*-dimethyltryptamine; 28 = 5-hydroxy-*N'N'*-diethyltryptamine; 29 = 5-hydroxy-*N'N'*-dipropyltryptamine; 32 = 5-hydroxy-*N'N'*-diisopropyltryptamine; 33 = 5-hydroxy-*N'N'*-dibutyltryptamine; 35 = 7-chloro-α-methyltryptamine; △ = imipramine; □ = methysergide. (From Born *et al.* 1972; reproduced by courtesy of *The British Journal of Pharmacology*.)

which included derivatives of tryptamine as well as of 5HT, turned out to be strong inhibitors of both the aggregating effect of 5HT and its uptake. When the inhibitory potencies of the analogues towards aggregation on the one hand and towards uptake on the other were plotted against each other (Fig. 4), no correlation emerged for 5-hydroxytryptamines whatever other substitutions they carried as well. But a remarkable feature emerged with the tryptamines: tryptamine itself was considerably more inhibitory towards aggregation than towards uptake. With increasing aliphatic substitution on the amino group the derivatives became increasingly potent inhibitors towards aggregation. The inverse relationship became even more striking when the inhibitory potencies of methysergide and imipramine were plotted on the same scale: methysergide as the most potent inhibitor of aggregation fell at one extreme of the tryptamine curve whereas imipramine as the most potent inhibitor of uptake fell at the other.

These results, in particular the very great differences in inhibitory potencies of methysergide and imipramine on the two processes, would be most straight-forwardly explained by assuming two different types of 5HT receptors on platelets, one mediating aggregation and the other uptake. However, it is worthwhile to consider this in the light of what is known or, rather, what is unknown about the modes of action of these inhibitors. Methysergide is a highly specific antagonist to the actions of 5HT on other cell types, including neurons, as well as on platelets and its antagonism is within limits competitive. This suggests that methysergide does indeed compete with 5HT for a receptor essential for initiating aggregation; this competition presumably depends on similarities in molecular structure (see Born 1970b). Imipramine, on the other hand, powerfully antagonizes not only the uptake by platelets and by trypt-aminergic neurons of 5HT but also that of noradrenaline, a very different molecule, by adrenergic neurons; furthermore, these inhibitory effects are non-competitive. It seems, therefore, that imipramine exerts its effect through something other than a direct competitive action on the 5HT receptor. The observation that increasing aliphatic substitution of tryptamine makes for an increasingly imipramine-like inhibition of uptake of 5HT by platelets and at the same time for decreasing inhibition of 5HT on aggregation suggests that these substances like imipramine do not compete with 5HT at the 'aggregation receptor' but have another, less specific reaction with the cell membrane which shows itself secondarily as the observed inhibition. These considerations also bring to mind the difference between the receptors for the catecholamines, because increasing aliphatic substitution on their amino group increases potency towards one type and decreases potency towards the other.

In low concentrations 5HT causes transient inhibition of aggregation induced not only by itself (see above) but also by ADP (Michal & Motamed 1975) (Fig. 5).

This supports the suggestion that one of the interactions of 5HT with the platelet membrane is sufficiently non-specific to affect the reactions of other receptors which are presumably entirely different to those for 5HT.

For 5HT, at least two different types of receptors have been known for a long time, located respectively on nerve and smooth muscle cells (for review see Born 1970b). One of these, the D-receptor of, for example, smooth muscle is specifically antagonized by methysergide and related compounds; and the receptor responsible for the effect of 5HT in causing platelet aggregation is apparently of this type (Michal 1969). The other type of receptor on platelets is, however, not analogous to the other classical receptor for 5HT (Gaddum & Hameed 1954; Rocha E Silva et al. 1953).

Clearly much remains to be discovered about the biochemical systems with

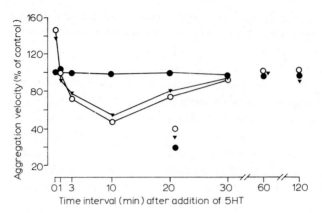

FIG. 5. Aggregation velocity of human platelets (expressed as percentage of control) produced by 1μM-ADP (○) at different time intervals after preceding addition of 5μM 5-hydroxy-tryptamine (5HT) in the presence of 0.1μM methysergide (●) or 0.5 μM imipramine (▼). Methysergide or imipramine were added 5 min before 5HT; all samples were incubated for 30 min at 37 °C before the addition of ADP. (From Michal & Motamed 1975; reproduced by permission of *The British Journal of Pharmacology*.)

which 5HT and its antagonists react to bring about transmembrane movement and aggregation. For some time past there have been hints that sialic acids bound to cell surface structures are required for the biological actions of 5HT (for review see Born 1967a). Recently it was shown that the enzymically catalysed incorporation of N-acetylneuraminic acid (NANA) into the platelet membrane accelerates platelet aggregation by 5HT (but not by ADP) as well as the influx of potassium that occurs during the accumulation of 5HT by platelets (Born 1967b; Mester et al. 1972; Michal et al. 1972). These results suggest that this sialic acid is a component of the 'aggregation receptor' for 5HT. It has now been established that such incorporation of NANA also accelerates the uptake of 5HT by human platelets, whether suspended in their own citrated plasma or in physiological saline (Szabados et al. 1975). Apparently, therefore, the sialic acid becomes a component of the receptor responsible for the active transport of 5HT through the platelet membrane.

Thus, incorporation of the same sialic acid can accelerate both reactions of platelets to 5HT, namely its uptake and the induction of aggregation. This again raises the question whether the two effects are mediated by the same receptor or by two different receptors. If there *are* two receptors, these latest observations imply that NANA is a component of both.

References

BAKER, R. V., BLASCHKO, H. & BORN, G. V. R. (1959) The isolation from blood platelets of particles containing 5-HT and ATP. *J. Physiol. (Lond.) 149*, 55P-56P

BAUMGARTNER, H. R. (1969) 5-HT uptake and release in relation to aggregation of rabbit platelets. *J. Physiol. (Lond.) 201*, 409-423

BAUMGARTNER, H. R. & BORN, G. V. R. (1968) Effect of 5-HT on platelet aggregation. *Nature (Lond.) 218*, 137-141

BAUMGARTNER, H. R. & BORN, G. V. R. (1969) The relation between the 5-HT content and aggregation of rabbit platelets. *J. Physiol. (Lond.) 201*, 397-408

BELAMARICH, F. A. & SIMONEIT, O. W. (1973) Aggregation of duck thrombocytes by 5-hydroxytryptamine. *Microvasc. Res. 6*, 229-234

BORN, G. V. R. (1956) Adenosine triphosphate (ATP) in blood platelets. *Biochem. J. 62*, 33P

BORN, G. V. R. (1958) Changes in the distribution of phosphorus in platelet-rich plasma during clotting. *Biochem. J. 68*, 695-704

BORN, G. V. R. (1965) Uptake of adenosine and of adenosine diphosphate by human platelets. *Nature (Lond.) 206*, 1121-1122

BORN, G. V. R. (1967a) Mechanism of platelet aggregation and of its inhibition by adenosine derivatives. *Fed. Proc. 26*, 115-117

BORN, G. V. R. (1967b) The effect of 5-hydroxytryptamine on the potassium exchange of human platelets. *J. Physiol. (Lond.) 190*, 273-280

BORN, G. V. R. (1970a) Observations on the change in shape of blood platelets brought about by adenosine diphosphate. *J. Physiol. (Lond.) 209*, 487-511

BORN, G. V. R. (1970b) 5-Hydroxtryptamine receptors. In *Smooth Muscle* (Bülbring, E., Brading, A. F., Kones, A. W. & Tomita, T., eds.), pp. 418-450, Edward Arnold, London

BORN, G. V. R. & BRICKNELL, J. (1959) The uptake of 5-HT by blood platelets in the cold. *J. Physiol. (Lond.) 147*, 153-161

BORN, G. V. R. & FEINBERG, H. (1975) Binding of adenosine diphosphate to intact human platelets. *J. Physiol. (Lond.)* in press

BORN, G. V. R. & GILLSON, R. E. (1959) Studies on the uptake of 5-HT by blood platelets. *J. Physiol. (Lond.) 146*, 472-491

BORN, G. V. R., INGRAM, G. I. C. & STACEY, R. S. (1958) The relationship between 5-HT and ATP in blood platelets. *Br. J. Pharmacol. Chemother. 13*, 62-64

BORN, G. V. R., JUENGJAROEN, K. & MICHAL, F. (1972) Relative activities on and uptake by human blood platelets of 5-hydroxytryptamine and several analogues. *Br. J. Pharmacol. 44*, 117-139

ERSPAMER, V. (1966) 5-Hydroxytryptamine and related indolalkylamines. In *Handbook of Experimental Pharmacology*, vol. 19 (Erspamer, V., ed.), Springer, Berlin

GADDUM, J. H. & HAMEED, K. A. (1954) Drugs which antagonise 5-hydroxytryptamine. *Br. J. Pharmacol. Chemother. 9*, 240-248

GRETTE, K. (1962) Studies on mechanism of thrombin-catalysed hemostatic reaction in blood platelets. *Acta Physiol. Scand. 56*, Suppl. 195

HUGHES, F. B. & BRODIE, B. B. (1959) A mechanism of 5-HT and catecholamine uptake by platelets. *J. Pharmacol. Exp. Ther. 127*, 96-103

MESTER, L., SZABADOS, L., BORN, G. V. R. & MICHAL, F. (1972) Changes in aggregation of platelets enriched in sialic acid. *Nature New Biol. 232*, 213-214

MICHAL, F. (1969) D-receptors for serotonin on blood platelets. *Nature (Lond.) 221*, 1253-1254

MICHAL, F. & MOTAMED, M. (1975) Time-dependent potentiation and inhibition by 5-hydroxytryptamine of platelet aggregation induced by ADP. *Br. J. Pharmacol. 54*, 221-222P

MICHAL, F., BORN, G. V. R., MESTER, L. & SZABADOS, L. (1972) Effect of 5-hydroxytryptamine on the potassium exchange of human platelets enriched in sialic acid. *Biochem. J. 129*, 977-978

MILLS, D. C. B. (1970) Platelet aggregation and platelet nucleotide concentration in different species. *Symp. Zool. Soc. Lond. 27*, 99-107

MITCHELL, J. R. A. & SHARP, A. A. (1964) Platelet clumping *in vitro. Br. J. Haematol. 10*, 78-93

PLETSCHER, A. (1968) Metabolism, transfer and storage of 5-HT in blood platelets. *Br. J. Pharmacol. Chemother. 32*, 1-16

PLETSCHER, A., DA PRADA, M. & TRANZER, J. P. (1969) Transfer and storage of biogenic monoamines in subcellular organelles of blood platelets. *Progr. Brain Res. 31*, 47-52

RAND, M. J. & REID, G. (1951) Source of serotonin in serum. *Nature (Lond.) 168*, 385

ROCHA E SILVA, M., VALLE, J. R. & PICARELLI, Z. P. (1953) A pharmacological analysis of the mode of action of serotonin (5-hydroxytryptamine) upon guinea-pig ileum. *Br. J. Pharmacol. Chemother 8*, 378-388

SEEMAN, P. (1972) The membrane actions of anaesthetics and tranquilizers. *Pharmacol. Rev. 24*, 583-655

SINAKOS, Z. & CAEN, J. P. (1967) Platelet aggregation in mammalians (human, rat, rabbit, guinea-pig, horse, dog): a comparative study. *Thromb. Diath. Haemorrh. 17*, 99-111

SNEDDON, J. M. (1973) Blood platelets as a model for monoamine-containing neurones. In *Progress in Neurobiology*, vol. 1, part 2 (Kerkut, G. & Phillis, J. W., eds.), pp. 151-198, Pergamon Press, Oxford & New York

SZABADOS, L., MESTER, L., MICHAL, F. & BORN, G. V. R. (1975) Accelerated uptake of 5-hydroxytryptamine by human blood platelets enriched in a sialic acid. *Biochem. J. 148*, 335-336

TRANZER, J. P., DA PRADA, M. & PLETSCHER, A. (1968) Electronmicroscopic study of the storage of 5-hydroxytryptamine in blood platelets. *Adv. Pharmacol. 6A*, 125-128

WHITE, J. G. (1970) A biphasic response of platelets to serotonin. *Scand. J. Haematol. 7*, 145

ZUZEL, M., IRVING, W. & BORN, G. V. R. (1976) Membrane transports of platelets present in plasma during clotting and lysis. In *Proceedings of the Vth Congress of the International Society of Thrombosis and Haemostasis*, Paris *(Thromb. Diath. Haemorrh.)* (Biggs, R., ed.) in press

Discussion

Crawford: There are several features about the part played by the platelet in the overall 5-hydroxytryptamine (5HT) dynamics of the body which I find irreconcilable. In man normal platelets contain between 150 and 600 ng/10^9 cells, with usually less than 30 ng/ml circulating in the plasma as free 5HT (Crawford 1965a, 1967, 1969). There is evidence that 5HT released from the enterochromaffin cells of the intestine is picked up by the platelets circulating through the mucosal capillaries (Toh 1956, in experiments with dogs). We have confirmed this finding (N. Crawford & B. N. Brooke, unpublished observations 1966) in studies involving the simultaneous sampling of human portal blood and systemic venous blood during surgery. The 5HT content of the portal blood platelets was consistently and significantly higher than in samples taken from peripheral sites (6–57% higher; mean 23%; 16 patients), with no difference in platelet counts or in the levels of plasma free 5HT (10–30 ng/ml). By similar simultaneous sampling of blood from the common pulmonary artery and from the pulmonary veins or left atrium we have also shown a gradient of platelet 5HT across the lungs in human subjects (Crawford 1965*b*) with decreases in platelet 5HT content of between 3% and 30%. Here again there was no significant difference in platelet counts or plasma free 5HT.

Since we were also unable to detect significantly increased levels of 5-hydr-oxyindoleacetic acid (5HIAA) in the portal blood samples and in the veins draining the lungs, and since the gastrointestinal tissue seems to be the major site of synthesis of 5HT, we have tentatively assumed that the urinary output of 5HIAA, which may amount to as much as 10 mg/day in normal subjects, is derived from the enterochromaffin cell 5HT and that the amine passes through the platelet system.

Pletscher: It might be metabolized in the enterochromaffin system itself.

Crawford: In that case you would expect to see an increased amount of 5HT metabolites in the portal blood, which we don't.

Born: It could also be metabolized in the liver and in other tissues.

Crawford: Yes but if it is metabolized by the liver it must have passed through the platelets.

Pletscher: 5HT is also metabolized in the brain, where the amine has a fast turnover.

Crawford: I think we can exclude the contribution from the brain, since by extrapolating from animal studies this probably represents only about 2% of the total body metabolism of 5HT. So we could have a situation where if we total the blood 5HT (free and platelet-bound) at any one moment in physiological time we find that it amounts to less than 1 mg. Now, if 5HT is only liberated from the platelets when they fulfill their normal haemostatic activity or when they are trapped out by the spleen, and if we assume a platelet lifespan of say five days, then one-fifth of the circulating platelet pool will turn over each day, releasing around 200 µg of 5HT. Yet we excrete 10 mg of the acid metabolite!

It seems to me that there must be a considerable influx and efflux of 5HT in and out of the platelet during its circulating lifespan. A number of earlier workers have attempted to examine this two-way transport across the platelet membrane, notably Born & Bricknell (1959), Born & Gillson (1957, 1959), Pletscher *et al.* (1965) and Pletscher (1968). Their findings, together with the more recent kinetic studies of Okuda & Nemerson (1971), strongly suggest that the maintenance of a steady-state equilibrium is due to the activity of an inward 5HT pump, counter-balancing passive diffusion out of the cell.

Born: As far as I know, the evidence is that some of the 5HT produced in the enterochromaffin cells finds its way into the blood. This blood goes through the portal system to the liver which removes most of that 5HT; only a minute proportion is taken up by platelets during each circulation through the intestinal microvessels and the portal venous tree. The uptake by platelets of 5HT, even at concentrations which saturate its active transport, is very slow. Far more may in fact pass at the same time into the red cells by simple diffusion (Born *et al.* 1967).

Crawford: As I said, there is less than 50 ng/ml free plasma 5HT in the portal blood, so it must be taken into the platelets fairly rapidly. The overall dynamics suggest to us a continuous two-way movement of 5HT across the platelet membrane. Whether this is by alterations in the activity of the 5HT pump-leak system or some other mechanism, I do not know. What worries me is that when conditions are used which alter the concentration of 5HT in the platelet either *in vivo* or *in vitro*, is one changing the kinetics of active uptake or altering the membrane protein configuration or molecular association to favour or inhibit the inward and outward passive fluxes? Zucker has pointed out, for example, that the half-life of 5HT in the platelet is dependent upon the pool size and that the more potential exchange there is between platelet 5HT and extracellular 5HT, the shorter the half-life of the platelet 5HT (Zucker *et al.* 1964).

Born: There is evidence against a rapid passive outflow and against a fast turnover of 5HT. In dogs, the rate at which labelled 5HT disappears from platelets *in vivo* is only slightly faster than the rate at which the platelets themselves, also labelled, disappear (Udenfriend & Weissbach 1958)—as if 5HT, once in the platelet, stayed there.

Crawford: I have taken 5HT by mouth (25 mg) many times and that amount is accountable by urinary excretion of 5HIAA in about three hours.

Born: That is not surprising.

Pletscher: Although you don't detect 5HIAA in the portal vein, there may be traces; the blood flow through the portal system is very substantial.

Crawford: One knows there are 5HT gradients across certain organs, the lungs for example. This is significant, and so there must be some metabolites of 5HT liberated from the platelets in the peripheral circulation.

Pletscher: Furthermore, the main metabolite of 5HT in the platelet is not 5-hydroxyindoleacetic acid, but 5-hydroxytryptophol (Bartholini *et al.* 1964; Da Prada *et al.* 1965).

Crawford: Dr Marcus suggested earlier (p. 284) that there may be some other forms of metabolic conversion of 5HT which change its structure in some way. How much should this be taken into account here?

Pletscher: The platelet contains monoamine oxidase and so 5HT is converted to the intermediate 5-hydroxyindolacetaldehyde by oxidative deamination. In a suspension of pure platelets, the main final metabolite is 5-hydroxytryptophol but if erythrocytes are present (which contain aldehyde dehydrogenase), 5-hydroxyindole acetic acid is the main major metabolite. So one cannot really say what is formed in the intact animal.

Born: I have always thought of 5HT as coming out of cells in the gut wall and entering a part of the blood circulation with very large volumes of flow. Nearly all this 5HT is taken up by liver cells and metabolized so that, as Dr Pletscher said, its breakdown products reappear in the blood in almost unmeasurably low concentrations and are excreted. The concentrations of 5HT and its metabolites are so minute because of the high blood flow volumes. It seems reasonable to suppose that platelets which, on the average, survive for up to nine days in the human circulation pick up very small quantities of 5HT each time they pass through the intestinal and portal circulations. It is probably possible to make some calculations to find out whether this proposition can account for the amounts of 5HT in a population of normal platelets.

Crawford: I would agree if one found elevated levels of free (non-platelet bound) 5HT in the portal blood, but we have never seen this. I should point out, however, that our studies in man (p. 298) were with patients undergoing abdominal surgery, and liver blood flow and transit times through the gut circulation may be altered. One has to be cautious about extrapolating such findings to the normal situation.

Shepro: When we pre-label platelets with [^{14}C]5HT and circulate them once through the dog lung or pump-perfuse a lung lobe, at least 75% of the [^{14}C]5HT is taken up by the lung (White *et al.* 1973, 1975).

Pletscher: How many of the platelets are destroyed?

Shepro: None. Not only do we recover, for all intents and purposes, all the platelets but in the healthy lung the transit times for platelets, red cells and plasma are almost identical (within one second). However, when the lung is unhealthy (with elevated venous resistance and physiological shunting, and low compliance) the platelet transit time is prolonged (over four seconds) and we see trapped platelets. In the latter situation we find no uptake of [^{14}C]5HT by the pulmonary tissues. The platelet: plasma [^{14}C]5HT ratio is higher in the effluent blood than in the injectate, so evidently the [^{14}C]5HT which is 're-leased' by the platelets and is normally removed by the pulmonary endothelium is simply taken up by the circulating platelet. It is our belief that endothelial cells throughout the circulatory system regulate 5HT levels in the plasma, since freshly isolated aortic endothelium and cultured endothelium also take up 5HT (Shepro *et al.* 1975).

Pletscher: I think you should double-label with a substance which really remains in the platelet. Tritiated reserpine has been shown to bind irreversibly to platelets.

Marcus: Professor Born, your experiments on *N*-acetylneuraminic acid might be even more informative if you knew where the incorporated sialic acid was localized. We know that 6% of the sialic acid in platelets is located in the glycolipids known as gangliosides (Marcus *et al.* 1972).

Born: The evidence so far suggests that the *N*-acetylneuraminic acid is incorporated into glycoproteins.

Marcus: There is another interesting 'compartment' in platelets which consists of non-releasable *N*-acetylneuraminic acid. Approximately 30% of the *N*-acetylneuraminic acid in platelets cannot be released with neuraminidase. It would be interesting to know whether the sialic acid which goes onto the platelets is releasable or not.

Born: It is released by neuraminidase.

Marcus: Therefore it may not be part of this compartment. It is of interest that recently Tamir & Huang (1974) have isolated a soluble protein from synaptosomes which has the capacity to bind 5HT.

Born: The systems are different, however. For one thing, synaptosomes are remarkably artifactual structures; and people seem to be using synaptosomes less now than more physiological preparations for similar kinds of experiments.

Sneddon: I have looked at the effects of neuraminidase on 5HT transport in rat platelets. Neuraminidase does not inhibit the accumulation of 5HT (unpublished observations). We have never measured the amount *N*-acetyl-neuraminic acid released into the supernatant, although a number of workers have demonstrated that neuraminidase treatment produces significant changes in the characteristics of platelet membranes (Davis *et al.* 1973; Nachman *et al.* 1973).

Nurden: There are also species differences in the type of sialic acid found (Adams *et al.* 1970). Not all neuraminidases hydrolyse all sialic acids, particularly if they have extra acetyl groups. I have also been looking at species differences in platelet glycoproteins, and they are considerable. The human platelet membrane glycoprotein pattern of three major glycoproteins of apparent molecular weights 155 000, 135 000 and 103 000 (Nurden & Caen 1974) is not reproduced in all mammals. For example, cat platelets, which show a relatively enhanced aggregation as induced by 5HT (Tschopp 1969), possess just two major membrane glycoproteins of approximate molecular weights 130 000 and 100 000.

With regard to the increase in platelet sialic acid after the incubation of platelets in the presence of CMP-*N*-[^{14}C]acetylneuraminic acid and a sialyl-transferase enzyme (Mester *et al.* 1972), the amount of sialic acid that is binding (an increase of up to 31% of the total sialic acid of the platelet) is so much that it would be remarkable if it were all going into the ganglioside fraction.

Probably molecular conformation changes are being induced on the surface of the platelet as a result of the increased sialic acid content of the membrane glycoproteins. This would perhaps tie in with the observed changes in the velocity of ADP-induced aggregation as well as 5HT-induced aggregation (Mester *et al.* 1972).

Born: One has to be careful in invoking conformation changes. It is certainly possible that the *N*-acetylneuraminic acid is incorporated into more than one type of site, presumably glycoprotein. Indeed it is an interesting thought which also applies to other cells: why is it possible to put extra *N*-acetylneuraminic acid onto a cell at all? Why are normal platelets and, possibly, other cells partially desialated? Is this functionally significant? The question is perhaps related to the role of sialic acids in the survival of glycoproteins in the plasma.

Nurden: Together with L-fucose, sialic acid is added last of all during the biosynthesis of glycoproteins, because of their terminal position on the oligo-saccharide chains. Recent evidence suggests that there is nearly always a certain degree of heterogeneity within glycoprotein structure with regard to the completeness of the addition of the monosaccharides as catalysed by the glycosyltransferase enzymes, at the time of the secretion of the glycoprotein molecules from the Golgi apparatus (Hughes 1973). In the case of the platelet it would seem that this would be most likely to occur within the megakaryocyte. This means that as galactose is nearly always the site of attachment of sialic acid within the glycoprotein, there will nearly always be a certain percentage of these sites available for sialylation.

Pletscher: Professor Born, you are assuming that the site of action of 5HT is the cell membrane. What is the evidence? All the drugs you showed are supposed to act on the cytoplasmic membrane, but all are basic compounds and also penetrate into the platelet; in fact an important site of their accumu-lation is the granular membrane. Imipramine and chlorpromazine accumulate at the granular level and this is true also for many amines.

Born: Imipramine inhibits the active transport of 5HT from the medium into the cytoplasm, on our evidence as well as your own. Therefore, that action must be at the outer membrane of the platelet. Whether it involves the actual accumulation of imipramine in that membrane is, as far as I am aware, not known. It seems unlikely, because, if it did, the inhibitory effect should in-crease with time; and there is no evidence for that. Incidentally, imipramine is just as effective in inhibiting the re-uptake of noradrenaline into nerve endings and all the evidence indicates that effect to be on the transport through the membrane. It is likely, of course, that very lipophilic drugs distribute themselves throughout the lipid phases of the cells, as anaesthetic agents do. I would have said that the most probable explanation—if you think of the sparrow rather than the flamingo—for the biological effects that we have seen is that they are due to an action of imipramine on the outer membrane. Do you not also believe that there is a membrane transport system plus the granule storage system?

Pletscher: I agree that there must be some kind of a carrier-mediated uptake which is energy-dependent in the cell membrane, but I was thinking of the interaction with the so-called receptor/acceptor.

Nachman: Does imipramine block shape change?

Smith: No; imipramine acts against the second wave of platelet aggregation (Mills & Roberts 1967).

Nachman: If, then, you work on the two-receptor premise, what happens if you pretreat platelets with imipramine and then add labelled 5HT? Can you demonstrate even a small amount of uptake, if you go through the same manipulation as you used for your ADP-binding studies? Has anybody looked for '5HT-binding', in the loose sense, in an imipramine-treated system?

Michal: In the whole platelet treated with imipramine we find a low, gradual increase in radioactivity under such conditions; we cannot say at this stage if this is passive diffusion, active accumulation or binding. Did you perhaps mean binding to subcellular fractions including isolated platelet membranes?

Nachman: No; without even going into subfractionation, just in a whole-cell system. A workable hypothesis is that there is a two-receptor system, and the first receptor is related to the binding which then mediates or is closely related to the shape change phenomenon. Then there is translocation to a second receptor which is related to storage. Could you approach this problem by trying to find some binding in an imipramine-treated system? We know that imipramine blocks uptake, but if you did some rapid wash experiments similar to those done by Dr Feinberg with ADP, could you find uptake?

Sneddon: I have done experiments that may help in this (unpublished, 1970). One problem in investigating 5HT binding to platelet membranes, or any other system, is the specific activity of commercially available radiolabelled compounds. We use [^{3}H]5HT from Amersham which has an activity of 500 mCi/mmol, and this may not be high enough. However, these experiments were done in cold buffered saline, so that there was little transport of 5HT during a two-minute incubation period. Using ^{14}C-labelled inulin as a measure of extracellular space I failed to demonstrate any decrease in the [^{3}H]5HT level of the centrifuged platelets either in the absence of Na$^+$ (which inhibits 5HT transport: Sneddon 1969) or in the presence of high concentrations of imipramine. I have always attributed the 'negative' results to the possibility that at the concentration of 5HT used (5×10^{-8} to 10^{-5}M), there was so much non-specific absorption onto the platelet surface that I was unable to demonstrate specific binding to the relatively small number of sites that may constitute the 'receptor' or 'carrier'.

Michal: We have some results (unpublished) which show a small pool of 5HT associated with the plasma membrane or membrane vesicles that can be labelled with radioactive 5HT. This may not be classed as specific binding but it is partially inhibited by imipramine and unaltered by methysergide.

Caen: You mentioned that sodium is necessary for the 5HT acceptor. If you change the amount of sodium outside the platelet, do you change the 5HT acceptor (and 5HT aggregation), in different species in which you have worked?

Born: We have not looked into that.

Packham: We have been examining various functions of neuraminidase-treated platelets using suspensions of washed rabbit or human platelets (Greenberg *et al.* 1975). We purify the neuraminidase extensively so that it does not cause release of the platelet granule contents. (We have been using *Clostridium perfringens* neuraminidase.) We have measured the amount of sialic acid (*N*-acetylneuraminic acid) removed by the enzyme and we believe that it is removed only from the surface, because there is no release reaction. We have been able to remove 40–60% of the total sialic acid using neuraminidase. When we tested the aggregation responses of neuraminidase-treated platelets, the only effect we observed was a slight enhancement of aggregation with ADP, collagen, thrombin, or 5HT (to study 5HT-induced aggregation we resuspended the platelets in citrated platelet-free plasma). Neuraminidase treatment also enhanced the release of [^{14}C]5HT from prelabelled platelets exposed to collagen, thrombin, or ADP (in citrated human plasma). Our preliminary experiments indicate that the uptake of 5HT is not changed by removing surface sialic acid in this way.

Caen: Have you also used the bovine factor VIII?

Packham: No. We used ristocetin and found a slight enhancement of aggregation when human platelets had been treated with neuraminidase. The platelets were treated with neuraminidase while they were suspended in an artificial medium so that we could quantify the amount of sialic acid removed. One cannot do an experiment with ristocetin in the artificial medium, however, so we resuspended the platelets in citrated platelet-free human plasma before examining their aggregation response to ristocetin.

Platelets from patients with the giant platelet syndrome (Bernard & Soulier 1948) do not aggregate on the addition of ristocetin, and have a low sialic acid content, and a shortened survival *in vivo* (Gröttum & Solum 1969; Howard *et al.* 1973; Caen *et al.* 1973). The inability of these platelets to aggregate when ristocetin is added has been attributed to a defect in the platelets, but our results indicate that this defect probably does not involve surface sialic acid. In our experiments, platelets from which sialic acid had been removed were rapidly cleared from the circulation (Greenberg *et al.* 1975) and it seems likely that the thrombocytopenia observed in patients with the Bernard-Soulier syndrome can be attributed to the abnormally low amount of sialic acid in the platelet membrane.

Mills: We have shown (Kirby & Mills 1975) that platelets digested with proteinase-free neuraminidase can lose 60% of their sialic acid without losing their ability to clump with bovine factor VIII or human factor VIII plus ristocetin.

References

ADAMS, E. P., NURDEN, A. T. & FRENCH, J. E. (1970) A comparative study of the bound carbohydrates in platelets, plasma and vascular endothelium. *Symp. Zool. Soc. Lond. 27*, 91-98

BARTHOLINI, G., PLETSCHER, A. & BRUDERER, H. (1964) Formation of 5-hydroxytryptophol from endogenous 5-hydroxytryptamine by isolated blood platelets. *Nature (Lond.) 203*, 1281-1283

BERNARD, J. & SOULIER, J. P. (1948) Sur une nouvelle variété de dystrophie thrombocytaire hémorragipare congénitale. *Sem. Hôp. Paris 24*, 3217-3223

BORN, G. V. R. & BRICKNELL, J. (1959) The uptake of 5-hydroxytryptamine by blood platelets in the cold. *J. Physiol. (Lond.) 147*, 153-161

BORN, G. V. R. & GILLSON, R. E. (1957) The uptake of 5-hydroxytryptamine by blood platelets. *J. Physiol. (Lond.) 137*, 82P-83P

BORN, G. V. R. & GILLSON, R. E. (1959) Studies on the uptake of 5-hydroxytryptamine by blood platelets. *J. Physiol. (Lond.) 146*, 472-479

BORN, G. V. R., DAY, M. & STOCKBRIDGE, A. (1967) The uptake of amines by human erythrocytes *in vitro*. *J. Physiol. (Lond.) 193*, 405-418

CAEN, J., LEVY-TOLEDANO, S., SULTAN, Y. & BERNARD, J. (1973) La dystrophie thrombocytaire hémorragipare (interaction des plaquettes et du facteur Willebrand). *Nouv. Rev. Fr. Hématol. 13*, 595-602

CRAWFORD, N. (1965a) Systemic venous platelet bound and plasma free serotonin levels in non-carcinoid malignancy. *Clin. Chim. Acta 12*, 274-281

CRAWFORD, N. (1965b) The lungs and serotonin metabolism: a study of the pulmonary arterio-venous levels of plasma free and platelet bound serotonin in man. *Clin. Chim. Acta 12*, 264-273

CRAWFORD, N. (1967) Serotonin absorption by normal and 'carcinoid' platelets. *Clin. Chim. Acta 18*, 297-307

CRAWFORD, N. (1969) Some observations on the blood serotonin levels in rheumatoid arthritis with a study of platelet serotonin absorption. *Clin. Chim. Acta 23*, 139-146

DA PRADA, M., BARTHOLINI, G. & PLETSCHER, A. (1965) Formation of 5-hydroxytryptophol by blood platelets after thrombin and reserpine. *Experientia 21*, 135-139

DAVIS, J. W., YUE, T. N. K. & PHILLIPS, E. P. (1973) The effect of neuraminidase on platelet aggregation induced by ADP, norepinephrine, collagen or serotonin. *Thromb. Diath. Haemorrh. 28*, 221-227

GREENBERG, J., PACKHAM, M. A., CAZENAVE, J.-P., REIMERS, H.-J. & MUSTARD, J. F. (1975) Effects on platelet function of removal of platelet sialic acid by neuraminidase. *Lab. Invest. 32*, 476-484

GRÖTTUM, K. A. & SOLUM, N. O. (1969) Congenital thrombocytopenia with giant platelets. A defect in the platelet membrane. *Br. J. Haematol. 16*, 277-290

HOWARD, M. A., HUTTON, R. A. & HARDISTY, R. M. (1973) Hereditary giant platelet syndrome: a disorder of a new aspect of platelet function. *Br. Med. J. 2,* 586-588

HUGHES, R. C. (1973) Glycoproteins as components of cellular membranes. *Progr. Biophys. Mol. Biol. 26,* 189-268

KIRBY, E. P. & MILLS, D. C. B. (1975) Interaction of human platelets with bovine factor VIII. *J. Clin. Invest.* in press

MARCUS, A. J., ULLMAN, H. L. & SAFIER, L. B. (1972) Studies on human platelet gangliosides. *J. Clin. Invest. 51,* 2602-2612

MESTER, L., SZABADOS, L., BORN, G. V. R. & MICHAL, F. (1972) Changes in the aggregation of platelets enriched in sialic acid. *Nature New Biol. 236,* 213-214

MILLS, D. C. B. & ROBERTS, G. C. K. (1967) Membrane active drugs and the aggregation of human blood platelets. *Nature (Lond.) 213,* 35-38

NACHMAN, R. L., HUBBARD, A. & FERRIS, B. (1973) Iodination of the human platelet membrane. Studies of the major glycoprotein. *J. Biol. Chem. 248,* 2928-2936

NURDEN, A. T. & CAEN, J. P. (1974) An abnormal platelet glycoprotein pattern in three cases of Glanzmann's thrombasthenia. *Br. J. Haematol. 28,* 253-260

OKUDA, M. & NEMERSON, Y. (1971) Transport of serotonin by blood platelets: a pump-leak system. *Am. J. Physiol. 220,* 283-288

PLETSCHER, A. (1968) Metabolism, transfer and storage of 5-hydroxytryptamine in blood platelets. *Br. J. Pharmacol. Chemother. 32,* 1-16

PLETSCHER, A., DA PRADA, M. & BARTHOLINI, G. (1965) Alterations of the 5-hydroxytryptamine outflux from blood platelets *in vitro. Biochem. Pharmacol. 14,* 1135-1139

SHEPRO, D., BATBOUTA, J. C., ROBBLEE, L. S., CARSON, M. P. & BELAMARICH, F. A. (1975) Serotonin transport by cultured bovine aortic endothelium. *Circ. Res. 36,* 799

SNEDDON, J. M. (1969) Sodium dependent accumulation of 5-hydroxytryptamine by rat blood platelets. *Br. J. Pharmacol. 37,* 680-688

TAMIR, H. & HUANG, Y. L. (1974) Binding of serotonin to soluble protein from synaptosomes. *Life Sci. 14,* 83-93

TOH, C. C. (1956) Release of 5-hydroxytryptamine (serotonin) and histamine from platelets by tissue extracts. *J. Physiol. (Lond.) 133,* 402-411

TSCHOPP, T. B. (1969) Aggregation of cat platelets *in vitro. Thromb. Diath. Haemorrh. 23,* 601-620

UDENFRIEND, S. & WEISSBACH, H. (1958) Turnover of 5-hydroxytryptamine (serotonin) in tissues. *Proc. Soc. Exp. Biol. Med. 97,* 748

WHITE, M. K., SHEPRO, D. & HECHTMAN, H. B. (1973) Pulmonary function and platelet lung interaction. *J. Appl. Physiol. 39,* 697-703

WHITE, M. K., HECHTMAN, H. B. & SHEPRO, D. (1975) Canine lung uptake of plasma and platelet serotonin. *Microvasc. Res. 9,* 131-143

ZUCKER, M. B., HELLMAN, L. & SUMOFF, B. (1964) Rapid disappearance of ^{14}C-labelled serotonin from platelets in patients with the carcinoid syndrome. *J. Lab. Clin. Med. 63,* 137-142

Interactions between 5-hydroxytryptamine and platelet lipid fractions

AARON J. MARCUS, LENORE B. SAFIER and HARRIS L. ULLMAN

Hematology Section, New York Veterans Administration Hospital, and the Department of Medicine, New York Hospital-Cornell Medical Center, New York

Abstract In contrast to other cells, platelets do not synthesize biogenic amines such as 5-hydroxytryptamine (5HT). Instead, preformed exogenous 5HT is actively taken up and stored in platelet granules. When platelets aggregate, 5HT is mobilized from membrane-bound storage granules, traverses the cytoplasm and penetrates the plasma membrane by an unknown mechanism. Implicit in this concept is the ability of a putative 5HT receptor to facilitate its passage through the granule and plasma membranes in an intact form. It has been demonstrated in several laboratories that certain phospholipids, cerebrosides and gangliosides can form complexes with biogenic amines. In the present studies partially purified extracts containing platelet gangliosides I, II and III (in addition to protein and phospholipid) were shown to take up [^{14}C]5HT as well as specific 5HT analogues, whereas other platelet lipid controls failed to do so. On the other hand, comparable ganglioside extracts prepared from human erythrocytes, brain and liver also bound 5HT, indicating that the phenomenon was not platelet-specific. 5HT binding was demonstrated by three techniques: (1) equilibrium dialysis; (2) uptake of unbound 5HT by platelet-rich plasma; and (3) ultracentrifugation of the incubation mixture. The interaction increased with time, and was retarded at 0 °C, slightly inhibited by cyanide (10^{-2} M), and uninfluenced by preheating (60 °C, 5 minutes). However, after boiling of the extract, binding was abolished. Inhibition of uptake was achieved by prior incubation of the extract with compounds such as non-radioactive 5HT, reserpine, 5-hydroxyindole, and 5-hydroxyindole acetic acid but not indole, indole acetic acid or tryptophan. Although the interaction appeared to have biochemical specificity, it was irreversible and retarded by antioxidants. The uptake of 5HT by crude ganglioside extracts does not appear to represent a receptor mechanism in the pharmacological sense. However, these extracts have the property of 'recognizing' hydroxyindole compounds and may contain the 'nonenzymic' portion of the 5HT receptor.

Platelets differ from the other blood elements in that they have a unique avidity for 5-hydroxytryptamine (serotonin, 5HT). The expression of this property is rapid uptake followed by storage. Current pharmacological thinking would tend to implicate a specific 5HT receptor on the plasma membrane of the platelet and the membrane of 5HT storage granules in the platelet cytoplasm. Although most receptors are thought to be predominantly protein in nature, there is also evidence that lipids such as gangliosides may be involved in receptor mechanisms. Van Heyningen *et al.* (1971) and Cuatrecasas (1973) have shown that gangliosides can bind cholera toxin and may be the membrane receptors for this substance. Woolley & Gommi (1965) had previously suggested that gangliosides were 5HT receptors. Marchbanks (1966) demonstrated that nerve ending particles prepared from rat brain could bind 5HT. Butanol extracts of such fractions contained material which could also take up 5HT. We have found radioactivity in butanol extracts of human platelets after they were labelled with [^{14}C]5HT.

For the past few years our laboratory has been involved in the isolation and biochemical characterization of human platelet gangliosides (Marcus *et al.* 1972). These studies were an integral part of our major research interests, which are concerned with the physiological properties of platelet membranes. Purification of these glycosphingolipids afforded the opportunity to evaluate their possible role and specificity as 5HT receptors. Although gangliosides comprise only 0.5 % of platelet lipids and account for 6 % of the total sialic acid in human platelets, their validation as membrane components (Lehninger 1968) and unique solubility properties (Ledeen 1966) suggest that they may play an important role in the chemistry of the cell surface.

HUMAN PLATELET GANGLIOSIDES

Table 1 summarizes the qualitative and quantitative composition of the non-lipid portion of gangliosides in human platelets. Ganglioside I (hematoside), the major platelet ganglioside, is also the major extraneural ganglioside. The carbohydrate and lipid composition of ganglioside I was not significantly different from that of gangliosides found in other tissues. Ganglioside II has also been described in bovine platelets (Etzrodt 1968). Although ganglioside III was identified as G_{3A}, thin layer chromatographic studies of concentrated material as well as the presence of hexosamine indicated the presence of at least one other ganglioside in trace amounts—possibly G_{D1a}. Additional chemical analysis of ganglioside III was logistically impractical.

The isolation of platelet gangliosides provided the opportunity to test the 5HT receptor hypothesis. An equilibrium dialysis system was chosen for this purpose. Platelet gangliosides were dialysed against [^{14}C]5HT. Controls consisted of gangliosides from other tissues and species as well as a variety of other platelet lipids. It was demonstrated that platelet gangliosides I and III

TABLE 1

Composition of human platelet gangliosides (non-lipid components)

	% of total gangliosides	Components (Molar ratio to glucose)				
		Galactose	Glucose	NANA[a]	Sphingosine	Hexosamine
I Hematoside (G_6)	92	1.07	1.00	1.07	1.06	0
II Lacto-N-neo-tetraose (G_{LNnT})	5	1.84	1.00	0.88	0.90	0.94
III Disialosyllactosyl ceramide (G_{3A})[b]	2	1.00	1.00	2.00	1.00	0

[a] N-acetylneuraminic acid.
[b] Theoretical values.

unequivocally bound small amounts of 5HT in an irreversible manner. The gangliosides that had taken up the 5HT could be pelleted by ultracentrifugation without loss of radioactivity. Other platelet lipids such as lecithin and cholesterol were negative for binding. Other gangliosides such as beef kidney G_{3A} were also capable of taking up 5HT. In a typical experiment with platelet ganglioside III examples of 24-hour counts were as follows: ganglioside III, 25 832 c.p.m./25 µl as against 23 150 c.p.m./25 µl in the opposite chamber. It was concluded that the uptake as observed was of insufficient magnitude to warrant the designation of platelet gangliosides as 5HT 'receptors'. Among the alternative explanations considered was that the gangliosides were indeed an intrinsic part of the 5HT receptor and that the purification procedure resulted in deletion of an essential fragment (Marcus et al. 1972).

An alternative methodological approach was considered which would accomplish the extraction of all platelet gangliosides, albeit in a relatively crude form, thereby retaining a cofactor(s) that may have been necessary for more effective 5HT binding. The method used is shown in Fig. 1; it is based on the procedure designed for brain tissue devised by Tettamanti et al. (1973). Ten grams of washed, frozen human platelets were extracted at a time with tetrahydrofuran. The tetrahydrofuran extract was partitioned first with ether, then with water. The organic phase of the partition mixture was discarded and the aqueous phase dialysed against distilled water. The dialysate was lyophilized and resulted in the recovery of approximately 7 mg of material. As depicted in Fig. 2, platelet gangliosides I, II and III were present in the final product. Some phospholipid and protein also passed into the aqueous phase of the partitioned system along with the gangliosides. No attempt was made to remove them since they may have included cofactor(s) necessary for efficient 5HT uptake. Thus the final lyophilized product contained 8% ganglioside, 66% phospholipid

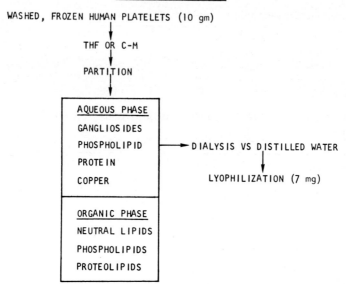

FIG. 1. 'Flow sheet' for extraction of ganglioside preparation which bound 5-hydroxy-tryptamine (5HT). The partitioning and dialysis steps were necessary prerequisites for the final product to take up [^{14}C]5HT. Lipids in the organic phase did not interact with 5HT. (THF, tetrahydrofuran; C-M, chloroform-methanol.)

and 14% protein. A comparable extract could be obtained by treating the platelets with chloroform-methanol 2:1 and then chloroform-methanol 1:2, according to Suzuki (1965). This was followed by a partitioning step essential for the purification of a product capable of binding 5HT. The final composition of the chloroform-methanol extract was similar to that of the tetrahydrofuran extract.

PLATELET SUPEROXIDE DISMUTASE

In concentrated form the tetrahydrofuran and chloroform-methanol extracts displayed a blue-green colour and were positive for copper by the benzoin oxime test (Feigl 1954). The colour was not due to ceruloplasmin, as ascertained by immunodiffusion against ceruloplasmin antibody.* The detection of copper also suggested the presence of the enzyme superoxide dismutase (Fridovich 1974). However, superoxide dismutase activity in the extracts was low and the

---

* Kindly performed by Dr Ralph Nachman, Cornell University Medical College.

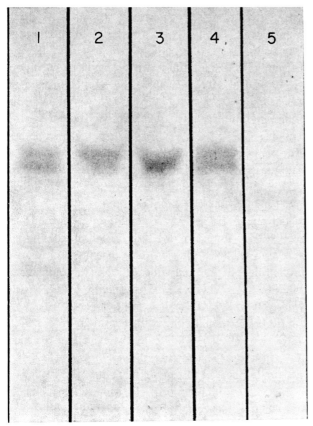

FIG. 2. Thin layer chromatogram of gangliosides in platelet extracts that bound 5-hydroxy-tryptamine.

Lane 1 – Total platelet ganglioside extract isolated as previously described (Marcus *et al.* 1972). *Top:* platelet hematoside (ganglioside I); *middle:* platelet ganglioside lacto-*N*-neotetra-ose (ganglioside II); *bottom:* ganglioside G_{3A} (ganglioside III).

Lane 2 – Gangliosides extracted from platelets with tetrahydrofuran.

Lane 3 – Gangliosides extracted by technique of Suzuki (1965), using chloroform-methanol 2:1 and 1:2.

Lane 4 – Purified platelet hematoside marker.

Lane 5 – Brain ganglioside GM_2 marker (not present in platelets). The thin layer plate was coated with silica gel G and developed in a solvent system consisting of chloroform: methanol: 2.5 N-NH_4OH, 60:40:9 (v/v/v). For colour development the plate was sprayed with resorcinol.

purified enzyme from bovine erythrocytes did not take up 5HT. On the other hand, polyacrylamide gel analysis of supernatants from sonified whole platelets demonstrated the presence of at least two bands containing superoxide dismutase activity. A possible role for this enzyme in platelet function is now under study in our laboratory.

UPTAKE OF 5HT BY CRUDE GANGLIOSIDE EXTRACTS

In the platelet-rich plasma (PRP) assay system the ganglioside extracts were incubated with [^{14}C]5HT, usually for one hour at room temperature. Aliquots of the incubation mixtures were then transferred to freshly prepared platelet-rich human plasma. Appropriate control mixtures were run simultaneously. The assay was based on the assumption that if the 5HT was bound by the extract it would not be accessible to the platelets in the plasma. The incubation mixtures were also tested for the presence of metabolic breakdown products of 5HT by high voltage electrophoresis, thin layer chromatography and a modified assay for monoamine oxidase activity (Kapeller-Adler 1971). No metabolic breakdown products were detected by these techniques.

In a typical experiment 0.5 mg of crude extract containing 33 nmoles of ganglioside were incubated with 0.4 nmole of [^{14}C]5HT. When aliquots of this incubation mixture were transferred to platelet-rich plasma, the uptake of 5HT averaged 7.5% of control values in nine experiments. Thus the ganglioside extract was capable of binding 92.5% of the [^{14}C]5HT with which it was incubated. When the extract was diluted a decrease in uptake was observed. For example, a fourfold dilution of the ganglioside extract resulted in reduction in binding from 92.5 to 47%. Uptake of [^{14}C]5HT by the extract also varied with time. When 0.05 mg of extract was incubated with 0.4 nmole of [^{14}C]5HT uptake continued to increase and appeared to reach a plateau at three hours.

Attempts to modify the uptake of 5HT by physical and chemical means were also made. The addition of cyanide resulted in slight inhibition of 5HT uptake by the ganglioside extract. Thus inhibition of platelet [^{14}C]5HT uptake by the extract was reduced from 93 to 81% in the presence of cyanide (10^{-2} M). Heating to 60 °C for 5 minutes had only a minimal inhibitory effect on the uptake of 5HT by the extract (reduction from 93 to 88%). In contrast, uptake was markedly retarded if the extract was incubated with 5HT at 0 °C (93 to 32%). If the extract was boiled, subsequent uptake of 5HT was abolished.

Several pure ganglioside preparations from platelets and other tissues as well as platelet lecithin, platelet sphingomyelin and platelet proteolipid did not bind [^{14}C]5HT under conditions of this assay. It was tentatively concluded that in contrast to the aforementioned controls the crude ganglioside extract, prepared and partitioned as described, was capable of 'recognizing' [^{14}C]5HT.

Additional binding studies were carried out using the equilibrium dialysis system previously devised for studies on purified gangliosides (Marcus *et al.* 1972). Since the ganglioside molecule has a non-polar portion, it retains its micellar form in aqueous media and does not traverse a dialysis membrane (above its critical micellar concentration). Incubations were carried out in subdued light on a rotating platform at room temperature. The 5HT control reached equilibrium in approximately 19 hours. At the conclusion of the incubation period 25 μl aliquots were withdrawn from each of the opposing chambers, placed in 'Aquasol' and counted for radioactivity. In 14 experiments platelet ganglioside extracts contained an average of 3003 c.p.m. as against 460 c.p.m. from the opposite chamber.

Crude ganglioside extracts were prepared from several other human tissues by the same techniques as those employed for platelets. These included 'dehaemoglobinized' erythrocytes (Dodge et al. 1963), brain, liver, and cultured lymphocytes (obtained commercially). These preparations were tested for their ability to take up [^{14}C]5HT in the equilibrium dialysis system, using the same quantity of platelet extracts for comparison. Under these conditions the platelet extract controls bound 71% of the available radioactivity. The liver, erythrocyte and brain extracts bound 67, 65 and 59% of the available radioactivity respectively. The lymphocyte preparation took up 37% of the available radioactivity. Thus the 5HT-binding capacity of crude ganglioside preparations cannot be considered a platelet-specific phenomenon. Although liver and brain are actively involved in uptake of biogenic amines, the phenomenon in erythrocytes is relatively passive (Born et al. 1967), and little is known of the interaction between lymphocytes and 5HT.

INTERACTION OF GANGLIOSIDE EXTRACT WITH 5HT ANALOGUES

The specificity of uptake of 5HT was examined by the use of compounds which are structurally related to it. The extracts were preincubated with the compound under study for one hour at room temperature in the dark. This was followed by the addition of [^{14}C]5HT, with subsequent incubation in the usual manner. The uptake was measured by equilibrium dialysis or the platelet-rich plasma assay technique. Analogues which blocked uptake of [^{14}C]5HT by the crude ganglioside extract are depicted in Fig. 3. At final concentrations of 10^{-3} M inhibition of 5HT uptake ranged from 65 to 90%. With the exception of reserpine the inhibitors have in common a hydroxyl group at position 5 of the indole ring system. Compounds which produced less than 10% inhibition of 5HT uptake by the ganglioside extract at a concentration of 10^{-3} M are shown in Fig. 4. These analogues differ from those shown in Fig. 3 in that the hydroxyl group is absent from position 5 of the indole ring system. In the case of indole and L-tryptophan, inhibition of 5HT uptake could be achieved at final concentrations of 10^{-2} M. It therefore appeared that uptake of 5HT by the platelet ganglioside extract showed a degree of biochemical specificity. Inhibition of [^{14}C]5HT uptake by non-radioactive 5HT was studied by ultra-

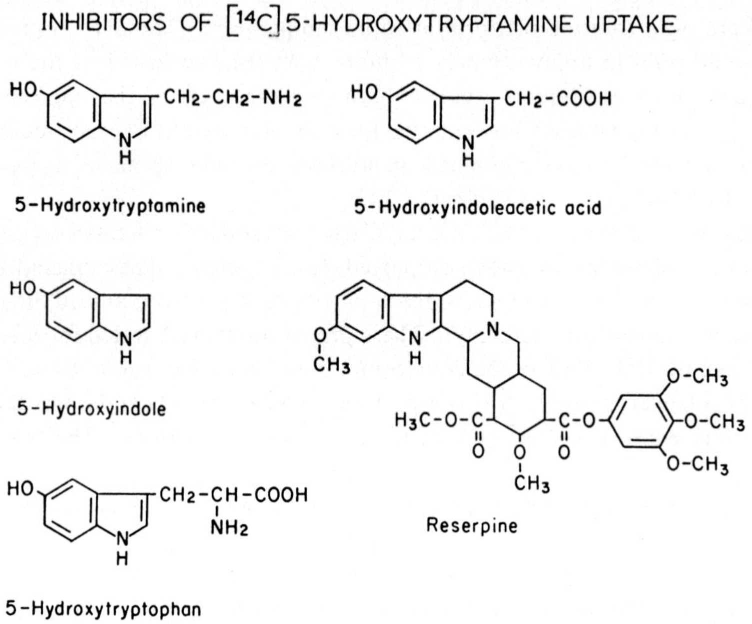

INHIBITORS OF [^{14}C]5-HYDROXYTRYPTAMINE UPTAKE

FIG. 3. When the above compounds were preincubated with the crude ganglioside extract at final concentrations of 10^{-3} M, there was inhibition of subsequent uptake of [^{14}C]5-hydroxy-tryptamine in the range of 65–90%. It was of interest that the addition of reserpine or non-radioactive 5HT after the extract had taken up [^{14}C]5HT did not release the bound [^{14}C]5HT. Note the presence of an -OH group at position 5 of the indole ring system (except in reserpine).

centrifugation of the incubation mixture. Preincubation of the ganglioside extract with cold 5HT resulted in a concentration-dependent decrease in the radioactivity recovered in the pellet as compared to control extracts incubated with [^{14}C]5HT alone. In the above experiments the concentration of [^{14}C]5HT was 2×10^{-6} M.

STUDIES ON THE IDENTIFICATION OF BOUND [^{14}C]5HT AND THE REVERSI-BILITY OF UPTAKE

At given intervals during the incubation period attempts were made to extract and identify the bound radioactivity. Among the procedures employed were: (*a*) extraction with perchloric acid followed by thin layer chromatography (t.l.c.) (Schick & Yu 1973); (*b*) direct t.l.c. in a chloroform:methanol:water solvent system; (*c*) treatment of the incubated radioactive extract with butanol-benzene (1:1) followed by extraction of the organic layer with 0.2 N-HCl and neutralization. Theoretically the released 5HT should have passed into the

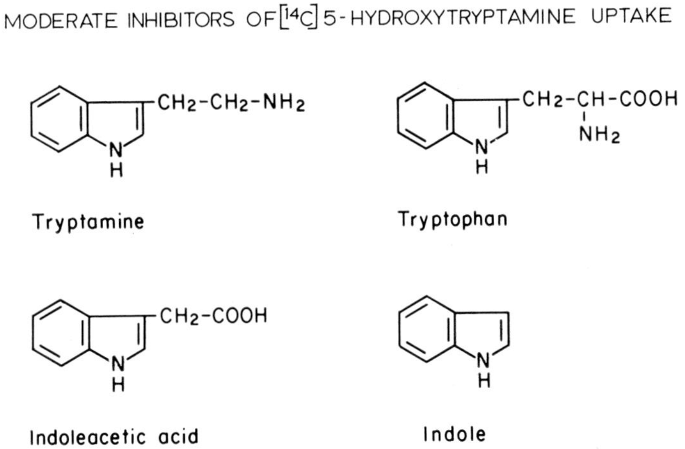

MODERATE INHIBITORS OF [^{14}C] 5-HYDROXYTRYPTAMINE UPTAKE

Tryptamine

Tryptophan

Indoleacetic acid

Indole

FIG. 4. In contrast to the compounds shown in Fig. 3, analogues of 5-hydroxytryptamine which lack an -OH group at position 5 of the indole ring system produce less than 10% inhibition of its uptake at concentrations of 10^{-3} M.

aqueous phase (Woolley 1958). Under the conditions of our experiments only 32% of the radioactivity was extracted into butanol-benzene and only 39% of this could be repartitioned into HCl. After neutralization the radioactive material in the HCl was evaporated to dryness and PRP was added. Whereas the PRP took up 69% of the counts in the 5HT control (which was carried through the procedure in the absence of ganglioside extract), only 4% of the counts in the test samples were taken up in PRP. Thus an insignificant amount of the bound radioactivity was extractable as free 5HT by this procedure. (d) The incubated extract was treated with ethyl acetate (pH 10) or ethyl ether (pH 1) in an effort to release the bound 5HT (Bartholini & Pletscher 1964). In neither of the latter procedures was the release of bound 5HT identifiable. (e) Pre- and post-incubation mixtures were examined by high voltage electrophoresis. The solvent system was pyridine:acetic acid:water (10:100:890). At 4500 volts (130 mA) complete separation of 5HT from 5-hydroxyindole acetic acid and 5-hydroxytryptophol could be obtained within 15 minutes. It was concluded from these experiments that free [^{14}C]5HT was clearly detectable until it became bound to the crude ganglioside extract. Concomitant with binding was the inability to remove and identify the bound radioactivity as 5HT or one of its metabolic breakdown products. In all of the time course experiments free 5HT decreased as the bound radioactivity increased.

It was not possible to detect reversibility by a variety of techniques. For example, after uptake had taken place in the equilibrium dialysis system, 800

nmoles of cold 5HT were added to the chambers. There was no change in the
amount of bound radioactivity under these circumstances. Bound radioactivity
was also unchanged after 10 changes of buffer in the opposing chamber. The
following chemical agents failed to induce reversal: reserpine, sodium chloride
(1 M) and guanidine hydrochloride (1 M).

INFLUENCE OF ANTIOXIDANTS ON UPTAKE OF [^{14}C]5HT

Since the 5-hydroxy group appeared to be involved in the uptake mechanism,
the influence of antioxidants and anaerobic conditions on the binding of
[^{14}C]5HT was evaluated. The antioxidants studied were sodium metabisulphite,
dithiothreitol, ascorbic acid and propyl gallate, all of which were added to the
crude ganglioside extract before incubation with [^{14}C]5HT in the equilibrium
dialysis system. In the presence of antioxidants (0.002-0.003 M final concentration) uptake of radioactivity by the platelet extract was reduced from a
control value of 73 % to an average of 30 %.

The platelet ganglioside extracts were examined for the presence of lipid
peroxidation (Marcus *et al.* 1962) since they contained a considerable amount
of phospholipid—especially phosphatidylserine and phosphatidylinositol. Lipid
peroxides were detectable and on this basis a crude ganglioside extract was
prepared under anaerobic conditions in the presence of the antioxidant butylated
hydroxytoluene (BHT), which in itself had no effect on the uptake of 5HT by
the ganglioside extract. When tested in the PRP assay system the anaerobically
prepared ganglioside extract took up 13.1 % of the labelled 5HT as compared
to the control value of 92.5 % for extracts prepared under aerobic conditions.
In contrast the anaerobically prepared extract displayed the same uptake
properties as the aerobic controls in the equilibrium dialysis assay. It is
possible that lipid peroxidation took place in the course of the dialysis procedure.
Comparable control experiments carried out with cultured lymphocyte extracts
demonstrated the same differences between the two assay systems. These
experiments have led to the tentative conclusion that the uptake of 5HT by the
tissue components we have studied is at least in part related to a peroxidative
change in their constituent phospholipids and that it was primarily an aerobic
process.

DISCUSSION

In recent years the identification and isolation of cell receptors for hormones
and pharmacological agents has received a great deal of attention. The methodological approaches and criteria for evaluation of results in this type of research
have recently been summarized by Cuatrecasas (1974). In most instances a cell

component is exposed to a radioactive ligand and subsequent binding interactions are evaluated by appropriate techniques. The binding should be specific
and the quantification of binding sites should approximate values associated
with the intact cell. In the case of intact platelets, quantitative data can be
obtained on the uptake and transport of 5HT, but studies on the interaction
between 5HT and subcellular platelet particles have so far been difficult to
carry out and interpret. For example, we found that isolated platelet membranes could take up [^{14}C]5HT but the quantity bound did not differ significantly from that bound by boiled membrane controls. Thus the specific
affinity of platelets for 5HT is apparently lost when platelets are disrupted.

Studies on the subcellular localization of a putative 5HT receptor remain a
difficult challenge at present. It is possible that even the most delicate disruption procedures result in damage to or loss of the 5HT receptor mechanism.
Historical precedents already cited stimulated an investigation of gangliosides
as 5HT receptors. It was possible to prepare a crude extract from human
platelets containing three gangliosides, in addition to protein and phospholipid,
which took up 5HT, in contrast to other appropriate controls. Since it is
generally accepted that gangliosides are cell membrane components, some
aspects of the uptake phenomenon were suggestive of a receptor mechanism,
whereas other aspects were not.

Under the experimental conditions used the uptake was irreversible. According to current concepts we should have been able to effect an exchange of
the bound radioactivity with non-radioactive 5HT or by repeated changes of
buffer in the opposite chamber of the equilibrium dialysis cell. In addition,
free radioactive 5HT could not be recovered by procedures which theoretically
disrupt hydrophobic or ionic bonds. Cuatrecasas et al. (1974), in studying the
binding of [^{3}H]noradrenaline to microsomes from liver, heart and adipose
tissue, found that the uptake was essentially irreversible. They suggested that
the binding may not have been related to a receptor mechanism but represented
a 'recognition' process for catechol moieties. It is possible that the platelet
ganglioside extracts we have studied have the property of 'recognizing' hydroxyindole compounds. Van Lenten & Ashwell (1972) have reported that the
binding of radioactive desialylated glycoproteins by plasma membranes from
rat liver was essentially non-dissociable even after the addition of an 80-fold
excess of non-radioactive asialo-orosomucoid. These investigators mentioned,
however, that the dissociation of the bound glycoprotein may be a slow process.
The above studies have been cited in order to point out that irreversible uptake
mechanisms between ligands and cell components are not without precedent.
The apparent irreversibility of uptake made it difficult to ascertain a valid
affinity constant in our experiments.

Some aspects of the uptake of [^{14}C]5HT by the platelet ganglioside extract indicated that the process had biochemical specificity. Preincubation with hydroxyindoles and reserpine appeared to block subsequent uptake of[^{14}C]5HT. This suggested that a finite number of binding sites may have been present in the extract. Reduction of uptake at 0 °C indicated that it was probably not a simple adsorption process. The extract may have contained an enzyme which was involved in the uptake of [^{14}C]5HT (as was postulated for the binding of [^{3}H]noradrenaline by microsomes [Cuatrecasas *et al.* 1974]). If so, the enzyme was insensitive to cyanide, stable at 60 °C for 5 minutes, and inactivated by boiling.

Since antioxidants reduced the uptake of 5HT and anaerobically prepared extracts were less efficient (in the PRP assay) than those prepared under the usual laboratory conditions, an oxidation process may have been involved in the binding of 5HT. The ganglioside extracts were found to contain a large amount of phosphatidylserine, which is rich in unsaturated fatty acids (Marcus *et al.* 1962). The 5HT (as well as the other hydroxyindole derivatives) could have been converted to an undetectable oxidized intermediate which subsequently formed a covalent bond with a component of the ganglioside extract. It can also be speculated that the compounds which inhibited 5HT uptake after prior incubation with the ganglioside extract may have served in part as 'antioxidants' and that unoxidized 5HT would not be taken up. On the other hand, platelet lecithin, which contains unsaturated fatty acids (Marcus *et al.* 1962), did not bind 5HT. In addition, the unpartitioned or undialysed crude ganglioside extract contained unsaturated fatty acids but did not interact with 5HT. Finally, the indole compounds which did not contain a potential oxidizable hydroxyl group blocked uptake of 5HT by the extract at higher concentrations.

ACKNOWLEDGMENTS

This study was supported by grants from the Veterans Administration, the National Institutes of Health (HL09070-11), the New York Heart Association, and the S. M. Louis Memorial Fund for Research in Thrombosis and Atherosclerosis.

References

BARTHOLINI, G. & PLETSCHER, A. (1964) Two types of 5-hydroxytryptamine release from isolated blood platelets. *Experientia* 20, 376-378

BORN, G. V. R., DAY, M. & STOCKBRIDGE, A. (1967) The uptake of amines by human erythrocytes *in vitro. J. Physiol. (Lond.)* 193, 405-418

CUATRECASAS, P. (1973) Gangliosides and membrane receptors for cholera toxin. *Biochemistry* 12, 3558-3566

CUATRECASAS, P. (1974) Membrane receptors. *Annu. Rev. Biochem. 43*, 169-214

CUATRECASAS, P., TELL, G. P. E., SICA, V., PARIKH, I. & CHANG, K. J. (1974) Noradrenaline binding and the search for catecholamine receptors. *Nature (Lond.) 247*, 92-97

DODGE, J. T., MITCHELL, C. & HANAHAN, D. J. (1963) The preparation and chemical characteristics of hemoglobin-free ghosts of human erythrocytes. *Arch. Biochem. Biophys. 100*, 119-130

ETZRODT, H. (1968) Über die Glycolipoide der Thrombozyten und die Funktion eines Thrombozytengangliosides als Serotonin-Rezeptor. Doctoral thesis, University of Köln

FEIGL, F. (1954) *Spot Tests*, vol. 1, *Inorganic Applications*, Elsevier, Amsterdam

FRIDOVICH, I. (1974) Superoxide dismutases. *Adv. Enzymol. 41*, 35-97

KAPELLER-ADLER, R. (1971) in *Analysis of Biogenic Amines and Their Related Enzymes* (Glick, D., ed.), *Methods of Biochemical Analysis*, supplemental vol., pp. 35-87, Wiley, New York

LEDEEN, R. (1966) The chemistry of gangliosides: a review. *J. Am. Oil Chem. Soc. 43*, 57-66

LEHNINGER, A. L. (1968) The neuronal membrane. *Proc. Natl. Acad. Sci. U.S.A. 60*, 1069-1080

MARCHBANKS, R. M. (1966) Serotonin binding to nerve ending particles and other preparations from rat brain. *J. Neurochem. 13*, 1481-1493

MARCUS, A. J., ULLMAN, H. L., SAFIER, L. B. & BALLARD, H. S. (1962) Platelet phosphatides: their fatty acid and aldehyde composition and activity in different clotting systems. *J. Clin. Invest. 41*, 2198-2212

MARCUS, A. J., ULLMAN, H. L. & SAFIER, L. B. (1972) Studies on human platelet gangliosides. *J. Clin. Invest. 51*, 2602-2612

SCHICK, P. K. & YU, B. P. (1973) Methylene blue-induced serotonin release in human platelets. *J. Lab. Clin. Med. 82*, 546-553

SUZUKI, K. (1965) The pattern of mammalian brain gangliosides – II. Evaluation of the extraction procedures, post-mortem changes and the effect of formalin preservation. *J. Neurochem. 12*, 629-638

TETTAMANTI, G., BONALI, F., MARCHESINI, S. & ZAMBOTTI, V. (1973) A new procedure for the extraction, purification and fractionation of brain gangliosides. *Biochim. Biophys. Acta 296*, 160-170

VAN HEYNINGEN, W. E., CARPENTER, C. C. J., PIERCE, N. F. & GREENOUGH, W. B. III (1971) Deactivation of cholera toxin by ganglioside. *J. Infect. Dis. 124*, 415-418

VAN LENTEN, L. & ASHWELL, G. (1972) The binding of desialylated glycoproteins by plasma membranes of rat liver. *J. Biol. Chem. 247*, 4633-4640

WOOLLEY, D. W. (1958) Serotonin receptors. I. Extraction and assay of a substance which renders serotonin fat-soluble. *Proc. Natl. Acad. Sci. U.S.A. 44*, 1202-1210

WOOLLEY, D. W. & GOMMI, B. W. (1965) Serotonin receptors. VII. Activities of various pure gangliosides as the receptors. *Proc. Natl. Acad. Sci. U.S.A. 53*, 959-963

Discussion

Shepro: Would you like to comment on the fact that the gangliosides extracted from various cell types all took up 5-hydroxytryptamine non-specifically, yet *in vivo*, only platelets or endothelial cells apparently take up the amine?

Marcus: It is known that liver cells and neurons are capable of taking up 5HT. Dr Born has shown that erythrocytes take up 5HT by passive diffusion (Born *et al.* 1967).

Born: It depends on what you mean by uptake.

Shepro: When we compared 5HT uptake between freshly harvested endothelial cells or cultured endothelial cells and autologous red cells, we observed that the endothelium removed at least six times more 5HT than the red cells. When imipramine was added to the incubating media the 5HT removed was almost identical to and quantitatively matched the 5HT removed by red cells, with or without imipramine.

Marcus: Oxyhaemoglobin is capable of oxidizing 5HT, so you cannot study that phenomenon using an incubation period of long duration (Blum & Ling 1959).

Born: We had no evidence for that (Born *et al.* 1967).

Shepro: You work with 10 g platelets; what is the smallest quantity with which one could run a similar assay?

Marcus: From 10 g of platelets we obtain about 7 mg of crude ganglioside extract. We calculated from this that 0.5 mg of extract—the quantity that we used in many of our experiments—can be obtained from 3×10^{10} platelets (0.7 g). Under our assay conditions 0.5 mg of extract binds 0.3 nmole 5HT in one hour. If the incubation is performed with increasing concentrations of 5HT, the binding can be increased several hundred-fold. We have also done experiments using 0.05 mg extract.

Feinberg: Can you predict how many molecules of 5HT might bind to a platelet, from the approximate surface area of the platelet and the ganglioside concentration?

Born: Have you done the following calculation? If your material were distributed over the surface of the cells, how many such gangliosides would there be on each platelet?

Marcus: If one makes several assumptions, the distribution of gangliosides on the platelet surface can be roughly calculated. However, it cannot be stated with certainty that gangliosides are the 5HT receptors of platelets. As we have just shown, platelet gangliosides in combination with protein and phospholipid have a greater affinity for 5HT than gangliosides alone. Although the evidence indicates that gangliosides are in some way involved in the uptake and transport of 5HT, we have been unable to obtain definitive proof that they are the 5HT receptor. The difficulties in this research are compounded by the inherent instability of 5HT.

There are approximately 146 mg of protein/10^{11} platelets. The membranes of a platelet homogenate account for about 9% of the total platelet protein. Thus there are about 13.4 mg membrane protein/10^{11} platelets. The lipid/protein ratio of platelet membranes is 0.58 (Marcus *et al.* 1969). There are thus 7.8 mg of membrane lipid/10^{11} platelets. Gangliosides make up approximately 0.5% of the platelet lipid and therefore it can be calculated that there is 0.039 mg of membrane ganglioside/10^{11} platelets. Using the approximate molecular weight of 1251 for hematoside (the major platelet ganglioside), we can obtain a figure of 31 nmoles of membrane ganglioside/10^{11} platelets. Using Avogadro's number, this can be converted to 18.7×10^4 molecules of membrane ganglioside per platelet.

A calculation can also be made on the basis of the fact that there are an average of 8.1 μg N-acetylneuraminic acid (NANA)/mg platelet protein. Multiplying by the figure of 13.4 mg membrane protein/10^{11} platelets we get 108.5 μg membrane NANA/10^{11} platelets. Since 6% of the platelet NANA is in the ganglioside fraction, we get 6.5 μg membrane ganglioside NANA/10^{11} platelets. Using the fraction 6500/309 (mol.wt. NANA), we get 21 nmoles membrane ganglioside NANA/10^{11} platelets, which is roughly equivalent to 12.6×10^4 molecules of membrane ganglioside per platelet.

Finally, calculating from the number of molecules of NANA obtained by surface charge measurements, a figure of 5.3×10^4 can be obtained.

Born: We made the estimate in two ways. First we measured the uptake of 5HT in the cold—that is, by diffusion only (Born & Bricknell 1959). At equilibrium there is a linear relationship between the 5HT concentrations inside and outside the platelets which does not pass through the origin but a small distance up the y axis. If you assume that this represents a high-affinity binding site for 5HT on the platelet surface, you arrive at the order of 10^4 such 5HT receptors per platelet. Then we tried to estimate the number of these receptors also with labelled imipramine, which inhibits the uptake of 5HT by platelets very specifically. Unfortunately the available imipramine did not have a high enough specific activity to give a wholly convincing result, but we did find that the uptake of labelled imipramine had two apparent K_m values; the low K_m step indicated the same order of imipramine uptake as we had found earlier with 5HT. This is interesting also in relation to Professor Pletscher's assertion that imipramine enters the platelets; that is consistent with our observation of imipramine uptake with two K_m steps.

Marcus: This brings up another problem in trying to characterize a 5HT receptor. It is possible that with the labelled 5HT we now have available, the specific activity may not be high enough to test for a small number of very high-affinity binding sites. We need a 5HT preparation with extremely high specific activity so that it can be used in a very low concentration and still be 'recognized' by a high-affinity binding site.

Pletscher: I enjoyed your paper very much, Dr Marcus; I also agree with your cautious conclusions. I doubt whether we should speak of receptors, however, because I don't think that a receptor will irreversibly bind the substance with which it reacts, otherwise we should be dead before we were born!

On the other hand, a good piece of evidence that you might be dealing with something like a receptor is your reserpine experiment, because reserpine selectively interferes with 5HT uptake. However, there are drawbacks to this. For instance, there is evidence that reserpine acts on the membrane of the organelles, but we did not find lysolecithin in this membrane.

Marcus: Lysolecithin accounts for about 13% of the lipid phosphorus in the extract. Remember that we were working with the aqueous phase of an extract prepared from whole platelets which has been partitioned with water. The high lysolecithin concentration is probably due to the fact that lysolecithin is soluble in water.

Pletscher: So it cannot come from the granular membrane. Of course, one can always argue that lysolecithin is formed during the process of uptake or release. But the other thing is your reserpine concentration; this was about 10^{-3} or 10^{-4}M, which is very high. Reserpine acts in much lower concentrations (10^{-6}–10^{-8}M). Do you see an effect in these conditions?

Marcus: The lowest concentration of reserpine which inhibited the binding of [^{14}C]5HT by the crude ganglioside extract was 1×10^{-5}M. In our experiments with whole platelets, 5×10^{-7}M-reserpine was the lowest concentration which inhibited the uptake of 5HT by platelets.

Pletscher: Another question: what are the fluorescence properties of 5HT in your bound material? Does it still have the same characteristics regarding the activation and fluorescence spectra?

Marcus: We have not yet done fluorescence studies with the extract.

Smith: There is a similarity between these studies and some work that Dr Born and I did several years ago (Born & Smith 1970). We found that radioactive adrenaline was taken up very slowly by human platelets, and that about half of the radioactivity in the platelets was present as a conjugate from which adrenaline was released by acid hydrolysis. The remainder of the radioactivity was intact adrenaline which was present in the granules, as it was released by thrombin. If one blocked transport into the granules with reserpine then all of the adrenaline taken up was conjugated. On the other hand, pyrogallol reduced the amount of adrenaline that was conjugated, but caused more adrenaline to enter the granules. I wonder if what Dr Marcus has described might be a carrier between the platelet membrane and the granule.

Marcus: We can say that the uptake we have studied favours the hydroxyindole configuration. It very well could represent a carrier in the cytoplasm, except that gangliosides are mainly found in membranes.

Michal: Dr Marcus has been concentrating on the 'outer' membrane; could not at least some of the material come from other compartments in the platelet?

Marcus: The extract we studied was prepared from whole platelets.

Born: Professor Pletscher showed clearly some time ago that reserpine inhibits the uptake of 5HT into the storage granules. When platelets take up 5HT in the presence of reserpine, 5HT breakdown products accumulate in the cytoplasm from which they diffuse into the medium.

Mills: We have a similar situation in platelets from patients with the storage defect. They take up 5HT in the normal way but they then rapidly lose it; radioactive 5-hydroxytryptophol and 5-hydroxyindole acetic acid appear in the plasma (Pareti *et al.* 1974).

Sneddon: The action of reserpine on the granule membrane raises the further question of what we mean either by the receptor (for example, that mediating 5HT-induced aggregation) or by the transport carrier. Most pharmacologists would agree that these two properties reside in the plasma membrane and would not be inhibited by reserpine.

Born: Exactly; reserpine does not interfere with the membrane transport of 5HT. The evidence indicates that. Whether the primary receptor site for 5HT, which is merely shorthand for the unknown chemical constituent to which it binds, is separate from the carrier that one has to postulate to explain the properties of the movement of 5HT through the membrane or whether they are one and the same molecule or molecular complex is one of the questions the answers to which are being sought in several systems, including neurons as well as platelets. I expect that the answer will come with techniques of specific affinity labelling, similar to those now being applied to the isolation and characterization of membrane receptors for other biologically active molecules such as acetylcholine or morphine. This is a complex undertaking requiring the synthesis of analogues which can become covalently bound to the receptor(s). There still remains the problem of proving specificity of binding; that is, the new analogue may bind (with similar affinities) to several sites only one of which is the receptor the activation of which initiates the biological effect. In the experiments I described (pp. 287–298) we have much to do before we shall know to what acceptor molecules the labelled NANA has become attached, and how the attachment affects them, conformationally or otherwise.

Marcus: In our hands, isolated platelet membranes do not aggregate on the addition of ADP. They do not bind more 5HT than a boiled membrane control. We have examined many platelet fractions, but the one I have just described is the only one which binds 5HT. Thus, we decided to study it in detail. Uptake of 5HT by the extract is reduced in the presence of antioxidants. If the extract is prepared under nitrogen, uptake is also reduced. This aspect of the phenomenon is reminiscent of the oxygen requirement for the formation of endoperoxide intermediates in the synthesis of prostaglandins in platelets, as already alluded to by Dr Smith in his paper (pp. 207–218).

Born: It seems to me that the demonstration of 5HT binding to a molecule under your conditions is very different from what probably happens in the living cell, where the duration of the molecular complex formed between 5HT and its receptor may well be, as I said, as short as 10^{-8} second. That is our problem.

Marcus: This is why platelet fractions are difficult to study under laboratory conditions! The 5HT uptake mechanism is lost when the platelet is fractionated. Binding by platelet fragments can only be considered as a model.

Lüscher: I would like to come back to the situation encountered when thrombin reacts with platelets. Much more thrombin combines with an inactive 'high-affinity' site than with the receptor which is responsible for triggering platelet activity (cf. Phillips 1974). Any attempt at characterizing a thrombin receptor which is based on the formation of a stable enzyme–receptor complex will invariably lead to the one which is not of direct significance for thrombin activity towards platelets. Of course, the 'high-affinity' receptor is nevertheless interesting, because it has the properties of an anti-thrombin which protects the platelet from being stimulated into activity by trace amounts of thrombin. All such combining sites are of interest; however, it is questionable whether they are of equal importance when the functional aspects are considered.

Born: That is exactly right. There are similar instances from straight pharmacology, where there are so-called silent receptors and non-specific receptors and all kinds of different binding sites for active amines.

References

BLUM, J. J. & LING, N.-S. (1959) Oxidation of serotonin and 5-hydroxyindoles during the denaturation of oxyhaemoglobin. *Biochem. J. 73*, 530-535

BORN, G. V. R. & BRICKNELL, J. (1959) The uptake of 5-hydroxytryptamine by blood platelets in the cold. *J. Physiol. (Lond.) 147*, 153-161

BORN, G. V. R. & SMITH, J. B. (1970) Uptake, metabolism and release of ^{3}H-adrenaline by human blood platelets. *Br. J. Pharmacol. 39*, 765-778

BORN, G. V. R., DAY, M. & STOCKBRIDGE, A. (1967) The uptake of amines by human erythrocytes *in vitro. J. Physiol. (Lond.) 193*, 405-418

MARCUS, A. J., ULLMAN, H. L. & SAFIER, L. B. (1969) Lipid composition of subcellular particles of human blood platelets. *J. Lipid Res. 10*, 108-114

PARETI, F. I., MILLS, D. C. B. & DAY, H. J. (1974) Nucleotide and serotonin metabolism in platelets with defective secondary aggregation. *Blood 44*, 789-800

PHILLIPS, D. R. (1974) Thrombin interaction with human platelets. Potentiation of thrombin-induced aggregation and release by inactivated thrombin. *Thromb. Diath. Haemorrh. 32*, 207-215

General discussion

Detwiler: The nomenclature of the release reaction is more than a question of semantics. Dr Holmsen, when you talk about release I and II, do you consider them as distinct phenomena and, if so, how do they differ?

Holmsen: They are both secretory mechanisms, but they can be clearly distinguished, as I tried to point out in my paper. They differ in: (1) time course, (2) inhibition pattern with aspirin, (3) requirement for metabolic ATP, and (4) dose–response patterns. Most important, the substances released during release I are stored in the dense granules while those released during release II are stored in the α-granules.

Detwiler: To my mind, the term 'secretion' is probably better than the word 'release' for these phenomena, because the term 'release' implies the wrong thing to a lot of people; it implies something passively leaking out.

Holmsen: According to Kirshner & Viveros (1972), secretion includes three steps or phases: induction, exocytosis, and recovery. The recovery step involves the filling up of the granules with the material that is to be secreted. Do platelets recover?

Mustard: They partly recover.

Holmsen: Perhaps it would be more descriptive to talk about dense granule secretion and α-granule secretion instead of release I and II!

Mustard: Dr Detwiler has a point. If we use the word 'secretion' it relates to a principle of cell biology and may avoid our complicating definitions.

Holmsen: This is all fine, but there is one important difference between platelets and 'normal' secretory cells: the circulating platelet does not *synthesize* and envelope into granules the substances that are to be 'secreted' or released. Platelets do, however, take up 5-hydroxytryptamine and store it in the dense granules, and they apparently are able to translocate adenine nucleotides slowly between cytoplasm and granules. But whether they can fill up empty granule bags after release, I really doubt.

ACTIVATION OF PLATELETS

Cohen: Platelets contain a contractile regulatory mechanism, and its physiological significance is that platelets may be able to relax. We may therefore imagine that *in vivo* when platelets are faced with a sub-threshold concentration of thrombin causing shape change and primary aggregation but not release, they subsequently relax, and aggregation and shape change become reversible. So far I agree with Dr Mustard; and in that case, platelets are not to be considered as disposable elements. In this specific case they can be used again for haemostatic purposes. On the other hand, if platelets are exposed to above-threshold concentrations of thrombin, release and platelet membrane damage occur, and the cells show irreversible features. We have illustrated this in an experiment using an isometric contractile system (Cohen & de Vries 1973).

We generate a platelet-rich plasma clot with thrombin (in the absence of EGTA) in a cylindrical tube. The clot is removed from the tube, put in Tyrode's solution and tied at both ends with a cotton thread. One extremity is tied to a rigid glass support, and the other tied to a force-displacement transducer. The whole system is immersed in a water bath at 37 °C. The advantage of this system is that we can change the composition of the incubation medium during the generation of force. Tension is developed under isometric conditions, since the clot is not allowed to shorten. The force generated is proportional to the cross-sectional area of the clot but is independent of its length. When a contracting clot had developed half its maximal tension, it could be relaxed by lowering the free Ca^{2+} concentration (by the use of an EGTA–calcium buffer) to 10^{-8}M. If we increase the Ca^{2+} concentration to 10^{-7}M, the clot continues to relax. Only at a Ca^{2+} concentration of 10^{-6}M is force generated again, similarly to the situation in muscle. Cycles of contraction and relaxation could be induced several times in the same clot by varying the Ca^{2+} concentration. Dr Detwiler asked earlier (p. 116) whether contractile proteins have any function whatsoever in platelets. The fact that platelets respond, by contracting or relaxing, to the same stimulus as muscle, constitutes a strong argument in favour of a function for the contractile system in platelets. Platelets in this case may be considered haemostatically normal.

On the other hand, when tension is generated in a platelet-rich clot, without any disturbance, it rises to a maximal value of about 2 g cm^{-2} (initial cross-sectional area) after 15 minutes. After a tension plateau had been maintained for about five minutes, the clot relaxed spontaneously and irreversibly, probably as a result of slackening of tension due to membrane damage. The clot remains insensitive to Ca^{2+} concentration after maximal tension is attained. Platelets in this case may have undergone far-reaching membrane alterations involving degranulation and cannot be considered haemostatically normal.

The question really is whether the release reaction is useless and harmless to platelets. This does not seem to be the case. In fact, the 'empty' platelets of storage pool disease are known to be haemostatically deficient (Holmsen & Weiss 1972).

Mustard: I would not disagree that the platelets have lost their granule contents. However, these platelets, as I have tried to emphasize, are not irreversibly aggregated or irreversibly damaged. The use of the term 'irreversible platelet aggregation' to describe the results of *in vitro* studies can lead to a misunderstanding of platelet function that is restrictive and hampers our understanding of thrombosis.

We know very little of the mechanisms in thrombosis that cause clinical complications in arterial disease. However, it has been fairly clearly demonstrated that mural thrombi form in the diseased bifurcation of the carotid artery and fragment. The emboli shower the microcirculation in the eye and the brain, causing transient attacks of blindness, weakness or paralysis (Gunning *et al.* 1964; Russell 1961). There is evidence that some forms of chronic renal disease in adults, and high blood pressure, may be caused by mural thrombi in the aorta above the renal artery showering the kidney with emboli (Moore & Mersereau 1968). Whether the process occurs in the coronary arteries and is associated with myocardial ischaemia and sudden death is more controversial (Mustard *et al.* 1974). When microemboli shower the microcirculation in the myocardium of pigs and dogs, arrhythmia and death can occur. Studies of thrombus formation in the microcirculation indicate that masses of platelets form at a site of vessel injury and then break up and a new mass forms. It seems reasonable to expect that the platelets in the emboli disperse when the fragments break up and that, unless these platelets are irreversibly damaged, they return to the circulation. I think there is good evidence that the platelets in these thrombi are not irreversibly damaged. They will have been exposed to ADP, thrombin, polymerizing fibrin and other stimuli and yet they do not appear to form irreversible aggregates. I find the use of the concept of irreversible platelet aggregation unsuitable in any attempt to understand the clinical manifestations of thrombosis.

It is certainly possible to demonstrate in animals that thrombin-induced platelet aggregates with fibrin around them can break up and the platelets can return to the circulation. In experiments with pigs we found that the infusion of thrombin induced thrombocytopenia with the formation of platelet aggregates in the microcirculation, and that there was fibrin around these platelet aggregates. After one to two hours the platelet count returned to normal. When the platelets had been labelled with diisopropyl fluoro[^{32}P]phosphate and ^{35}S, the same platelets that were present in the circulation before the thrombin infusion were observed to return to the circulation. Furthermore, the platelets that returned to the circulation survived normally (Mustard *et al.* 1966). In these experiments the fibrin presumably was lysed by activation of the fibrinolytic mechanism by the endothelial cells of the small vessels in which the platelet–fibrin masses formed. When the fibrin lysed, the platelets could rapidly deaggregate and return to the circulation. As I indicated earlier (p. 96), the degranulation of platelets by thrombin does not irreversibly damage them. They show a normal response to ADP and circulate normally in an animal when reinfused.

A further problem in the study of platelets and thrombosis is that the only test of platelet function which seems to bear some relationship to arterial disease and its complications is platelet survival (Mustard *et al.* 1974). So far, no-one has been able to demonstrate that tests of the effects of aggregating stimuli can be related to changes in platelet survival. Drugs which restore platelet survival to normal are used in concentrations which do not affect the response of the platelets to aggregating agents. The interaction of platelets with stimuli such as thrombin or ADP does not appear to influence platelet survival. If these aggregating agents caused irreversible aggregation one would expect them to shorten platelet survival. The answer to the question 'What influences platelet survival?' may be very important in understanding the role of platelets in arterial thrombosis. However, the answer is not be found in a concept of irreversible platelet aggregation developed from *in vitro* studies.

Born: I agree with you. Dr Skaer described the growth of haemostatic plugs *in vivo* (p. 250), asked how it occurred, and suggested that it was not exponential. Dr Nicola Begent and I caused thrombi of platelets to grow on the walls of little venules by applying ADP microiontophoretically to the outside of the vessels (Begent & Born 1970). These platelet thrombi did grow exponentially; this fact has given rise to much thinking about the mechanism of thrombus growth *in vivo*. It is more difficult to determine the growth rate of haemostatic plugs. Recently, however, it has been shown that platelet thrombi forming in vessels damaged by a laser beam also grow exponentially (Afors *et al.* 1975).

Lüscher: I would like to comment on the significance of the phenomenon called 'irreversible aggregation' or, perhaps better, 'second-phase aggregation'. It is an interesting question whether release is the trigger mechanism for second-phase aggregation, or whether it is the other way round. I feel strongly that it *is* the other way round, because release is the consequence of membrane fusion, and this in turn is the result of far-reaching alterations in the membrane structure. It seems reasonable to assume that such an altered membrane lends itself to second-phase aggregation.

Mills: There is a situation in which one can demonstrate classical second-phase aggregation in the aggregometer with no release; this is during aggregation by factor VIII. How it does it I don't know, but in the presence of inhibitors of the release reaction, the second wave occurs normally, with no release. I am sure Dr Lüscher is right and there are other processes going on, therefore, not directly related to feedback from released substances.

Smith: When Dr Mustard and I were discussing membrane contact and prostaglandin formation earlier (p. 221) we should, of course, have acknowledged the suggestion by Massini & Lüscher (1971, 1972) that contact is a stimulus for the release reaction. So contact may be the stimulus for both release and prostaglandin formation.

Holmsen: We have recently shown (unpublished) that the calcium ionophore A23187 gives a biphasic aggregation in which the second phase is not attributed to release of ADP. The ionophore induces complete release of ADP within 2–3 seconds after its addition to platelet-rich plasma, but a biphasic aggregation response is seen, with the secondary aggregation displayed about $1\frac{1}{2}$ minutes after the addition of ionophore.

Born: The second phase—the second, fast increase in light transmission—is due mainly to an increase in tight packing of the platelets in the aggregates (Born & Hume 1967).

Mustard: Can anybody consistently demonstrate two waves of aggregation in a system that does not contain citrate?

Mills: Yes; with adrenaline (Macfarlane & Mills 1965).

Mustard: What is the first light transmission change with adrenaline? Have you looked at it morphologically?

Mills: It looks like loose end-to-end aggregates of discoid platelets.

Mustard: Is there anything else which will do it in a non-citrate system? To study platelets in citrated plasma may be a useful method for answering some questions, but what is the biological relevance of the second wave of aggregation that is induced by ADP in citrated platelet-rich plasma?

Mills: Most of the *in vitro* investigations of platelet pharmacology and biochemistry have been done in citrated plasma, and citrate, as Dr Mustard has shown, has distinct effects that are responsible for biphasic aggregation with ADP. I am not saying that this phenomenon is not reproducible or interesting, but there is no doubt that it is an artifact.

Detwiler: Two points to Dr Cohen: first, I didn't, of course, intend to imply that the contractile proteins have no function! Secondly, is it implicit in your experiment that the intracellular ionized calcium is at the same concentration as the extracellular ionized calcium? If so, that would be very surprising.

Cohen: Once platelets are treated with thrombin, they behave like glycerinated or skinned muscle fibres. They become, unlike intact muscle, permeable to EGTA and Ca^{2+}, and probably identical concentrations of Ca^{2+} outside and in the cytoplasmic compartment are attained.

Detwiler: I am not convinced that thrombin does do this, but even if it did, that does not say that the concentration of ionized calcium is what you put outside, because in the platelet you have a very large number of calcium-binding sites.

Cohen: I use a high concentration of EGTA, about 10 mM, in my buffer system, which I presume is enough to chelate the usual amount of calcium present in the cytoplasmic compartment.

Born: It occurs to me that, depending on how platelets act in a clot, how they pull it together, and how the platelets are attached to the fibrin fibres, another possible explanation is that calcium is needed for attachment of the platelet spikes to the fibrin. Then the difference in concentration that you introduce may increase that interaction in some way. Pictures of clotted plasma show platelets at separate points in the fibrin network without, apparently, even their longest projections touching each other. However, nothing much is known about this.

Mustard: Niewiarowski studied polymerizing fibrin (Niewiarowski *et al.* 1972*a*, *b*); some of the experiments were done with EDTA and EGTA and the results indicated that pig and rabbit platelets will not bind to polymerizing fibrin in the absence of calcium. Your point is significant, because once fibrin is fully polymerized it is difficult to demonstrate platelet adherence to it, whereas while the fibrin is polymerizing, platelets adhere to the fibrin. If this binding is disturbed in any way, it would have a major effect on platelet retraction of fibrin.

Feinberg: Does anyone consider that actin and myosin in the resting platelet are in continuous interaction and that inhibition of that interaction is the basis of the platelet shape change? This concept has been suggested earlier; Dr Holmsen's paper seems to be a variant and it is consistent with Dr Detwiler's comment that he knew of no convincing evidence for *activation* processes.

Adelstein: Two major problems facing investigators working on contractile proteins in non-muscle cells such as platelets are: (*a*) where are these proteins located in the cell? (*b*) what is their function? In regard to their location, there is a consensus by a number of workers that actin may be attached to the inside of the cell membrane, and recent work by Burridge & Phillips (1975) suggests that it may also be attached to the secretory granules of the adrenal medulla. The location of myosin in non-muscle cells has been more elusive. Although a number of authors claim to have produced antibodies to non-muscle myosin which they have used to locate myosin, only Willingham *et al.* (1974) have been rigorous in doing the necessary controls. Their work shows that in mouse fibroblasts, some of the myosin appears to be attached to the outside surface of the cell membrane (see p. 104). Most of the myosin, which was not visualized in this study, is located inside the cells, but just where is not clear.

Numerous roles have been postulated for actin and myosin in non-muscle cells: (1) secretion, (2) cell division, (3) cell motility, and (4) specialized functions such as clot retraction in platelets and phagocytosis in polymorphonuclear leucocytes. So far, though, there is only circumstantial evidence that actin and myosin are responsible for these processes. Puszkin & Kochwa (1974) presented evidence that actin and myosin in the brain play a role in neurotransmitter release and Schroeder (1973) showed that actin filaments are present in the contractile ring of a dividing HeLa cell. Polymorphonuclear leucocytes isolated from a patient suffering multiple infections were found by Boxer *et al.* (1974) to migrate abnormally and ingest particles at a slower rate than controls. The authors isolated actin from these cells and found that it was defective in its ability to polymerize.

All these studies, as mentioned above, suggest, but do not prove, that actin and myosin are involved in these cell processes. They do point to the possibility, though, that cytoplasmic actin and myosin may be involved in different processes, under various circumstances, in any one cell.

What experiments are needed to firmly establish the role of actin and myosin in non-muscle cells? I would summarize some of these as follows: (1) Complete characterization of the various contractile proteins thought to be involved in cell motility. Troponin, kinases and possible co-factors would be high on the list. (2) The *in situ* identification of the various proteins by using antibodies made to highly purified proteins and shown to be specific for these proteins by a number of criteria. (3) Identification of a specific inhibitor of actin–myosin interaction which can be used *in vivo* as well as *in vitro*. The cytochalasins do not at present fit this requirement. (4) The use of cells with defects in motility, secretion, etc. to look for abnormalities in the various contractile proteins. The list of course is incomplete, but one hopes that progress in these areas will aid in understanding the role of actin and myosin in platelets.

Cohen: On Dr Feinberg's question of whether one sees cross-linking between actin and myosin in platelets, as in muscle, and bearing in mind Dr Adelstein's remarks about the localization of the contractile elements, one sees actin filaments in platelets, especially after activation, but one cannot really see any myosin filaments. Noteworthy are Pollard's findings (1975) on the peculiar assembly properties of platelet myosin molecules. These aggregate in physiological conditions into 'small' thick filaments. Whereas in skeletal muscle myosin, the thick filaments measure 1500 nm by 30 nm, in the same conditions platelet myosin aggregates into filaments only 300 nm long and 10 nm wide. When these filaments are dehydrated during preparation for electron microscopy, the platelet 'thick' myosin filaments show a width of about 8–9 nm, being very similar to the 6–8 nm of actin thin filaments. Dr Pollard interprets this as meaning that the thick filaments in platelets look like thin filaments and this may be why you cannot see thick filaments.

Adelstein: Returning to your experiments, Dr Cohen, didn't Niewiarowski replace platelets with fibroblasts and produce clot retraction?

Cohen: Yes.

Born: The geometry of what happens there is easily understood.

Cohen: The amazing thing is that fibroblasts respond to exactly the same stimuli as platelets do.

Mustard: They also have nucleosidediphosphate kinase on their surface membrane!

Haslam: I would like to return to the question of what, if anything, can be deduced from the effects of cytochalasin B on platelet function. There has been a tendency in the literature to assume that every action of cytochalasin B can be interpreted in terms of effects on microfilaments or more generally on contractile mechanisms. It has been claimed that cytochalasin B interacts directly with *actin* filaments, at least in the absence of tropomyosin (Spudich 1972). On the other hand, Puszkin *et al.* (1973) have reported that cytochalasin D, which hypothetically acts by the same mechanism, competes with actin for binding sites on platelet *myosin*. So there are suggestions of at least two interactions with the contractile protein system. Moreover, cytochalasin B has also been shown to be a potent inhibitor of the membrane transport of glucose and nucleosides in many cell types. In some preliminary experiments, I have observed these effects with blood platelets. Therefore, naturally, one wonders if it is possible to explain these widely different effects by a single mechanism. In this connection, Spooner (1973) has suggested that cytochalasin B may not so much affect actomyosin within the cytoplasmic compartment as interfere with the attachment of actin filaments to the membrane by binding to specific membrane sites, and that it may also inhibit membrane transport processes at these same sites. Even if the membrane binding sites turn out to be on a component of the contractile protein system, there may often be some ambiguity as to whether a particular functional effect is due to an action on contractile protein *per se* or on, for example, glucose transport.

Born: I fully agree with you. Dr E. Cunliffe in my department is engaged in fascinating work on why antibiotic-producing organisms do not commit suicide. Cytochalasins are produced by moulds; why are they not killed by these products which are so toxic to other organisms? Presumably such potentially self-destructive agents are synthesized, stored and released in ways which prevent their coming in contact with metabolically essential cell constituents with which they could react, rather as hydrolytic enzymes are kept *incommunicado* in normal cells.

Haslam: I don't know; but in answering a question like that one might find out how cytochalasin B works.

Born: Of course, in this symposium we have not even touched on the questions that arise about trying to apply our *in vitro* knowledge about platelet function to conditions *in vivo*. For example, there is a whole set of questions about the influence of the vessels; their geometry; the bloodflow; the distribution within it of platelets, and the influence of other cells on them. About all of these we know practically nothing. Several years ago, Dr Mustard and his co-workers began to provide information on this in experiments with extra-corporeal flow chambers (Murphy *et al.* 1962); and more recently we have started to investigate the kinetics of platelet thrombogenesis in living vessels (Begent & Born 1970). But there is a long way to go before we understand these processes and the relevance of most of the *in vitro* observations to thrombus formation is very uncertain still.

OXIDATIVE PHOSPHORYLATION

Holmsen: Dr Detwiler claimed that the yield of ATP from the oxidation of glucose in mitochondria is very small. Professor Mustard says that when he tries to restore aggregating activity in substrate-depleted rabbit platelets by adding glucose, the recovery is markedly reduced when antimycin is present. We have done some experiments on the effect of antimycin and deoxyglucose on platelet adenine nucleotides in platelets isolated by different means. When antimycin and deoxyglucose are added to platelets, isolated by all methods, the ATP level drops and hypoxanthine accumulates. When antimycin is added alone to platelet-rich plasma (PRP) in amounts that completely inhibit electron transport, nothing happens; the ATP levels remain constant for hours. When antimycin (alone) was added to platelets, washed with EDTA-containing saline without glucose but suspended in this saline *with* glucose, there was a very fast drop in the ATP level followed by a transient formation of IMP and accumulation of hypoxanthine. To me this indicates that in these washed platelets, the mitochondrial contribution of ATP is of great importance, and glycolysis does not readily compensate for the ATP production from mitochondria that was suddenly switched off. In platelet-rich plasma glycolysis does compensate right away, and the difference between platelet-rich plasma and the washed platelet must reside in the treatment induced by the washing procedure.

Mills: Can I interpret your point, Dr Holmsen, as being a question of what this procedure does to platelets that is deleterious? Has anybody any information on what EDTA does to platelets?

Schneider: To investigate this point, we incubated platelets isolated from blood of the same donor containing increasing amounts of EDTA and resuspended them to the same platelet count in the same synthetic medium. During an incubation period of one hour at 37 °C oxygen consumption was measured manometrically and at the end of the incubation period the ATP content of the platelets as well as their lactate and pyruvate production was estimated in the perchloric acid extracts. Increasing the amounts of EDTA in the blood from the donor results in a highly significant decrease of oxygen consumption in spite of the fact that all platelets are immediately resuspended in the same synthetic medium. The decrease in oxygen consumption is followed by a significant decrease in ATP content of the platelets, whereas lactate and pyruvate production as an indicator of the glycolytic flow rate are less severely affected (Fig. 1, p. 337).

In spite of the significant decrease in oxygen consumption there was no increase in lactate production, as an indication of a Pasteur effect, so one can say that only a short period of 20–30 minutes of preincubation with higher amounts of EDTA results in a significant inhibition of oxygen metabolism and in a lesser inhibition of glycolysis.

May I come back to the question of citrate-induced artifacts? White (1974) has recently described how platelets do not transform to spheres if they are incubated in citrate before EDTA is added, and in spite of EDTA they maintain their disk shape. Dr E. Morgenstern in Homburg has recently confirmed this. Has anybody an explanation for the fact that citrate is able to prevent the shape changes induced by EDTA?

Born: I have none. When we made optical measurements on the shape change of platelets in human citrated plasma and added EDTA to prevent aggregation, after the rapid initial effect of ADP or 5HT there was a slow but continuing increase in optical density, as if the cells were changing in some progressive way (Born 1970).

Feinberg: If EGTA or EDTA operate as a calcium 'sink' and platelets lose calcium from their surface or from the platelet interior, shape change might

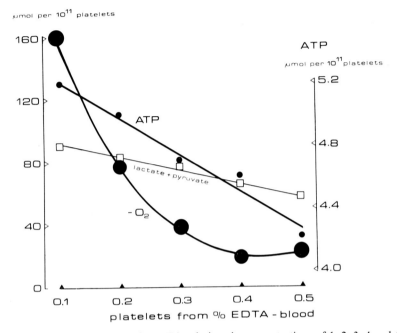

μmol per 10^{11} platelets

FIG. 1 (Schneider). Isotonic EDTA solutions in concentrations of 1, 2, 3, 4 and 5% (pH = 7.4) were mixed (1 + 9) with human blood from the same donor. The blood was immediately centrifuged, and the platelets were isolated from platelet-rich plasma and resuspended in the same synthetic medium containing sodium, potassium, and magnesium but no calcium at a final concentration of 10^9 platelets per ml. Oxygen consumption was measured manometrically, and lactate and pyruvate production as well as ATP content were estimated in the perchloric acid extract after 1 hour of incubation at 37 °C. The decrease in oxygen consumption and the lack of a Pasteur effect demonstrate that glycolysis as well as oxygen metabolism must be affected by short preincubation with increasing amounts of EDTA, resulting in a decrease in ATP content.

be explained by the loss of calcium needed for activation of reactions associated with the maintenance of the disk shape.

Adelstein: EDTA is much more effective in chelating Mg^{2+}.

Feinberg: Does EGTA induce the same shape change as does EDTA?

Mustard: No. If suspensions of washed human or rabbit platelets are incubated with EDTA or EGTA at equimolar concentrations at 37 °C the EDTA–platelets will lose their shape over a period of 2–3 hours, but the EGTA–platelets will not. The suspending medium contains apyrase which will degrade any ADP that accumulates in the suspending fluid. This is necessary if the platelets are not to become refractory to ADP. Apyrase is active in the presence of EGTA (if the concentration is not excessive) but will not act in the presence of EDTA because the enzyme needs either calcium or magnesium. If the EDTA-treated platelets are resuspended in a fresh medium without EDTA, their disk shape will return. I think the loss of shape in the presence of EDTA at 37 °C is due to the accumulation of traces of ADP in the suspending fluid which the apyrase cannot break down.

Mills: Ardlie & Han (1974) have recently claimed an obligatory role for thrombin generation on the platelet surface for the aggregating action of such agents as ADP, but I think this is wrong, as Mustard *et al.* (1975) and we (Macfarlane *et al.* 1975) have demonstrated aggregation and release in citrated platelet-rich plasma with heparin or hirudin added to block the effects of thrombin. Ardlie also claims that EDTA treatment reduces the amounts of various clotting factors that are retained on the surface of the platelets during washing procedures. Using Walsh's method of spinning platelets into an albumin density gradient, we have tested this theory and do not find any evidence to confirm it (Macfarlane *et al.* 1975).

Mustard: With respect to the citrate effect, we had for years been concerned about why we could not induce a suspension of washed human platelets to undergo a secondary wave of aggregation and release when the platelets were stimulated with ADP. We tested almost every plasma protein but none of them, when added in its natural state to the suspending fluid, would restore the platelets' sensitivity to secondary aggregation. We were doing unrelated experiments examining the effect of magnesium and calcium on the release reaction in suspensions of washed human platelets when we found that if ADP were added to platelets in a medium containing magnesium but no added calcium, they went through a primary wave and a secondary wave of aggregation. It became apparent that the plasma factor was probably citrate. If we used a suspension of washed human platelets containing calcium and magnesium and added citrate, the addition of ADP would now induce the secondary wave of platelet aggregation and the release reaction (Mustard *et al.* 1975).

Mills: We have known for a long time that you do not see the secondary phase if you use heparinized plasma; however, I have found release of 5HT induced by ADP in heparinized plasma on some occasions—it is an irregular phenomenon. This leads to an appraisal of the action of aspirin, because its primary and most obvious effect *in vitro* is the correction of the citrate artifact; that is, abolition of the second phase of aggregation induced by ADP. But of course aspirin also inhibits collagen-induced aggregation both in heparinized and in citrated plasma. So there is at least one *in vitro* correlate to the *in vivo* effect of aspirin.

Mustard: In our experience with heparin, if there is some sticking of the platelets to the surface of the containers, the platelet preparation is usually unsatisfactory. I don't know why heparin causes this.

Mills: Different batches of heparin are very diverse. Some of them accelerate the release reaction induced by ADP and citrate; others inhibit it.

Mustard: Some batches of heparin can be used to replace fibrinogen to support ADP-induced aggregation in suspensions of washed human platelets. This may be due to some of the effects of heparin on platelets.

Haslam: It has been claimed that 50% of the heparin in blood may be associated with platelets (Horner 1974), so this may not be an unreasonable suggestion.

PRIMARY AGGREGATION BY 5HT, VASOPRESSIN AND THROMBIN

Mills: Haslam (1964) demonstrated that the release reaction induced by thrombin and fatty acids involved an aggregation which could be prevented by enzyme systems that selectively convert ADP to ATP. I want to refer to the situation in platelet-rich plasma where several agents, including 5HT, vasopressin and thrombin, cause primary aggregation, as well as the secondary aggregation which is correlated with the release of ADP. Using purified ATP as a specific antagonist of ADP we have shown (Macfarlane & Mills 1975) that the first phase of aggregation by 5HT, thrombin and vasopressin is not affected, though aggregation by ADP is blocked. This we find to be convincing evidence that these compounds are aggregating agents in their own right and that the ADP common pathway, though a valid concept in relation to the release reaction, should not obscure the fact that other agents besides ADP can cause aggregation.

Haslam: There is no doubt about the truth of that now. One can also argue very strongly from the effects of different aggregating agents on platelet cyclic AMP levels in the presence of PGE_1. If agents like vasopressin or 5HT released much ADP during primary aggregation, this would lower the cyclic AMP levels in the same way as added ADP. This does not happen, so there is no question that these agents have a primary action of their own, which is unrelated to the ADP mechanism. However, having said that, often during so-called primary aggregation, a small amount of ADP appears to be released, perhaps because the release reaction begins relatively early in a small proportion of platelets. For this reason one can usually inhibit primary aggregation slightly by enzymes which remove ADP. This is a small effect, and does not detract from the fact that a variety of pharmacological agents can elicit the same physiological response, namely platelet aggregation, via independent receptors.

Born: That makes good sense. The primary interaction of each agent is presumably with a receptor specific for it on the outer membrane of platelets, just as on those of other tissues such as smooth muscle or nerve cells; otherwise it is difficult to imagine how their effects are initiated at all. One would hardly expect that 5HT would have to rely on a second *external* messenger, as it were, in order to produce an effect on platelets.

When one recalls the origin of platelets, which are formed through the break-up of the cytoplasm of megakaryocytes, it is surprising that receptors for so many different endogenous agents should be present on the platelets' surfaces. Presumably these receptors must have been produced already by the megakaryocytes, perhaps during their complicated maturation and disintegration. It is interesting to think of this in relation to how cell membranes are formed. This brings to mind also the question of whether any of the agents, such as the biogenic amines, which act on cells from the outside, also have *intracellular* functions.

Marcus: This may explain why we have difficulty reproducing interactions with platelet membranes that are so easily elicited with membranes from other cells. If one postulates that the platelet membrane arises intracellularly in the megakaryocyte, perhaps one can speculate that this is the reason for differences between platelet membranes and those from other cells.

Mills: A claim has recently been made by Professor Caen and his associates (Izrael *et al.* 1974) that rapid removal of ADP by the creatine phosphate and creatine kinase system inhibits aggregation by all agents, suggesting that ADP is responsible for the primary aggregation by these other agents. However, I don't think the controls are adequate to justify the conclusions.

Mustard: Have you looked at collagen in this context as well?

Mills: Yes. Collagen is an entirely different situation.

Mustard: Surely collagen has two components in respect to shape change and aggregation. Degranulated rabbit or human platelets which no longer have significant pools of releasable material in the 5HT granules will show a shape change and an increase in light transmission when exposed to collagen. This effect can be blocked with aspirin. With normal platelets you can produce some inhibition of collagen-induced aggregation with creatine phosphate–creatine kinase. Its combined use with aspirin inhibits collagen-induced shape change and aggregation with normal platelets. Although the mechanism with collagen may be different, it is similar to thrombin in that it induces a shape change which appears to be independent of released ADP.

Mills: It differs because there is a much greater inhibition of this effect of collagen by anti-inflammatory agents, and the shape change which occurs in human citrated platelet-rich plasma on the addition of collagen is delayed by several seconds, whereas these other agents act immediately.

Smith: That is an example, if not *the* example, of the fact that collagen-induced aggregation is an 'irreversible' aggregation which is dependent both on ADP release and on the formation of prostaglandins. You can block either, and thereby block collagen-induced aggregation.

References

AFORS, K.-E., COCKBURN, J. S. & GROSS, J. F. (1975) Measurement of growth rate of laser-induced intravascular platelet aggregation and the influence of blood flow velocity. *Microvasc. Res.* in press

ARDLIE, N. G. & HAN, P. (1974) Enzymatic basis for platelet aggregation and release: the significance of the 'platelet atmosphere' and the relationship between platelet function and blood coagulation. *Br. J. Haematol. 26,* 331-356

BEGENT, N. & BORN, G. V. R. (1970) Growth rate *in vivo* of platelet thrombi produced by iontophoresis of ADP, as a function of mean blood flow velocity. *Nature (Lond.) 227,* 926-930

BORN, G. V. R. (1970) Observations on the change in shape of blood platelets brought about by adenosine diphosphate. *J. Physiol. (Lond.) 209,* 487

BORN, G. V. R. & HUME, M. (1967) Effects of the number and sizes of platelet aggregates on the optical density of plasma. *Nature (Lond.) 215,* 1027-1029

BOXER, L. A., HEDLEY-WHYTE, T. & STOSSEL, T. P. (1974) Neutrophil actin dysfunction and abnormal neutrophil behavior. *N. Engl. J. Med. 291,* 1093-1099

BURRIDGE, K. & PHILLIPS, J. H. (1975) Association of actin and myosin with secretory granule membranes. *Nature (Lond.) 254,* 526-529

COHEN, I. & DE VRIES, A. (1973) Platelet contractile regulation in an isometric system. *Nature (Lond.) 246,* 36-37

GUNNING, A. J., PICKERING, G. W., ROBB-SMITH, A. H. T. & RUSSELL, R. R. (1964) Mural thrombosis of the internal carotid artery and subsequent embolism. *Q. J. Med. (N.S.) 33,* 155-195

HASLAM, R. J. (1964) Role of adenosine diphosphate in the aggregation of human blood platelets by thrombin and by fatty acids. *Nature (Lond.) 202,* 765-768

HOLMSEN, H. & WEISS, H. J. (1972) Further evidence for a deficient storage pool of adenine nucleotides in platelets from some patients with thrombocytopathia—'storage pool disease'. *Blood 39,* 197-209

HORNER, A. A. (1974) Demonstration of endogenous heparin in rat blood. *FEBS. Lett. 46,* 166-170

IZRAEL, V., ZAWILSKA, K., JAISSON, F., LEVY-TOLEDANO, S. & CAEN, J. (1974) Effect of a fast removal of plasmatic ADP by the creatine phosphate and creatine phosphokinase system on human platelet function *in vitro.* In *Platelets: Production, Function, Transfusion, and Storage* (Baldini, M. G. & Ebbe, S., eds.), pp. 187-196, Grune & Stratton, New York

KIRSHNER, N. & VIVEROS, O. H. (1972) The secretory cycle in the adrenal medulla. *Pharmacol. Rev. 24,* 385-398

MACFARLANE, D. E. & MILLS, D. C. B. (1975) Effect of aspirin on the platelet release reaction in different anticoagulants. *Clin. Res. 23,* 278A (abstr.)

MACFARLANE, D. E., WALSH, P. N., MILLS, D. C. B., HOLMSEN, H. & DAY, H. J. (1975) The role of thrombin in ADP-induced platelet aggregation and release: a critical evaluation. *Br. J. Haematol. 30,* 453-459

MASSINI, P. & LÜSCHER, E. F. (1971) The induction of the release reaction in human blood platelets by close cell contact. *Thromb. Diath. Haemorrh. 25,* 13-20

MASSINI, P. & LÜSCHER, E. F. (1972) On the mechanism by which cell contact induces the release reaction of blood platelets; the effect of cationic polymers. *Thromb. Diath. Haemorrh. 27*, 121-133

MOORE, S. & MERSEREAU, W. A. (1968) Microembolic renal ischemia, hypertension and nephrosclerosis. *Arch. Pathol. 85*, 623-630

MURPHY, E. A., ROWSELL, H. C., DOWNIE, H. G., ROBINSON, G. A. & MUSTARD, J. F. (1962) Encrustation and atherosclerosis: the analogy between early *in vivo* lesions and deposits which occur in extracorporeal circulations. *Can. Med. Assoc. J. 87*, 259-274

MUSTARD, J. F., ROWSELL, H. C. & MURPHY, E. A. (1966) Platelet economy (platelet survival and turnover). *Br. J. Haematol. 12*, 1-24

MUSTARD, J. F., KINLOUGH-RATHBONE, R. L. & PACKHAM, M. A. (1974) Recent status of research in the pathogenesis of thrombosis. *Thromb. Diath. Haemorrh.* Suppl. 59, 157-188

MUSTARD, J. F., PERRY, D. W., KINLOUGH-RATHBONE, R. L. & PACKHAM, M. A. (1975) Factors responsible for ADP-induced release reaction of human platelets. *Am. J. Physiol. 228*, 1757-1765

NIEWIAROWSKI, S., REGOECZI, E.. STEWART, G. J., SENYI, A. F. & MUSTARD, J. F. (1972a) Platelet interaction with polymerizing fibrin. *J. Clin. Invest. 51*, 685-700

NIEWIAROWSKI, S., REGOECZI, E. & MUSTARD, J. F. (1972b) Platelet interaction with fibrinogen and fibrin: comparison of the interaction of platelets with that of fibroblasts, leukocytes, and erythrocytes. *Ann. N.Y. Acad. Sci. 201*, 72-83

POLLARD, T. D. (1975) Functional implications of the biochemical and structural properties of cytoplasmic contractile proteins. In *Molecules and Cell Movement* (Inoue, S. & Stephens, R. E., eds.), pp. 259-285, Raven Press, New York

PUSZKIN, S. & KOCHWA, S. (1974) Regulation of neurotransmitter release by a complex of actin with relaxing protein isolated from rat brain synaptosomes. *J. Biol. Chem. 249*, 7711-7714

PUSZKIN, E., PUSZKIN, S., LO, L. W. & TANENBAUM, S. W. (1973) Binding of cytochalasin D to platelet and muscle myosin. *J. Biol. Chem. 248*, 7754-7761

RUSSELL, R. R. (1961) Observations on the retinal blood vessels in monocular blindness. *Lancet 2*, 1422-1428

SCHROEDER, T. E. (1973) Actin in dividing cells: contractile ring filaments bind heavy meromyosin. *Proc. Natl. Acad. Sci. U.S.A. 70*, 1688-1692

SPOONER, B. S. (1973) Cytochalasin B: toward an understanding of its mode of action. *Dev. Biol. 35*, f13-18

SPUDICH, J. A. (1972) Effects of cytochalasin B on actin filaments. *Cold Spring Harbor Symp. Quant. Biol. 37*, 585-594

WHITE, J. G. (1974) Physicochemical dissection of platelet structural physiology. In *Platelets: Production, Function, Transfusion, and Storage(* Baldini, M. G. & Ebbe, S., eds.), pp. 235-252, Grune & Stratton, New York

WILLLINGHAM, M. C., OSTLUND, R. E. & PASTAN, I. (1974) Myosin is a component of the cell surface of cultured cells. *Proc. Natl. Acad. Sci. U.S.A. 71*, 4144-4148

Index of contributors

343

Indexes compiled by William Hill

Subject index

345